Minimally Invasive Fracture Repair

Editors

KARL C. MARITATO
MATTHEW D. BARNHART

VETERINARY CLINICS OF NORTH AMERICA: SMALL ANIMAL PRACTICE

www.vetsmall.theclinics.com

January 2020 • Volume 50 • Number 1

ELSEVIER

1600 John F. Kennedy Boulevard ● Suite 1800 ● Philadelphia, Pennsylvania, 19103-2899
http://www.vetsmall.theclinics.com

**VETERINARY CLINICS OF NORTH AMERICA: SMALL ANIMAL PRACTICE Volume 50, Number 1
January 2020 ISSN 0195-5616, ISBN-13: 978-0-323-75430-9**

Editor: Colleen Dietzler
Developmental Editor: Laura Kavanaugh

Veterinary Clinics of North America: Small Animal Practice (ISSN 0195-5616) is published bimonthly by Elsevier Inc., 360 Park Avenue South, New York, NY 10010-1710. Months of issue are January, March, May, July, September, and November. Business and Editorial Offices: 1600 John F. Kennedy Blvd., Ste. 1800, Philadelphia, PA 19103-2899. Customer Service Office: 3251 Riverport Lane, Maryland Heights, MO 63043. Periodicals postage paid at New York, NY and additional mailing offices. Subscription prices are $348.00 per year (domestic individuals), $705.00 per year (domestic institutions), $100.00 per year (domestic students/residents), $451.00 per year (Canadian individuals), $876.00 per year (Canadian institutions), $488.00 per year (international individuals), $876.00 per year (international institutions), $100.00 per year (Canadian students/residents), and $220.00 per year (international students/residents). To receive student/resident rate, orders must be accompanied by name of affiliated institution, date of term, and the *signature* of program/residency coordinator on institution letterhead. Orders will be billed at individual rate until proof of status is received. Foreign air speed delivery is included in all *Clinics* subscription prices. All prices are subject to change without notice. **POSTMASTER:** Send address changes to *Veterinary Clinics of North America: Small Animal Practice*, Elsevier Health Sciences Division, Subscription Customer Service, 3251 Riverport Lane, Maryland Heights, MO 63043. Customer Service (orders, claims, online, change of address): Elsevier Periodicals Customer Service, Elsevier Health Sciences Division Subscription **Customer Service 3251 Riverport Lane Maryland Heights, MO 63043. Tel: 1-800-654-2452 (U.S. and Canada); 314-447-8871 (outside U.S. and Canada). Fax: 314-447-8029. E-mail: journalscustomerservice-usa@elsevier.com (for print support); journalsonlinesupport-usa@elsevier.com (for online support).**

Reprints. For copies of 100 or more of articles in this publication, please contact the Commercial Reprints Department, Elsevier Inc., 360 Park Avenue South, New York, NY 10010-1710. Tel.: 212-633-3874; Fax: 212-633-3820; E-mail: reprints@elsevier.com.

Veterinary Clinics of North America: Small Animal Practice is also published in Japanese by Inter Zoo Publishing Co., Ltd., Aoyama Crystal-Bldg 5F, 3-5-12 Kitaaoyama, Minato-ku, Tokyo 107-0061, Japan.

Veterinary Clinics of North America: Small Animal Practice is covered in *Current Contents/Agriculture, Biology and Environmental Sciences, Science Citation Index, ASCA, MEDLINE/PubMed (Index Medicus), Excerpta Medica, and BIOSIS.*

Contributors

EDITORS

KARL C. MARITATO, DVM
Diplomate American College of Veterinary Surgeons; Department of Surgery, MedVet Medical and Cancer Centers for Pets, Cincinnati, Ohio, USA; Department of Surgery, MedVet Medical and Cancer Centers for Pets, Dayton, Ohio, USA

MATTHEW D. BARNHART, DVM, MS
Diplomate, American College of Veterinary Surgeons, MedVet Medical and Cancer Centers for Pets, Worthington, Ohio, USA; Surgery Specialty Leader, Department of Surgery, MedVet, Columbus, Ohio, USA

AUTHORS

MATTHEW D. BARNHART, DVM, MS
Diplomate, American College of Veterinary Surgeons, MedVet Medical and Cancer Centers for Pets, Worthington, Ohio, USA; Surgery Specialty Leader, Department of Surgery, MedVet, Columbus, Ohio, USA

ALESSANDRO BOERO BARONCELLI, DVM, PhD
Clinica Albese per Animali da Compagnia, Cuneo, Italy

BRIAN BEALE, DVM
Diplomate, American College of Veterinary Surgeons; Gulf Coast Veterinary Specialists, Houston, Texas, USA; Department of Surgery, The Beale Clinic, Sugar Land, Texas, USA; Beale Veterinary Specialist and Emergency, Victoria, Texas, USA

EMANUELE CASTELLI, DMV
Vetsuisse Faculty, University of Zurich, Zurich, Switzerland

GRAYSON COLE, DVM
Diplomate, American College of Veterinary Surgeons-Small Animal; Department of Surgery, Gulf Coast Veterinary Specialists, Houston, Texas, USA

LOÏC M. DÉJARDIN, DVM, MS
Diplomate, American College of Veterinary Surgeons, Diplomate, European College of Veterinary Surgeons; Professor, Head of Small Animal Orthopaedic Surgery; ACVS Founding Fellow MIS Orthopaedics SA; Director, Collaborative Orthopaedic Investigations Laboratory, Department of Small Animal Clinical Sciences, College of Veterinary Medicine, Michigan State University, East Lansing, Michigan, USA

LAURENT P. GUIOT, DVM, MS
Diplomate of the American College of Veterinary Surgeons, Diplomate of the European College of Veterinary Surgeons; ACCESS Bone & Joint Center, ACCESS Specialty Animal Hospital, Culver City, California, USA

CALEB C. HUDSON, DVM, MS
Diplomate, American College of Veterinary Surgeons-Small Animal, Staff Surgeon, Gulf Coast Veterinary Specialists, Houston, Texas, USA

STANLEY E. KIM, BVSc, MS
Diplomate, American College of Veterinary Surgeons; Associate Professor Small Animal Surgery, Department of Small Animal Clinical Sciences, College of Veterinary Medicine, University of Florida, Gainesville, Florida, USA

MICHAEL P. KOWALESKI, DVM
Diplomate, American College of Veterinary Surgeons, and European College of Veterinary Surgeons; ACVS Founding Fellow, Minimally Invasive Surgery, Professor of Orthopedic Surgery, Cummings School of Veterinary Medicine, Tufts University, North Grafton, Massachusetts, USA

DANIEL D. LEWIS, DVM, MS
Diplomate, American College of Veterinary Surgeons, ACVS Founding Fellow Minimally Invasive Surgery, Small Animal Orthopedics; Professor, Small Animal Surgery, Jerry and Lola Collins Eminent Scholar, Canine Sports Medicine and Comparative Orthopedics, Department of Small Animal Clinical Sciences, College of Veterinary Medicine, University of Florida, Gainesville, Florida, USA

KARL C. MARITATO, DVM
Diplomate, American College of Veterinary Surgeons; Department of Surgery, MedVet Medical and Cancer Centers for Pets, Cincinnati, Ohio, USA; Department of Surgery, MedVet Medical and Cancer Centers for Pets, Dayton, Ohio, USA

CHARLES S. McBRIEN Jr, DVM, MS
MedVet Cleveland West, Cleveland, Ohio, USA

RYAN McCALLY, DVM
Veterinary Specialty, Center of Tucson, Tucson, Arizona, USA

BRUNO PEIRONE, DVM, PhD
Professor, Department of Veterinary Science, University of Turin, Turin, Italy

KAREN L. PERRY, BVM&S, CertSAS, MRCVS
Diplomate, European College of Veterinary Surgeons; Department of Small Animal Clinical Sciences, College of Veterinary Medicine, Michigan State University, East Lansing, Michigan, USA

LISA ADELE PIRAS, DVM, PhD
Department of Veterinary Science, University of Turin, Turin, Italy

ANTONIO POZZI, med Vet
Diplomate, American College of Veterinary Surgeons, Diplomate, European College of Veterinary Surgeons, Diplomate, American College of Veterinary Sports Medicine and Rehabilitation, ACVS Founding Fellow, Minimally Invasive Surgery, Small Animal Orthopedics, Professor, Department for Small Animals, Clinic for Small Animal Surgery, Vetsuisse Faculty, University of Zurich, Zurich, Switzerland

SIMON ROE, BVSc, PhD
Diplomate, American College of Veterinary Surgeons; Professor, Small Animal Orthopaedics, Department of Clinical Sciences, College of Veterinary Medicine, North Carolina State University, Raleigh, North Carolina, USA

GIAN LUCA ROVESTI, DVM
Diplomate, European College of Veterinary Surgeons; Department of Orthopedics, Clinica
Veterinaria M.E. Miller, Cavriago, Reggio Emilia, Italy

PHILIPP SCHMIERER, med Vet
Diplomate, European College of Veterinary Surgeons; Department for Small Animals,
Vetsuisse Faculty, University of Zurich, Zurich, Switzerland

JAMES TOMLINSON, DVM, MVSc
Diplomate, American College of Veterinary Surgeons; Professor Emeritus of Small Animal
Orthopedic Surgery, Department of Veterinary Medicine and Surgery, College of
Veterinary Medicine, University of Missouri, Columbia, Missouri, USA

DIRSKO J.F. VON PFEIL, DVM
Diplomate of the American College of Veterinary Surgeons; European College of
Veterinary Surgeons, & American College of Veterinary Sports Medicine and
Rehabilitation; Sirius Veterinary Orthopedic Center, Omaha, Nebraska, USA

Contents

Biomechanics of Fracture Fixation   1

Simon Roe

> This article reviews the biomechanical parameters of fracture repair that influence construct stiffness and strength. The stiffness influences the relative motion between fracture fragments, known as gap strain, and, thus, callus development. Construct strength determines the magnitude and number of load events that the repair can resist before failure. Surgeons must optimize these parameters in order to achieve satisfactory outcomes for the patients.

Pitfalls of Minimally Invasive Fracture Repair   17

Matthew Barnhart

> Minimally invasive fracture repair (MIFR) is the ultimate culmination of current osteosynthesis concepts that emphasize the preservation and enhancement of the biologic components of fracture healing. Although the "less is more" approach to tissue dissection and fracture exposure and handling that defines MIFR has numerous reported advantages over more traditional open surgical treatments, it does present some unique challenges and important considerations for the surgeon. This article describes some of the general MIFR challenges a surgeon may encounter.

Minimally Invasive Plate Osteosynthesis Fracture Reduction Techniques in Small Animals   23

Bruno Peirone, Gian Luca Rovesti, Alessandro Boero Baroncelli, and Lisa Adele Piras

> Indirect fracture reduction is used to align diaphyseal fractures when using minimally invasive fracture repair. Indirect reduction achieves functional fracture reduction without opening the fracture site. The limb is restored to length and spatial alignment is achieved to ensure proper angular and rotational alignment. Fracture reduction can be accomplished using a variety of techniques and devices, including hanging the limb, manual traction, distraction table, external fixators, and fracture distractors.

Perioperative Imaging in Minimally Invasive Osteosynthesis   49

Laurent P. Guiot and Loïc M. Déjardin

> Peri-operative imaging using various appropriate modalities is critical to the successful planning and performance of any orthopedic surgery. The use of intra-operative imaging, while not an absolute prerequisite for long bone fractures, considerably facilitates the smooth and effective execution of minimally invasive osteosynthesis of articular fractures. One

must keep in mind, however, that the risk of overexposure to radiation with fluoroscopy and conventional radiology is real, particularly when considering its insidious effect over time. Strict adherence to the "As Low As Reasonably Achievable" (ALARA) principles is critical to mitigate the deleterious effect of radiation exposure while optimizing surgical outcome.

Reviews of clinical outcomes led to the foundation of a new approach in fracture management known as biological osteosynthesis. As intramedullary rods featuring cannulations and locking devices at both extremities, interlocking nails are well suited for bridging osteosynthesis. Unique biological and mechanical benefits make them ideal for minimally invasive nail osteosynthesis and an attractive, effective alternative to plating, particularly in revisions of failed plate osteosynthesis. Thanks to a new angle-stable locking design, interlocking nailing indications have been expanded to osteosynthesis of epi-metaphyseal fractures, including those with articular involvement and angular deformities such as distal femoral varus and associated patellar luxations.

This article describes the technique of percutaneous pinning in dogs and cats. Only acute fractures evaluated within the first 48 hours after trauma are selected for percutaneous pinning. Reduction is performed with careful manipulation of the fracture to minimize the trauma to the growth plate. After ensuring the fracture is reduced anatomically, smooth pins of appropriate size are inserted through stab incisions or through large-gauge needles. Depending on the anatomic location, the pins are cut flush with the bone or bent over. The main advantages of this technique are the minimal surgical trauma and lower perioperative morbidity.

A thorough knowledge of humeral anatomy is critical to performing minimally invasive techniques. Fluoroscopy, when available, is invaluable in optimizing fracture repair with minimally invasive techniques. Minimally invasive approaches decrease morbidity and allow an earlier return to function. Minimally invasive fracture repair is performed using implant systems similar to open approaches.

Minimally invasive plate osteosynthesis (MIPO) is a biologically friendly approach to fracture reduction and stabilization that is applicable to many radius and ulna fractures in small animals. An appropriate knowledge of the anatomy of the antebrachium and careful preoperative planning are essential. This article describes the MIPO technique, which entails stabilization of the fractured radius with a bone plate and screws that are applied without performing an extensive open surgical approach. This technique results in good outcomes, including a rapid time to union and return of function.

A thorough working knowledge of the anatomic landmarks of the femur facilitates anatomic alignment during minimally invasive osteosynthesis (MIO). A variety of fixation techniques, including plate, plate-rod, and interlocking nail, are well suited for stabilization of femoral shaft fractures with MIO techniques. Axis and torsional alignment can be assessed with various intraoperative techniques to ensure that anatomic alignment is obtained.

Fractures of the tibia and fibula are common in dogs and cats and occur most commonly as a result of substantial trauma. Tibial fractures are particularly amenable to treatment using minimally invasive fracture repair (MIFR) techniques that preserve blood supply to comminuted fracture fragments, accelerating bone callus production and speeding fracture healing. Treatment of tibial fractures using MIFR techniques has been found to reduce surgical time, reduce the time for fracture healing, and to decrease patient morbidity, while at the same time reducing complications compared with traditional open reduction and internal fixation.

A concise review of the history of meta-bone fracture repair is provided. The relevant surgical anatomy, available instrumentation, and execution of preoperative, intraoperative, and postoperative surgical care using minimally invasive plate osteosynthesis are discussed in detail. A short discussion that touches on future directions for care of meta-bone fractures follows.

Articular fractures are common injuries in veterinary medicine. The principles of articular fracture repair are anatomic reduction and rigid fixation in order to optimize joint function. Fluoroscopy and arthroscopy are tools commonly used to allow for anatomic reduction with a minimally invasive approach. Minimally invasive techniques can decrease morbidity and promote an early return to function. Different types of articular fractures and options for minimally invasive repair are reviewed in this article.

VETERINARY CLINICS OF NORTH AMERICA: SMALL ANIMAL PRACTICE

SERIES OF RELATED INTEREST

Veterinary Clinics of North America: Exotic Animal Practice
https://www.vetexotic.theclinics.com/

THE CLINICS ARE NOW AVAILABLE ONLINE!
Access your subscription at:
www.theclinics.com

Preface

Minimally Invasive Fracture Repair

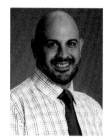
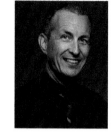

Karl C. Maritato, DVM   Matthew D. Barnhart, DVM, MS
Editors

Throughout the history of fracture repair, there are numerous descriptions of minimally invasive repair implants and techniques that have fallen in and out of favor. In 1886, Carl Hansmann invented the first plate and screws (which were locking) for use in humans. They were placed externally with the plate above the skin and the screws going through the skin into the bone, ultimately an early example of minimally invasive fracture repair (MIFR). Eventually the plates and screws made their way under the skin, and over time the preferred techniques of fracture repair involved opening the fracture site and precise anatomic reduction. Through research and education, the biologic fracture environment came into focus in the late 1980s, and in 1990, the limited contact dynamic compression plate was introduced, with the goal of minimizing the plate damage to the periosteum. This led to the resurgence of locking implant use in the mid 1990s with further emphasis put on reducing damage to the periosteum and disturbance of the perifracture environment.

The concept of minimally invasive plate osteosynthesis (MIPO) was first introduced in 1997 by Christian Krettek and Harald Tscherne and revealed rapid bone healing and larger callus formation. In 2008, published research into plate biomechanics and MIPO entered the veterinary literature and, over the past decade, continued attention to MIFR techniques and implants has occurred.

In this issue of the *Veterinary Clinics of North America: Small Animal Practice*, the authors have built upon the excellent 2012 MIFR issue. The editors are grateful to the contributing authors for their time and efforts to ensure that the most up-to-date research and information available are included and summarized effectively in the following articles.

MIFRs are technically more demanding, and a thorough working knowledge of anatomy and the implants to be used is of paramount importance. Understanding bone healing and biomechanics is also important in the decision-making process when

Vet Clin Small Anim 50 (2020) xiii–xiv
https://doi.org/10.1016/j.cvsm.2019.10.001
0195-5616/20/© 2019 Published by Elsevier Inc.

choosing between fracture repair techniques. In the early articles of this issue, we focus on fracture biomechanics and biology as well as techniques for reduction and general guidelines of MIFR. We then focus on regional skeletal systems and techniques unique to those systems. Since the majority of the literature published on this topic is focused on the canine, we end this issue with an article on the important MIFR differences for the feline.

Karl C. Maritato, DVM
MedVet Medical and Cancer Centers for Pets Cincinnati
3964 Red Bank Road, Fairfax, OH 45227, USA

MedVet Medical and Cancer Centers for Pets Dayton
2714 Springboro West Road, Moraine, OH 45439, USA

Matthew D. Barnhart, DVM, MS
MedVet Medical and Cancer Centers for Pets
300 East Wilson Bridge Road
Worthington, OH 43085, USA

E-mail addresses:
kmaritato@medvet.com (K.C. Maritato)
mbarnhart@medvet.com (M.D. Barnhart)

Biomechanics of Fracture Fixation

Simon Roe, BVSc, PhD

KEYWORDS

- Biomechanics • Area moment of inertia • Stiffness • Yield strength • Fatigue
- Direct and indirect bone healing • Gap strain • Working length

KEY POINTS

- Because accurate reduction is harder to achieve in minimally invasive osteosynthesis, most constructs are bridging.
- Fracture callus development and maturation are influenced by the mechanical environment of the fracture gap.
- The structural properties of the implants and the bone-implant constructs determine the mechanical environment.
- Construct stiffness is influenced by the structural properties and the working length of the bridging implants.
- Construct strength and durability are influenced by the structural properties of the implant, the relative single-cycle and repetitive loads applied by the patient, and the rapidity of callus development and maturation.

INTRODUCTION

Understanding the mechanical principles that determine the performance of implants, how the implants and bone interact, and the subsequent mechanical environment of the fracture is essential for successful fracture fixation and uneventful healing. The outcome is influenced by the material and geometry of the implants; how they are attached to the bone; and the loads that the patient applies, both singly and repetitively during healing. In this introductory article, the biomechanical terms that are commonly used in fracture fixation are explained, followed by a review of how the mechanical environment of the fracture can influence the biology of bone healing. Based on a solid understanding of these principles, this article outlines how these factors are applied during surgical decision making for a specific fracture and implant choice.

Small Animal Orthopaedics, Department of Clinical Sciences, College of Veterinary Medicine, 1052 William Moore Drive, Raleigh, NC 27607, USA
E-mail address: sroe@ncsu.edu

Vet Clin Small Anim 50 (2020) 1–15
https://doi.org/10.1016/j.cvsm.2019.08.009
0195-5616/20/© 2019 Elsevier Inc. All rights reserved.

vetsmall.theclinics.com

BIOMECHANICAL PRINCIPLES OF ORTHOPEDIC MATERIALS AND IMPLANTS
Material Properties

The ability to describe the mechanical properties of a material in a way that is independent of any geometric parameters is important for understanding how implants made from that material will perform when a load is applied. In orthopedics, this allows the comparison of the expected properties of 2 implants of the same dimension, but made with different materials; for example, stainless steel and titanium. It also is important for understanding implants made of the same materials that have the same composition (ie, 316L stainless steel) but in which the material has been altered by processing techniques (ie, cold working) for different use scenarios. Orthopedic wire, bone plates, screws, and pins are all made of the same material, but, through a process of cold working, the yield strength is increased. Note that the elastic nature of the material (defined as the elastic modulus; discussed later) does not change with cold working.

The primary terms used to describe the properties of implant materials are stress, strain, and elastic modulus. These properties are calculated from mechanical tests on specimens with defined geometry. Most commonly, for materials used in implants, tensile tests are used, although bending, compressive, and torsional tests are helpful for some scenarios. Stress is calculated from the load applied divided by the cross-sectional area of the specimen. The most common units are Newton per millimeter squared.

Stress = Load (N)/cross-sectional area (mm^2) N/mm^2 or pascals (Pa)

Strain is calculated as the change in length as a percentage of the original length. It is expressed as a percentage and is, therefore, dimensionless.

Strain = Change in length (mm)/Original length (mm) %

The elastic modulus (often termed the Young modulus) describes the relationship between stress and strain, and is the most useful parameter for comparing materials. It is calculated from the slope of the stress versus strain curve (**Fig. 1**). It has the same units as stress (N/mm^2) because strain has no dimensions. A single value assumes a linear relationship, which is true for metals (until their yield point; discussed later). The elastic modulus of implant stainless steel is usually 188 GPa[a], pure titanium is 116 GPa[b], and titanium alloy (Ti-6Al-4V) is 113 GPa.[c]

The yield stress is defined as the stress that can be resisted by a material before there is permanent deformation. Before that stress, the material behaves elastically; it returns to its original shape after the stress is removed. After the yield stress is surpassed, the material is permanently deformed, and does not assume its original shape when the stress is removed; this is the plastic phase of its response. After a period of plastic deformation, most materials break or fail; this is failure stress, or ultimate stress. The nature of the plastic response is described as brittle if there is little plastic

---

[a] http://www.matweb.com/search/datasheet.aspx?matguid=29a84d10fada4e4fa3ebe3986e52d848&ckck=1.

[b] http://www.matweb.com/search/DataSheet.aspx?MatGUID=66a15d609a3f4c829cb6ad08f0dafc01.

[c] http://www.matweb.com/search/DataSheet.aspx?MatGUID=a0655d261898456b958e5f825ae85390.

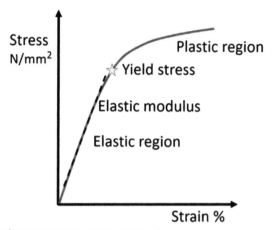

Fig. 1. Representative stress versus strain curve. This curve is produced following a tensile test of a defined sample of a material. The stress and strain are calculated from the dimensions of the specimen. The initial linear portion of the curve is the elastic region. No permanent changes occur in the region. The slope of the curve is the elastic modulus, and is a parameter used to compare materials. As the stress increases, the yield stress is reached, and permanent deformation of the sample is present. The curve moves into the plastic region, and the stiffness is usually reduced.

deformation before failure (eg, bone or ceramics) or ductile, if there is a long plastic phase. Metals are generally compared based on their ultimate tensile stress (UTS). The UTS of medical-grade stainless steel (316L) ranges from around 500 MPa in its annealed (unworked) state to 1100 MPa for 60% cold worked, and up to 1300 MPa for highly worked material.[d] The UTS of titanium is 220 MPa,[e] and a common titanium alloy - Ti-6Al-4V - is 950 MPa.[f]

The bending strength of orthopedic materials affects the utility and performance of implants. Because bending induces tensile and compressive stresses in the material, bending strength is related to the tensile yield strength, which is the parameter most commonly reported for materials. Cold working improves the molecular packing in steel and results in an increase in yield strength and, thus, bending strength. Orthopedic wire is not worked, and, as such, has a low bending strength. This property allows it to be easily conformed and manipulated. However, because the security of wire relies on the unbending properties of wire, cerclage and tension band devices loosen when the yield strength is exceeded. Steel used in bone plates is moderately worked so that it resists bending forces, but they are still ductile enough to allow contouring. The steel for pins and screws is more highly worked because they do not need to be contoured and, therefore, they are able to resist bending well. The degree of cold working is considered proprietary by most manufacturers. The yield strength ranges from 250 MPa for annealed material, to 880 MPa for 60% cold worked, and up to

---

[d] https://www.upmet.com/products/stainless-steel/316lslvm.

[e] http://www.matweb.com/search/DataSheet.aspx?MatGUID=66a15d609a3f4c829cb6ad08f0dafc01.

[f] http://www.matweb.com/search/DataSheet.aspx?MatGUID=a0655d261898456b958e5f825ae85390.

945 MPa for highly worked material.[9] The yield strength for titanium is 140 MPa,[h] and for Ti-6Al-4V is 880 MPa.[i]

Structural Properties

The structural properties of an implant or a bone-implant construct have more clinical relevance because surgeons can compare actual implants or simulations of fracture repair scenarios. These simulations are determined by placing a specimen in a testing machine and simulating the loads or displacements that might be experienced in the patient. The load and displacement are recorded simultaneously and analyzed to aid understanding of a particular repair scenario. The structure may be tested in bending, compression or torsion, or a combination of loads to provide a full understanding of biomechanical performance. Bending tests are generally considered most clinically relevant. The way in which bending is applied (3-point, 4-point, or cantilever) is dictated by the particular hypothesis being investigated. When implants are eccentrically positioned relative to the loading axis, which occurs in many fracture simulation models, axial loading or compression of the specimen causes bending of the implant. Some clinical scenarios are best emulated using a combination of forces. Static compression followed by progressive rotation is the most common combination for fracture fixation assessment. Testing in multiple directions may help reveal specific weaknesses of some implants.

These tests produce a load versus deformation curve (**Fig. 2**), which has similar regions to the stress-strain curve discussed earlier, but with different terminology.

Load

Load is measured by the load cell of the testing machine, and is usually reported in Newtons.

Displacement

Displacement can be measured in a variety of ways. If the position of the crosshead or actuator of the testing machine is used, it represents the global behavior of the whole specimen (as well as any machine compliance). This method is suitable for simple specimens but is less meaningful for more complex constructs. Deformation at the site of interest (ie, the fracture gap) often provides a better understanding of the situation and has more relevance. Contact (extensometers or linear variable-displacement transducers) or noncontact (single-plane video tracking, three-dimensional motion) methods can be used. In some experiments, implant strain (the microdeformations on the surface) is measured using either strain gauges adhered to the implant at the predicted site of interest[1] or, more recently, using video analysis of speckled surface markings.[2]

Stiffness

Stiffness is the slope of the load versus deformation curve and is commonly reported as Newtons per millimeter (N/mm). By reporting a single value, there is an assumption that the response is linear. If the response is not linear, the method for calculating stiffness must be described. The crudest approximation is assuming linearity from the beginning of loading to the yield load. Another approach is to select the most linear

---

[9] https://www.upmet.com/products/stainless-steel/316lslvm.

[h] http://www.matweb.com/search/DataSheet.aspx?MatGUID=66a15d609a3f4c829cb6ad08f0dafc01.

[i] http://www.matweb.com/search/DataSheet.aspx?MatGUID=a0655d261898456b958e5f825ae85390.

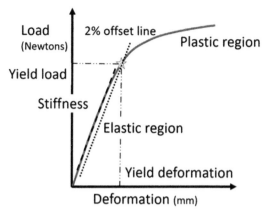

Fig. 2. Representative load versus deformation curve. The response of a structure to an applied load is shown in relationship with the measured deformation. The elastic region is the portion of the curve before any yield of the structure. The slope of the response curve is the stiffness of the structure. In this stylized curve the response is linear, but biological systems may display nonlinear behavior. The yield load is the load at which permanent changes develop in the construct. In tests of metal, the slope of the curve changes gradually, so this point is often defined by the 2% offset method. A line is drawn parallel to the slope, but is offset to the right by 2%. The load value at the point where the offset line intersects the response curve is considered the yield load. The shape of the plastic region determines whether the structure has a ductile or brittle response.

portion of the curve, or define a load range that is consistent, or clinically relevant, for all specimens. The assumption is that this response is elastic.

Yield load and yield displacement
The yield point is where the response transitions from elastic to plastic. From that point onward, there is permanent deformation and, if the load is removed, the specimen does not return to its original shape. This point is very clinically relevant because it implies that there is a change in the specimen from its intended shape. However, it can also be difficult to accurately detect from the response curve of metal implants because the transition is gradual. In linear systems, a 2% offset method is often used (**Fig. 2**). In more complex systems, a test method that uses incrementally increasing load-unload cycles may be required to detect the true yield point.

Peak load and failure load are also often reported, but, because they usually occur well past the point that would be considered clinical failure, they are not as clinically relevant.

Because many constructs are weakest in bending, the bending stiffness is often the most clinically relevant parameter. This value is dictated by the elastic modulus of the material and the area moment of inertia (AMI) *in the direction of bending* of the weakest portion of the construct. AMI is the parameter that surgeons can influence by the choice of implants. It is also influenced by whether the fractured bone is reconstructed or not. When fracture reduction achieves direct contact of the main bone fragments, especially on the side of the bone opposite the implant, the AMI, and thus the bending stiffness, is greatly increased because the implant and bone both contribute to the calculation. However, in many minimally invasive approaches to shaft fractures, accurate reduction is not achieved, and AMI, and thus construct stiffness, is dictated solely by the implants chosen.

Area moment of inertia

AMI is a geometric parameter that is calculated based on the dimensions of the structure in the direction of bending. For a circular implant (eg, a pin or interlocking nail), the direction is not relevant, and the formula is $1/4.\pi.r^4$. Note that the radius is raised to the fourth power, so small increases in diameter have a large impact on the bending stiffness. For example, the AMI of a 2.4-mm pin (3/32 inch) is 1.6 mm^4 and that of a 3.2-mm (1/8 inch) pin is 5.1 mm^4; 3 times larger. The AMI of solid rectangular structures is calculated using formula $1/3.b.h^3$, where b = width, and h = the height in the direction of bending. The thickness of a plate is, therefore, an important parameter, because this dimension is cubed. However, the situation is much more complex for bone plates because of the presence of the holes for the screws. The AMI of a bone plate at a screw hole is usually less than half the value that would be calculated from its outer dimensions. If the direction of bending is known, the surgeon can also use this understanding of AMI to consider alternate plate locations. The classic example of this is for distal radius fractures. If the primary direction of bending is considered to be in the craniocaudal plane, a 2.7-mm LC-DCP (Limited Contact - Dynamic Compression Plate) placed on the medial aspect will have a higher AMI (solid section approximately 111 mm^4) than a 3.5-mm LC-DCP placed on the cranial aspect (30 mm^4), because the height of the 2.7 mm plate in the direction of bending is 8 mm, compared with 3.3 mm for the 3.5-mm plate (**Fig. 3**).

Working length

Because bridging implants are frequently used in minimally invasive fracture management, the length of the portion that spans the fracture gap (working length) influences the deflection of the construct. This deflection determines the movement of fracture fragments, and this influences tissue differentiation and maturation. For implants with the same AMI, the amount of deflection is related to the span length cubed. As an example, if a 300-N load is applied to a 3.5-mm plate (AMI = 15 mm^4) with a working length of 2 cm there will be approximately 0.3 mm of deflection. If the working length is increased to 4 cm, the deflection would be approximately 2.3 mm.[j] Working length is also an important factor in external fixator frame design. The working length of a fixation pin is the distance from the bone to the clamp. The working length of the frame is the length of the connecting bar segment(s) that span the fracture. Reducing the pin and/or connecting bar lengths increases the stiffness of the frame.

Fatigue

Few orthopedic implants or constructs fail clinically because of a single incident of applied load, so understanding cyclic loading and fatigue is important for guiding implant selection. The factors that influence fatigue failure are the magnitude of the applied load (which generates stress within the implant), the geometry, the material and how it was handled and manufactured, and the local environment. The surgeons' primary role is to anticipate the applied load and select a geometry (and maybe material) that will be adequate in a particular situation. The fatigue behavior of a material is determined experimentally by developing an S versus N curve, where S = applied stress, and N = number of cycles to failure (plotted on a logarithmic scale). If a stress is applied that is greater than the yield stress, the number of cycles to cause failure will be small (like the repeated bending of a paper clip). As the applied stress is reduced,

---

[j] Derived using https://www.amesweb.info/StructuralBeamDeflection/CantileverBeamStressDeflection Calculator.aspx.

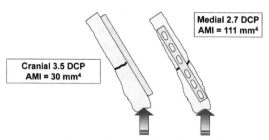

Fig. 3. Impact of plate orientation on AMI. If loading of a distal radial fracture is simplified to a single vector in the caudocranial direction, the AMI of a 3.5 DCP placed on the cranial surface is 30 mm⁴. The AMI of a 2.7 DCP placed on the medial surface is 111 mm⁴ because the height in the direction of bending is much greater.

the number of cycles to cause failure increases. The endurance limit is the stress level at which the material will not fail, no matter how many cycles are applied. For most metals, the endurance limit is around 50% of the ultimate tensile stress.

The fatigue behavior of a structure (eg, a bone plate) can be characterized using a similar process using a load vs number curve (**Fig. 4**). After determining the yield load, a progressively decreasing peak load series is established. Specimens are cycled until a defined failure point (breakage, or reduced stiffness, indicating partial failure) is detected and the number of cycles required to reach that point recorded. This number increases as the applied load is reduced. There is a load at which failure does not occur, similar to the endurance limit for a material. An implant's performance may also be considered adequate if it survives a clinically relevant number of cycles, often set at 10^6. This type of study is not done frequently because the number of cycles can be very large, and thus it takes a long time to complete each test. The response curve for structures may be more complicated because geometry, material, and manufacturing factors may all interact. Some geometries, such as screw holes in a plate, may cause local stress concentrations that accelerate fatigue. The degree of cold working and even the purity of the manufacturing process may vary between different suppliers of similar products. Very small imperfections and cracks can be initiating factors in the failure cascade. Surgeons should also be aware that small notches on the surface of a structure can significantly decrease the endurance limit, because they cause local stress concentration.

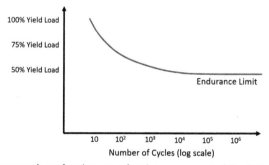

Fig. 4. A load versus number of cycles curve for the assessment of the fatigue response of an implant or construct. At 100% of yield load, the structure fails after a small number of cycles. As the load reduces, the number of cycles to failure increases. For metal structures, when the applied load reduces to around 50% of the yield load, fatigue failure does not occur. This point is termed the endurance limit.

In a clinical situation, surgeons can help avoid fatigue failure by selecting implants of appropriate strength; minimizing notching; and, through good client education, reducing the magnitude and frequency of the applied loads. Optimizing the rate at which the fracture gap consolidates also helps avoid fatigue failure because stress in the plate decreases as the healing bone is able to support more of the applied load.

BIOMECHANICS OF FRACTURE HEALING

Bone and the tissues of the callus that develop through the phases of healing are able to sense and respond to the local mechanical environment. The progression of bridging of a fracture is influenced by many factors, but the primary ones are the adequacy of local blood supply and the amount of motion present between fracture fragments.

The theory of interfragmentary strain has been proposed to provide a framework of understanding of how local tissues respond to movement of fracture fragments.[3] If there is no movement, and no gap, direct healing occurs. Small gaps (<1 mm) are filled by induction and conduction of osteogenic precursors bought to the damaged regions as the local blood supply is reestablished. When movement is present, the amount of strain that the local tissues experience influences the stages of differentiation. In this situation, the gap strain is defined as the change in gap width divided by the original gap width. If the gap between 2 fragments was 3 mm, and the fragments moved apart 0.3 mm, the gap strain would be 10%. If the fragments only moved 0.03 mm, the gap strain would be 1%.

Based on this understanding, the goal of the surgeon is to provide the appropriate amount of stability such that the biology of healing can proceed with little impediment. The 2 main modes of bone healing, and the role fracture stability plays in their progression, are outlined next.

Direct Bone Healing

Direct bone healing occurs when bone fragments are in direct contact and there is absolute stability. The fracture line is remodeled by progression of bone remodeling units or cutter cones from one fragment into the other as the osteonal repair processes remove and replace the damaged bone that is adjacent to the fracture (**Fig. 5**). Because these units have a complex and microscopic structure, any motion between the fragments disrupts them and bridging of the fracture does not occur.

A bone remodeling unit begins with a group of osteoclasts that tunnel through cortical and lamellar bone. A fine blood vessel is adjacent to them to fuel their activity. The local release of minerals and cytokines induces osteoblast formation immediately behind the osteoclasts, and they produce osteoid, which is then mineralized as the cavity made by the osteoclasts is filled in behind them with viable healthy bone. The osteoblasts become osteocytes as they are surrounded by mineralized matrix, and a new osteon is formed.

These units are not able to traverse gaps and perfect reduction is impossible to achieve. When there is absolute stability and the gap is small (<1 mm), blood vessels are able to penetrate these gaps and, because of the close apposition of conductive and inductive surfaces and availability of osteogenic cells, the space is filled by intramembranous ossification. The filled gap is then remodeled by the cutter cones. It is important to understand that it can take many months for sufficient remodeling to return the bone to its original strength, and that the healing process can be difficult to assess radiographically, other than by the gradual loss of sharpness of any visible fracture lines.

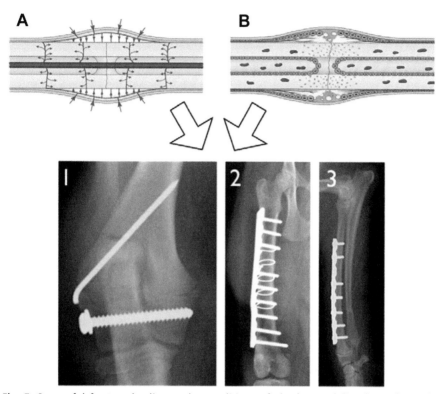

Fig. 5. Successful fracture healing under conditions of absolute stability depends on the mechanical conditions at the fracture gap and the presence of an adequate blood supply. As shown in (A) with the arrows directed toward the fracture, the blood supply originates from the peripheral soft tissue. Fixation providing absolute stability eliminates motion at the fracture site, as shown in these fractures stabilized with a lag screw and Kirschner wire (1), cerclage wires and neutralization plate (2), and compression plate (3). Limited callus formation as depicted in (B) is expected under these mechanical conditions. (*From* P. Chao, D. D. Lewis, M. P. Kowaleski, A. Pozzi. Biomechanical Concepts Applicable to Minimally Invasive Fracture Repair in Small Animals. Veterinary Clinics: Small Animal Practice 2012;42;5:861-62; with permission.)

Absolute stability of a fracture is achieved by firm compression of fragments that are accurately reduced. Cerclage wire, lag screws, or plates applied with compression are devices that can maintain the required pressure and intimate contact. When the appropriate conditions are met, healing progresses with minimal to no visible callus.

Indirect Bone Healing

If motion is present between fracture fragments, the bone and the surrounding tissues respond with a more stepwise process that is termed indirect healing. Immediately after the fracture, a hematoma develops and the soft tissues around the bone become swollen and inflamed. Over the following few days to weeks, the periosteum, endosteum, and other adjacent soft tissues proliferate to form a soft callus around the fragments. These tissues begin to become more firm on the periphery, with osteoblasts depositing osteoid, and then mineralization, and the formation of woven bone. As the callus stiffens, fragment movement reduces, and, given the right conditions, the proximal and distal responses connect across the fracture, and clinical union occurs. The woven bone of this bulky immature callus is then remodeled as the cortical structure is rebuilt (**Fig. 6**).

There are several factors that are needed to make this process successful, and surgeons can influence many of these. The type of tissue that develops in the soft callus is influenced by the blood supply and the relative movement between the fragments, also known as interfragmentary strain. To understand this principle, it helps to simplify the role of strain in tissue differentiation. When there is

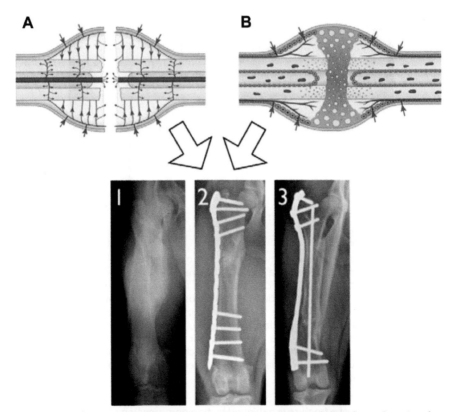

Fig. 6. Successful fracture healing under conditions of relative stability, shown here in a fracture that healed by the process of secondary bone healing, depends on maintaining adequate circulation to the fracture and appropriate gap motion. Immediately after the fracture is sustained (A), there is hematoma formation caused by disruption of blood vessels. The fracture hematoma is gradually replaced by granulation tissue. Under conditions of controlled gap motion, soft callus is progressively replaced with hard callus (B). As shown by the arrows directed toward the callus (A and B), the major source of blood vessels supporting the callus formation is the surrounding soft tissues. Secondary bone healing noted in 3 diaphyseal femoral fractures healed under conditions of relative stability: (1) femoral functional malunion healed without surgical fixation, (2) femoral fracture stabilized with bridging plate (3.5 broad locking compression plate), (3) femoral fracture stabilized with plate-rod combination (4.5 narrow dynamic compression plate and 5-mm intramedullary pin). (*From* P. Chao, D. D. Lewis, M. P. Kowaleski, A. Pozzi. Biomechanical Concepts Applicable to MinimallY Invasive Fracture Repair in Small Animals. Veterinary Clinics: Small Animal Practice 2012;42;5:861-62; with permission.)

considerable motion between fragments, the gap strain is high. Because granulation tissue is soft and flexible, it can sustain high strains (maybe as much as 100%) without damage. The strain in the periphery of the callus is less, so fibrous tissue is able to develop. It can tolerate strains around 10%. With increasing callus stiffness, fragment motion decreases, and the interfragmentary strain diminishes further. Osteoblasts are induced and mineralized callus forms in the periphery. If the strain at the gap diminishes to a low level (<2% is usually quoted), the mineralized tissues on either side of the fracture can join, and clinical union is achieved. The bulky immature woven bone is then remodeled to a more dense, stiffer tissue, with eventual reformation of the cortical structure.

Exactly what happens in the fracture gap, and what factors play a role in how tissues develop, is only partially understood. There are mechanical theories based on tensile strains, shear strain, fluid flow or pressures, or complex interactions of these, and then a biological aspect is added on top of these. Blood supply and, thus, oxygenation are important factors in the cell infiltration and differentiation processes.[4] What is important for surgeons is to know that the amount of motion that occurs and the size of the gap (or gaps) greatly influence the progression of indirect bone healing.

APPLIED BIOMECHANICS
Choosing the Type of Plate: Locking Versus Nonlocking

Regular bone plates (often termed nonlocking) are secured to bone using screws such that, as the screw is tightened, the plate is compressed onto the surface of the bone. As a general rule, if 3 screws that engage both the near and far cortices are placed, the fixation is considered secure. For the plate-bone attachment to remain rigid throughout healing, the screws must remain tight. It is important that the plate be in direct contact with the bone, which requires complete elevation of the periosteum. The initial tightness of the screw depends on the quality of the bone into which it is placed, so bones with thin cortices, or patients with poor bone quality (osteoporosis), have greater chance of screw loosening and fixation failure. These plates also necessitate accurate contouring before application because the final alignment of the fragments will be determined by the shape of the plate.

Locking plates use a different method of attachment to bone. Although a screw is still placed into the bone, the head of the screw locks into the plate and holds it rigidly in position, rather than pulling it to the bone. The most common method for locking is a threaded screw head engaging a threaded hole in the plate. The SOP (string of pearls) system (Orthomed, Inc, United Kingdom) captures the head of a regular screw in the "pearl" in order to create the lock. The Fixin system (Intrauma, Rivoli, Italy) uses a threaded conical bushing to lock the screw head. With most threaded systems, the screw must be aligned perpendicular to the plate, so the surgeon must consider carefully the direction of all the screws when deciding on plate shape and position. There are several advantages of using a locking system. Because the plate is not compressed to the bone, the periosteum does not need to be elevated. This technique should help maintain the vascularity of the bone. Also, the plate does not need to be accurately contoured, because the fragments are held in their reduced position, not pulled to the plate. However, because the plate is slightly offset from the bone, the bending and shear forces on the screws are much greater. In recognition of these increased stresses, locking screws generally have a larger core diameter and, thus, a larger AMI. However, it is still advised to keep the bone-plate distance less than 2 mm, whenever possible, to reduce the chance of screw breakage.[5] Another advantage of locking screws is that they are at a fixed angle to the plate and thus work together to keep the plate attached to the bone. This property is particularly helpful when the quality of the bone engaged is weak, or the fragment is small. It has also been proposed that 2 well-seated locked screws provide a mechanically safe attachment to a fragment.[5]

Several systems allow either regular or locking screws to be placed in the plate, and there are situations that are described later in which this may be advantageous. If this is done, it is important to place the regular screws first so that the plate is in contact with the bone, and then place any locked screws.

For some reducible fracture configurations, absolute stability can be achieved by compressing fragments to one another. Several plate systems have screw holes that are sloped hole such that, when the screw is placed at the high end of the hole, and then tightened, the fragment that it is engaging is compressed onto the opposite fragment. In some systems, the plate hole has been designed to accommodate either a regular screw in either compression or neutral position, or a locking screw. Many locking systems do not have this dual function. The compression mode of plate application is not used often with minimally invasive approaches.

Although the minimum plate length is defined by the need to achieve the minimum number of screws required for secure fragment purchase, the optimal plate length, and the number of screws needed, has had much discussion.[6] The current approach is to choose longer plates that span much of the bone, but to not fill all of the screw holes. When a plate is loaded in bending, the pullout load resisted by the screws is greatly reduced when they are further from the fracture. Screw density (number of screws divided by the number of holes) has been used to guide how many screws should be placed. Because this number is usually applied to the whole plate, it may not be as applicable for highly comminuted fractures in shorter animal bones. Mechanically, there seems to be little advantage to more than 4 screws in a fragment. Within a fragment, there should be 1 screw close (near) to the fracture and 1 at the very end of the plate (far), and then a minimum of 2 additional screws spaced evenly over the remaining span. Further screws add no mechanical security but do add to the surgical damage to the bone.

Factors Affecting Stiffness and Failure of the Construct

All of the material in this article is required to understand this issue, because it is the key to how the choices the surgeon makes influence the mechanical environment of the fracture. The primary factors affecting stiffness are the modulus of the material used, the AMI of the construct, and the span across the fracture (the working length). The factors influencing gap strain are the width of the gap and the amount of motion between the fragments. The factors affecting fatigue failure are the yield bending strength of the construct and the cumulative load/number of cycles that are applied.

For bone plates, most are made from medium worked stainless steel, although some are available in titanium, which reduces the stiffness. The AMI is determined by the size of the plate that the surgeon chooses, and how it is oriented relative to the bending loads. A plate with no empty holes has a higher AMI than one with unfilled holes, but this generally requires that there be no fracture gap. When there is a fracture gap, the plate must span the gap. For most styles of plate, there are unfilled holes, and a significantly lower AMI, which also reduces the yield bending strength of the construct, thus decreasing the fatigue life. Because the size of the bone limits the size of plate that is appropriate for a particular patient, the AMI and yield bending strength are usually augmented by the addition of other implants. The most common approach is to add an intramedullary (IM) pin. Based on the reduction in strain in the plate, an IM pin that is approximately 30% of the medullary diameter of the bone is usually selected.[2] Another option is to add a second plate, particularly if this is placed orthogonal to the first, but this usually has a greater impact on the biology of the fracture, so is usually only used in very large patients.

The span of the plate across a fracture, the working length, is an important consideration for bridging of nonreconstructable fractures. As discussed earlier, the stiffness of the construct is inversely related to the working length cubed. When the working length is longer, the yield bending strength may also be reduced, depending on the length of the moment arm that is present when bending is applied. The longer the bending moment arm, the lower the applied load that will cause the plate to yield and have a permanent bend. The working length of a plate is influenced by the type of plate and the direction of bending. The classic discussion is for the femur, where the plate is placed laterally, and, because of eccentric loading, the plate bends medially (**Fig. 7**). For a regular plate that is in contact with the bone, the working length is the segment of plate that spans from one fracture end to the other. For a locking plate, particularly if the plate is not in contact with the bone, the working length is from the screw closest to the fracture in the proximal fragment to the screw closest to the fracture in the distal fragment,[7] because the bone and plate do not bend together. However, if bending were to occur in the opposite direction, then the working length

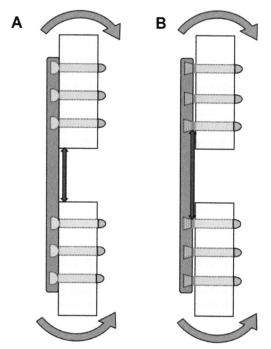

Fig. 7. The working length of a bridging plate is influenced by the type of plate, and the interaction of the plate with the bone. (*A*) A regular plate is held to the bone by regular screws. When bending occurs, the plate and bone act together, and the working length is the unsupported length of the plate. (*B*) A locking plate spans the same gap but, because the plate is not in direct contact with the bone, the working length is the distance between the 2 screws closest to the fracture. It is important to understand that, if bending occurred in the opposite direction, the working length would be the same for both plates.

would be the same for the regular and locking plates, because, with bending in this direction, the regular plate is not supported by the bone.

In some discussions of working length, it has been suggested that creating a construct with a longer working length (ie, placing screws more distant from the fracture ends) will reduce the stress in the plate, making it less likely to fail by fatigue. This suggestion is not correct, and several studies have shown that, for the same applied load, the measured strain beside a plate hole is similar for constructs with 1 hole unfilled compared with 3 or 4 holes unfilled.[2] In an early biomechanical study of locked plates,[8] a reduction in plate stress was found when working length was increased, but this was only for a model that had a small fracture gap. In that model, the reduced stiffness of the long working length construct resulted in closure of the gap and contact between the proximal and distal fragments across from the plate. The bone then resisted further bending, thus protecting the plate. In that same study, when there was a large fracture gap and, therefore, no bone contact and a larger working length, the construct was less stiff, the displacement greater for the same load, the yield load was reduced, and the fatigue life reduced.

The stiffness of external fixators is influenced by the diameter of the pin and connecting bars chosen, the frame configuration, and the length of the span across the fracture. The least stiff external fixator is a unilateral linear frame with 2 pins in each fragment. However, with appropriate-sized pins, minimization of the connecting bar-to-bone distance, and a short span across the fracture, even a simple frame can achieve a clinically acceptable level of stiffness. Stiffness can be increased by adding a second unilateral frame in another plane, or by using full pins to construct a bilateral frame, with connecting bars on both sides of the limb. External fixators are used less commonly in bones where only unilateral configurations are possible, and where large muscle mass means that the connecting bar-to-bone distance is long. Failure of external fixator pins may occur if they are too small in diameter, or there are too few per fragment (3 is optimal).

Interlocking nails are mechanically very robust. Because they are round, centrally located, and have a high AMI, they counter bending loads in all directions. The bolts proximally and distally resist compressive and rotational forces. The veterinary nail that has bolts that lock into the nail does provide superior resistance to rotational forces.[9] The stiffness of the construct is primarily determined by the AMI and the span between the bolts.

The Uncertainties Around Optimizing Gap Strain

The concept that there is an optimal gap strain that results in the perfect mechanical environment for the early callus tissues to rapidly differentiate to osteogenic capabilities is general accepted. However, even in a very defined experimental model, in which those strains are controlled and measured, exactly what the optimal amount should be is still unknown. In addition, the in vivo situation is much more complicated, particularly in bridging osteosynthesis, in which there are multiple fracture lines with complex geometries. When a load is applied and the construct deforms, fragment motion could lead to narrowing, widening, or shearing of the fracture gaps. Some might move a lot, and others very little. The load magnitude in patients is very variable, depending on comfort, activity, and need to use a limb. This variability produces a complex cycle history for the implants. The load direction likely varies with different phases of gait, leading to potential changes in direction of fragment movement. The stiffness of the construct changes over time as the soft callus matures such that the strain levels in a weaker construct are reduced, and a potential fatigue failure is averted. However, another scenario might be that healing is slow, because of either biological or mechanical factors, and a weak construct fails before clinical union is achieved.

Despite not knowing what the optimal environment around the fracture fragments is, surgeons must make decisions regarding the strength and stiffness of the fixation for each patient. Fixation that is too stiff seems to result in slow development of bridging callus. Fixation that is too weak may deform if a single large load is applied, or fail by fatigue if high strains persist over time. In the end, it comes down to clinical judgment. This judgment is often based on personal and reported experiences. The surgeon assesses the mechanical and biological factors of a particular fracture, applies a fixation based on an understanding of how it will perform mechanically, and then attempts to optimize the postoperative loading factors that produce the optimal gap strains to induce rapid development of callus and bridging of the fracture gap.

SUMMARY

Surgeons must understand the biomechanical principles associated with orthopedic implants, fracture healing, and their interaction. By using this understanding of AMI and working length, the stiffness of a construct is estimated. The stiffness influences the development of the callus by affecting gap strain. Optimal gap strain allows vascular ingrowth and tissue differentiation along the osteogenic pathway. The yield strength of the construct is also influenced by AMI and working length. The higher the yield strength, the greater the load magnitude and events that can be resisted before failure. An important part of the postoperative assessment of constructs is for surgeons to use their understanding of these mechanical parameters to predict the weakest point and have this guide patient management decisions.

REFERENCES

1. Hulse D, Hyman W, Nori M, et al. Reduction of plate strain by the introduction of an intramedullary pin. Vet Surg 1997;26:451–9.
2. Pearson T, Glyde MR, Day RE, et al. The effect of intramedullary pin size and plate working length on plate strain in locking compression plate-rod constructs under axial load. Vet Comp Orthop Traumatol 2016;29:451–8.
3. Perren SM, Cordey J. The concept of interfragmentary strain. In: Stahl E, Uhthoff HK, editors. Current concepts in internal fixation of fractures. New York: Springer; 1980. p. 63–77.
4. Betts DC, Muller R. Mechanical regulation of bone regeneration: theories, models and experiments. Front Endocrinol (Lausanne) 2014;5:211.
5. Gautier E, Sommer C. Guidelines for the clinical application of the LCP. Injury 2003; 34 Suppl 2:SB63–76.
6. Cronier P, Pietu G, Dujardin C, et al. The concept of locking plates. Orthop Tramatol Surg Res 2010;96S:S17–36.
7. Chao P, Conrad BP, Lewis DD, et al. Effect of plate working length on plate stiffness and cyclic fatigue life in a cadaveric femoral fracture gap model stabilized with a 12-hole locking compression plate. BMC Vet Res 2013;9:125.
8. Stoffel K, Dieter U, Stachowiak G, et al. Biomechanical testing of the LCP - how can stability of locked internal fixators be controlled? Injury 2003;34 Suppl 2:SB11–9.
9. Dejardin LM, Cabassu JB, Guilluo RP, et al. In vivo biomechanical evaluation of a novel angle-stable interlocking nail design in a canine tibial fracture model. Vet Surg 2014;43:271–81.

Pitfalls of Minimally Invasive Fracture Repair

Matthew Barnhart, DVM, MS*

KEYWORDS

- Minimally invasive fracture repair (MIFR) • Fracture healing
- Intraoperative fluoroscopy

KEY POINTS

- Minimally invasive fracture repair (MIFR) is the ultimate culmination of current osteosynthesis concepts that emphasize the preservation and enhancement of the biologic components of fracture healing.
- Although the "less is more" approach to tissue dissection and fracture exposure and handling that defines MIFR has numerous reported advantages over more traditional open surgical treatments, it does present some unique challenges and important considerations for the surgeon.
- This article describes some of the general MIFR challenges a surgeon may encounter.

INTRODUCTION

Minimally invasive fracture repair (MIFR) is the ultimate culmination of current osteosynthesis concepts that emphasize the preservation and enhancement of the biologic components of fracture healing. Although the "less is more" approach to tissue dissection and fracture exposure and handling that defines MIFR has numerous reported advantages over more traditional open surgical treatments, it does present some unique challenges and important considerations for the surgeon. This article describes some of the general MIFR challenges a surgeon may encounter. The potential difficulties associated with the application of specific implants used in MIFR are described elsewhere in this issue.

PLANNING

Perhaps one of the biggest differences between MIFR and original guidelines set forth by the Arbeitsgemeinschaft für Osteosynthesefragen (AO) group is the need for more extensive presurgical planning and awareness. The original AO goal of direct open surgical visualization of all fracture components to facilitate complete anatomic

The author has nothing to disclose.
Department of Surgery, MedVet, Columbus, OH, USA
* 300 East Wilson Bridge Road, Worthington, OH, 43085.
E-mail address: Matthew.Barnhart@medvet.com

Vet Clin Small Anim 50 (2020) 17–21
https://doi.org/10.1016/j.cvsm.2019.08.001

reconstruction requires less planning because little is left to the imagination. Less concern for hematoma preservation and minimizing soft tissue and bone fragment manipulation makes fracture repair easier in many ways compared with when great care is taken to avoid such things. Simply put, not being able to see what you're doing when one is used to visualizing everything is a radical change. One of the best ways to combat this daunting difference is with preoperative planning.

Planning: Know Your Anatomy

All surgeons know that a thorough knowledge of regional anatomy is critical for minimizing patient morbidity and facilitating fracture repair. However, it is even more important when structures such as arteries, veins, and nerves cannot be visually identified and protected directly. Awareness of "safe" and "unsafe" MIFR zones/corridors for MIFR implant placement is vital.[1] In addition, knowing where to place an implant to maximize screw or pin bone purchase must be more highly considered during MIFR. For example, placing a plate on the caudal one-third of the proximal tibia will to help to ensure optimal screw or pin purchase compared with implants placed in the cranial two-thirds of the bone at the level of the cranial tibial fossa (**Fig. 1**). Moving a plate to a different position because you are unhappy with your screw placement is simple during an open approach but is far more difficult through a small MIFR incision.

Planning: Preparing the Implant

Although presurgical planning for determining implant size is a known requirement of interlocking nail use in both traditional open reduction and MIRF applications, it is less of a consideration when using plates. During traditional open reduction repairs plates can be placed on the bone, contoured, replaced, and contoured some more, and so on, until they are deemed anatomically appropriate by the surgeon. This is contrary to the goal in MIFR cases. In minimally invasive plate osteosynthesis (MIPO) applications, sliding a plate in and out of a created soft corridor multiple times to contour it

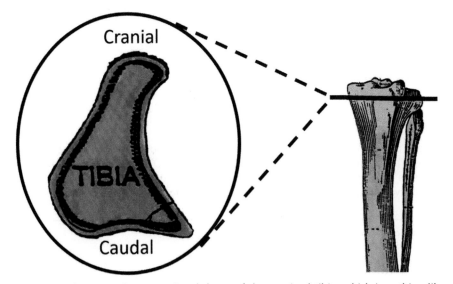

Fig. 1. Note the unusual cross-sectional shape of the proximal tibia, which is nothing like the classic "cylindrical" shape of a long bone diaphysis. Implants placed cranially will engage much less bone than implants placed caudally.

will cause unnecessary trauma to soft tissue and the often-tenuous blood supply to bone fragments and disrupt hematoma, all of which are contrary to the goal. Preoperative planning based on radiographs of the normal contralateral bone allows for predetermining plate size, length and precontouring plates can eliminate the aforementioned issues and greatly reduce surgery time. Procedural technique is detailed in Bruno Peirone's article, "Minimally Invasive Plate Osteosynthesis Fracture Reduction Techniques in Small Animals," elsewhere in this issue.

ANCILLARY CONSIDERATIONS
The Basics

Excellent lighting may seem like a basic operating room necessity, but it is a particularly important requirement in MIFR cases. Visualizing implants and anatomy through small stab incisions requires more focused lighting than does an open approach. As such, I believe that a high-quality headlamp is a necessity for any surgeon preforming MIFR. In addition, having a supply of instruments to facilitate MIFR will greatly reduce hardships. An ample supply and assortment of different-sized right-angled Gelpi retractors, soft tissue protection drill sleeves, extra-long Metzenbaum scissors (for creating tissue tunnels along the bone), and long drill bits will allow the surgeon to maintain the smallest incisions possible with proper retraction and tissue protection. Additional helpful MIFR-specific instrumentation is discussed in the Bruno Peirone's article, "Minimally Invasive Plate Osteosynthesis Fracture Reduction Techniques in Small Animals"; and Laurent P. Guiot and Loïc M. Déjardin's article, "Peri-operative Imaging in Minimally Invasive Osteosynthesis," elsewhere in this issue.

Timing is Everything

Performing MIFR earlier versus later is important to help facilitate bone alignment and reestablish limb length. Delays in fracture repair can make otherwise good MIFR applications very difficult to anatomically align, reduce, and bring out to length without requiring more invasive surgical dissection and reduction methods. Overcoming muscle contraction and managing early callus formation, all while attempting to minimize soft tissue dissection and fracture handling, is highly challenging and may make MIFR impossible.

Choose Your Battles

Multi-fragmentary fractures of the diaphysis and metaphysis are most suitable for MIFR. Articular fractures should be considered on a case-by-case basis but are generally better candidates for open reduction so that reestablishment of articular surface continuity can be definitively confirmed. Simple diaphyseal fractures are potential candidates for MIFR, but the advantages over interfragmentary compression in these applications is debatable.

Last, a well-executed open surgical fracture repair is a far better alternative than a well-intentioned but poorly performed MIFR. Surgeons should never resist converting to an open approach if they are not confident in their MIFR. The biologic advantages offered by MIFR are immediately negated by poor mechanical fixation and stability or injury to nonvisualized anatomic structures.

Fluoroscopy Is Often but Not Always Required

Intraoperative fluoroscopy (C-arms) is viewed by some a necessity when performing MIFR. However, repeated use of such equipment potentially exposes surgeons and staff to high cumulative levels of radiation. In addition, C-arm units and radiolucent operating room tables are expensive and the required radiation shield-ing equipment for personnel is cumbersome and gets very hot. Fortunately, a sur-geon interested in MIFR should not be discouraged if he or she does not have access to intraoperative imaging because many types of MIFR can be performed without fluoroscopic guidance with great success. External skeletal fixator place-ment using MIFR techniques often can be accomplished without imaging. In addi-tion, tibia fractures are particularly amenable to MIPO applications without need for a C-arm (**Fig. 2**), and intramedullary implants can be inserted in the humerus and femur without direct visualization of the fracture site and little to no direct frac-ture site palpation (**Fig. 3**). Throughout the articles in this journal, there are

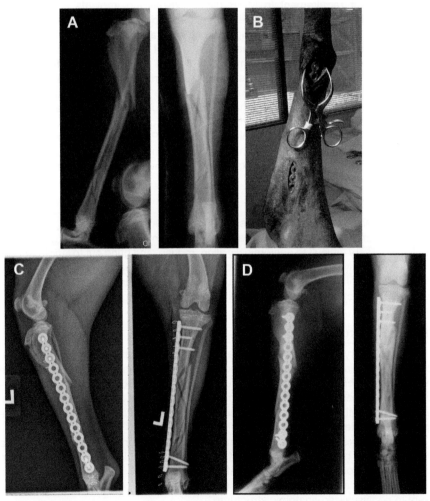

Fig. 2. (*A*) Lateral; and AP projection Preoperative radiographs of a tibial fracture highly amenable to MIPO methods without the assistance of intraoperative imaging. Note the fib-ula is intact. (*B*) Intraoperative view of hanging leg technique for maintaining reduction and limb alignment during plate placement. (*C*) Immediate lateral and AP projection postoper-ative radiographs. (*D*) AP and lateral projection Radiographs 5 weeks following surgery demonstrate bridging callus formation.

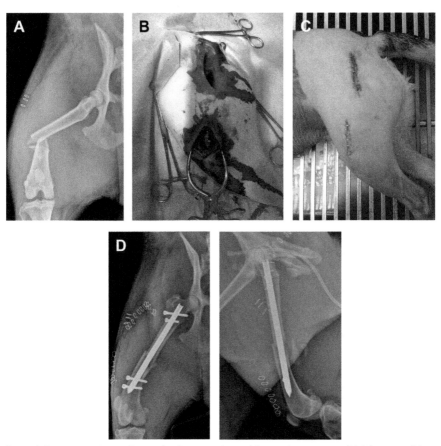

Fig. 3. (*A*) Preoperative radiograph of a comminuted femur fracture was highly amenable to minimally invasive interlocking nail stabilization without the assistance of intraoperative imaging. (*B*, *C*) Note that the soft tissue region over the fracture site is untouched. "Blind" normograde passage of this nail was possible with guidance by gentle digital palpation at the fracture site via the distal incision, while distraction was achieved at the proximal and distal incisions. (*D*) Immediate AP and lateral projection postoperative radiographs.

numerous methods and tricks described for fracture reduction and implant placement that can be performed without fluoroscopic guidance.

REFERENCE

1. Palmer RH. External fixators and minimally invasive osteosynthesis in small animal veterinary medicine. Vet Clin North Am Small Anim Pract 2012;42(5):913–34.

Minimally Invasive Plate Osteosynthesis Fracture Reduction Techniques in Small Animals

Bruno Peirone, DVM, PhD[a], Gian Luca Rovesti, DVM[b],
Alessandro Boero Baroncelli, DVM, PhD[c],
Lisa Adele Piras, DVM, PhD[a],*

KEYWORDS

- MIPO • Fracture • Reduction • Alignment • Traction • Distractor

KEY POINTS

- Anatomic fracture reduction is not typically achieved with minimally invasive fracture repair in small animals.
- Indirect fracture reduction is used with minimally invasive plate osteosynthesis to restore limb's length and alignment.
- Indirect fracture reduction preserves soft tissue attachment to fracture fragments, speeding healing and reducing complications.
- Many techniques are available to facilitate fracture reduction, including intramedullary pinning, hanging the limb, manual traction, distraction table, external fixators, and a fracture distractor.

INTRODUCTION

Minimally invasive plate osteosynthesis (MIPO) in small animals involves the application of a bone plate, typically in a bridging fashion, without performing a surgical approach to expose the fracture site.[1]

Treatment of a diaphyseal fracture with MIPO does not usually require the anatomic reduction of the fracture. Functional reduction is the goal; it restores bone length and

Disclosure Statement: Dr G.L. Rovesti owns shares of the Ad Maiora company. The other authors have nothing to declare.

The article is an update of "Peirone B, Rovesti GL, Baroncelli AB, et al. Minimally invasive plate osteosynthesis fracture reduction techniques in small animals. Vet Clin North Am Small Anim Pract 2012;42(5):873-95."

[a] Department of Veterinary Science, University of Turin, Largo Paolo Braccini 2-5, Grugliasco, Turin 10095, Italy; [b] Clinica veterinaria M. E. Miller, Via della Costituzione 10, Cavriago, Reggio Emilia 42025, Italy; [c] Clinica Albese per Animali da Compagnia, Alba, Cuneo, Italy

* Corresponding author.

E-mail address: lisa.piras@unito.it

correct alignment in the frontal, sagittal, and axial planes. Indirect reduction is used to obtain functional fracture reduction without opening the fracture site. This method allows the fracture fragments to remain connected to the adjacent soft tissues. This is the key to improve bone healing, because viable bone rapidly unites by callus formation.[2]

Indirect reduction is the "blind" repositioning of bone fragments using some form of distraction and translation. This method relies on aligning fragments and restoring bone length by distracting the bone ends instead of manipulating the fracture site. It is achieved using a remote instrument so there is no disturbance of the soft tissues around the fracture site. Indirect reduction may require exposure to apply the reduction devices, but not for visualization of the fracture site.

The general principle involved in indirect reduction is the use of the soft tissue envelope to help stabilize and reduce the fracture fragments indirectly. This goal can be achieved through forces applied either on the adjacent bone segments or on the epiphyseal or metaphyseal regions of the fractured bone. The former is commonly referred to as ligamentotaxis.[3] Traction table and limb hanging techniques are prime examples. In the latter, the tension on the soft tissues surrounding the fracture site guides the fragments into alignment as the bone ends are distracted. Intramedullary (IM) pinning, temporary application of a linear or circular external skeletal fixator, bone-holding forceps, bone distractor, or the plate itself are examples of this. These techniques can be used as a sole method of reduction or in any combination.

Fracture reduction can be accomplished completely closed or with the help of small incisions (portals). Proximal and distal incisions are needed to insert the plate and screws when using the MIPO technique. A small third portal (observation portal) can be used to view the fracture zone to facilitate placement of an IM pin (discussed elsewhere in this article). It should be emphasized that manipulation of the fracture fragments should be avoided when using an observation portal. If fracture reduction is unsuccessful using the following techniques, the surgeon should consider using a technique described by Hulse as "open but don't touch."[4] A long incision is made over the length on the bone, but the fracture fragments are not manipulated. This more generous approach allows an improved view of the fracture, facilitating indirect reduction of the fracture.

SKELETAL TRACTION TABLE

Traction tables are commonly used for human trauma patients and standardized reproducible techniques are routinely used for fracture reduction. These techniques include proper patient positioning, specific instrumentation, and application of intraoperative skeletal traction (IST).[5,6] The rationale behind fracture reduction by IST is counteracting the muscle contraction and regaining the original limb length. In this way, the bone segments are not overlapped and easily fit each other. When fragmentation is present, the fragments are pulled back in the area they came from by their muscular attachments, which exert a centripetal force. This philosophy of reduction, called ligamentotaxis, has the main objective of achieving fracture reduction by a minimally invasive or closed approach.

Recently, a skeletal traction table (Ergomed 99, Ad Maiora, Cavriago, Italy) was specifically designed for veterinary traumatology.[7] This table allows IST to be consistently applied in small animals with safe application of opposition and anchorage points.[8]

The opposition points are defined as the points on the body where stabilization can be applied to counteract the traction forces and avoid translation, without injuring the patient. Anchorage points are defined as the points where traction can be applied distal to the fractured skeletal segment, without damaging the bone or the soft tissues (**Fig. 1**).

Indications

The veterinary traction table has been used to apply IST and reduce different fracture patterns of the appendicular skeleton.[7] It is mandatory to thoroughly follow the suggested steps in applying the technique. It is a powerful technique that can be potentially dangerous if applied incorrectly.

Application of Intraoperative Skeletal Traction with a Traction Table

The anchorage devices used for application of traction are represented by anchorage belts for the antebrachium and tibia and a traction stirrup attached to a transcondylar Kirschner wire (K-wire) in the humerus and femur. The belts are coupled to evenly distribute the traction forces to both sides of the limb and then applied in the metacarpal or metatarsal area. The traction stirrup is used in conjunction with a transosseous K-wire through the condylar region of the humerus or the femur, in a position that is compatible with the site of fracture and the proposed osteosynthesis technique. The wire ends are connected to the stirrup arms by means of bolts. Once secured, the wire is tensioned by the stirrup lever mechanism. This tensioning avoids wire bending and prevents soft tissues from being cut by the bent wire.

Traction is exerted by means of a micrometric traction bar that can be lengthened by up to 20 cm. The traction bar has an L shape: the long component has a micrometric movement that allows bar elongation. One end of the bar is attached to the table rails with a clamp. The short component has 3 pins that allow connection to either of the belts or the stirrup.

Traction is applied progressively and incrementally increased at a rate of about 50 N every 2 minutes. More traction is applied as needed to maintain the scheduled force. The amount of load applied is related to patient body weight, muscular strength, and

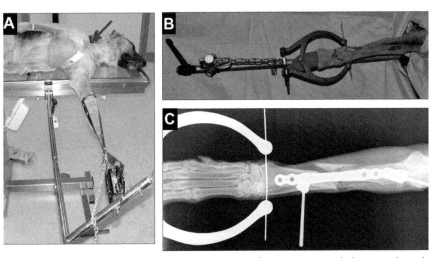

Fig. 1. Skeletal traction table and patient positioning for the craniomedial approach to the antebrachium in a cadaver. The dog's body is held in position by 2 nylon belts crossed over the sternum (*red arrow*). (A) Traction is applied via coupled belts connected to the traction bar, (B) or by means of a tensioned K-wire inserted in the distal radius and connected to an arch. (C) Intraoperative radiograph with the K-wire parallel to the carpal joint.

time between trauma and surgery, but especially to the quality of fracture alignment obtained. The fracture distraction and alignment achieved can be judged by palpation of the fractured site and or with intraoperative imaging.

During the application of traction, the maximal traction load is measured using a dynamometer. For safety reasons, the maximum load applied to each limb is never allowed to exceed 250 N. If the reduction is not achieved with this amount of load, some kind of interference should be suspected. A reduced approach to the fracture area can be considered to help in the reduction process by local direct manipulation. The duration of traction should be recorded. A shorter traction time reduces the potential damage to tissues subjected to traction.

The positioning for the traction of each bone segment is as follows.

Patient Positioning

Antebrachium

The animal is positioned in lateral recumbency with the affected limb lowermost and the contralateral forelimb maintained against the thoracic wall with the shoulder flexed. The neck is extended. The limb that is to be subjected to traction is positioned with the midshaft of the humerus at the edge of the table. The traction bar is attached to the table caudal to the forelimb, with the short component oriented cranially so that traction can be exerted with the craniomedial region of the radius remaining completely unobstructed.

Opposition points

Two belts are crossed over the sternum. A dorsal stabilizer is used on the dorsal area of the neck. The belt crossing the upper side surface of the neck region is passed over the stabilizer so that excessive pressure on the base of the neck by this belt is avoided.

Anchorage points

For this traction technique, traction belts applied to the carpometacarpal region of the forelimb are usually used. A transosseous K-wire can also be inserted through the distal epiphyseal region of the radius or through the metacarpal bones for anchorage in the case of older, displaced, or overriding fractures.

Humerus

Lateral plate application The animal is positioned in lateral recumbency with the affected limb uppermost. The contralateral forelimb is flexed at the elbow and secured with the carpus under the animal's muzzle. The traction bar is placed caudal to the forelimb with the short component oriented caudally to exert axial traction on the humerus.

Opposition points A single belt is passed circumferentially around the thorax in the region caudal to the axilla. Sometimes the application of a second K-wire and traction stirrup to the proximal metaphysis of the humerus is required. This approach is adopted because humeral traction applied with a single distal stirrup causes significant distal translation of the scapula without obtaining satisfactory alignment of the fracture segments.

Anchorage points For this technique, the traction stirrup is used. A K-wire is inserted with lateromedial direction across the condylar region or, instead, across the proximal ulna just following the humeral axis. Traction exerted with the belt applied to the carpometacarpal region can damage the distal structures before exerting a useful traction on the humerus because the musculature surrounding the humerus is usually very strong.

Medial and caudomedial plate application
The patient is positioned similar to that used for the antebrachium. The body of the patient is slightly tilted by interposition of sand bags between the thorax and the table. In all other respects, traction bar position and opposition points are the same as for the antebrachium (**Fig. 2**).

Anchorage points These are the same as described for the humeral lateral approach.

Tibia
Medial plate application: Lateral recumbency The animal is positioned in lateral recumbency with the affected limb lowermost and the contralateral hindlimb secured caudally with the stifle flexed and the hip extended. The limb that is to be subjected to traction is positioned with the midpoint of the femoral diaphysis overlying the border of the table. The traction bar is positioned caudal to the limb, with the shorter component of the bar oriented cranially, to keep the craniomedial aspect of the tibia completely unobstructed.

Medial plate application: dorsal recumbency This positioning is very useful because it allows a better assessment of the limb alignment on the frontal plane. The animal is positioned in dorsal recumbency. The limb being subjected to traction is extended caudally, with a support placed in the popliteal region. The contralateral hindlimb is positioned in abduction with the joints flexed and secured such that the calcaneus

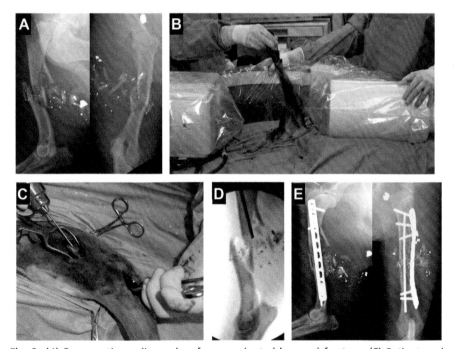

Fig. 2. (*A*) Preoperative radiographs of a comminuted humeral fracture. (*B*) Patient positioning in dorsal recumbency and C-arm position for intraoperative imaging. (*C*) IM pin: insertion into the cranioproximal aspect of the humerus, directed distally and medially. (*D*) Adjust the direction of IM pin with the fluoroscopic images. (*E*) Immediate postoperative radiographs after plate stabilization on the lateral side. (*Courtesy of* A. Pozzi, DVM, MS, DACVS, DECVS, DACVSMR, Zurich, Switzerland.)

is as close as possible to the ischiatic tuberosity. The traction bar is connected to the end of the table. Usually, a dorsal positioner is put underneath the thoracic region to maintain this position during traction.

Opposition points For the craniomedial approach to the tibia, 2 nylon bands are applied. One belt is passed over the uppermost ilium, across the inguinal region, and under the scrotum of male animals, and then secured to the table caudodorsally. It is useful to add a protective polyurethane cushion to this belt to prevent any harm to the patient. The second belt is passed circumferentially around the caudal region of the abdomen and both ends are secured to the table dorsally.

For the craniomedial approach with dorsal recumbency, the oppositional forces are applied to the caudal part of the thigh by means of a limb rest placed in the popliteal region.

Anchorage points A traction belt applied to the tarsometatarsal region of the limb for traction to evenly distribute the forces along the longitudinal axis of the tibia. The traction stirrup can be anchored to a transosseous K-wire inserted in the distal epiphysis of the tibia (**Fig. 3**) or to the metatarsal bones in cases of distal, overriding fractures.

Femur
The animal is positioned in lateral recumbency with the limb being subjected to traction uppermost. The contralateral limb is secured to the table caudally with the stifle flexed and the calcaneus positioned close to the ischiatic tuberosity. The traction bar is attached to the table cranial to the limb, with the shorter component oriented caudally to exert the traction along the longitudinal axis of the femur. A limb rest is used to support the tarsus to maintain the limb in a horizontal plane.

Opposition points A stabilization belt is passed across the abdomen caudally, just under the iliac wing, then across the inguinal region and under the scrotum of male animals. It is useful to add a protective polyurethane cushion to this belt to prevent any harm to the patient. The belt is secured caudodorsally to table. A second belt is passed around the caudal region of the abdomen and both ends of this belt are secured to the table dorsally.

Anchorage points For this traction technique, the traction stirrup anchored to a transcondylar K-wire placed at distal end of the femur is used, because of the strength of the thigh muscles.

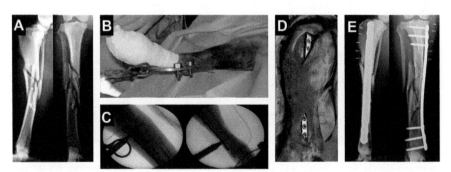

Fig. 3. (*A*) Preoperative radiographs of a comminuted tibial fracture. (*B*) IST. (*C*) Intraoperative fluoroscopy images showing the indirect reduction of the fracture and plate temporary fixation. (*D*) Plate insertion in a MIPO fashion. (*E*) Immediate postoperative radiographs.

Procedure technique Traction modalities vary in each case, mostly based on fracture location. Usually, the animals affected by radius–ulna and tibia closed fractures are positioned on the traction table and traction is applied before the limb is scrubbed. Once the fracture segments are realigned, the fracture reduction is confirmed by digital palpation, radiology, fluoroscopy, or a combination of these techniques. In this setting, the reduction procedure is performed without scrubbing of the limb. Once the fracture is satisfactorily realigned, the limb is maintained in traction, scrubbed, and prepared for surgery as usual. With this traction modality, the traction devices are nonsterile and are not included in the surgical field.

For open fracture stabilization, the limb is prepared for surgery, as usual, and traction is applied in a sterile surgical field.

For fractures of the humerus and femur, the limb is first scrubbed and prepared for surgery as usual. After performing the surgical approaches, the transcondylar K-wire is inserted and the sterile traction stirrup is applied and then connected to the micrometric traction bar with a small sterile chain. The end of this chain connected to the stirrup is kept sterile, and the end connected to the dynamometer and distraction bar becomes contaminated. An unscrubbed operating room assistant, who sets the load on the surgeon's request, applies the load required to distract the fracture segments. Contamination of the surgical field is avoided, because the assistant can set the traction bar from its top, far from the surgical field, while the portion of the traction bar close to the surgical field remains covered by sterile towels.

Correction of malalignment
Correction of intraoperative angular malalignment of fractures is performed entirely by the unscrubbed assistant who moves the traction bar under the direction of the surgeon, as described elsewhere in this article.[6] Correction of varus or valgus malalignment is achieved by rotating the short portion of the traction bar in a clockwise or counterclockwise direction, after temporarily loosening the lock of the clamp holding this bar. In this way, the tip of the bar is moved higher or lower than the starting point. For example, elevation of the tip of the bar results in correction of a valgus malalignment of the tibia with the animal in lateral recumbency and the operated limb in the lowermost position. However, the direction of the correction in relation to the animal's position should be evaluated. For example, when the animal is in dorsal recumbency, the correction of valgus or varus deformity is performed by loosening the clamp and sliding the entire traction bar along the lateral rail of the table, either in a medial or lateral direction.

To correct procurvatum or recurvatum malalignment, for all the positions but for the tibia with the animal in dorsal recumbency, the clamp is loosened and the entire traction bar is pushed horizontally along the lateral rail of the table. The clamp and the connected traction bar are pushed toward the cranial part of the animal for the correction of procurvatum and toward the caudal part for the correction of recurvatum. For the approach to the tibia with the animal in dorsal recumbency, the upward or downward rotation of the shorter part of the traction bar is used for the correction of procurvatum and recurvatum malalignment, respectively.

Potential Complications

This system of skeletal traction for fracture reduction has some elasticity that is inherent to the animal's tissues and the anchoring and opposition belts, which renders the process nonlinear during the initial stages. Although the application of opposition and anchorage belts is relatively simple, slippage of these belts may also contribute to this problem[7] or result in local tissue injury. In contrast, traction applied with a traction stirrup results in negligible elastic drop and does not cause any compressive soft tissue injury. It is important to use the opposition points that were developed from the cadaver study[7] and to monitor the duration and magnitude of the loading force to avoid any tissue damage.

Excessive traction also potentially results in compromise of the nervous and vascular systems. In circumstances in which an elevated load must be applied, it may be prudent to minimize its duration to decrease the likelihood of complications. When the procedure cannot be completed in a sufficiently brief period, it is preferable to consider temporary stabilization of the fracture (ie, long oblique fracture) with either a point reduction forceps or a K-wire applied percutaneously, releasing the traction to allow tissues to be better perfused, and then resuming traction after a short period.

Proper patient positioning and the use of skeletal traction are easily learned techniques that can rapidly become standard procedure. Although the time required for setting up the table, positioning the patient, and performing traction is somewhat lengthy, this time is regained during the osteosynthesis phase. In fact, plate application in an MIPO fashion is greatly simplified once the desired reduction is achieved because the osseous segments are steadily maintained in correct alignment for the necessary amount of time.

However, the technique may be potentially dangerous and, therefore, should be applied cautiously to avoid iatrogenic trauma. It is imperative that the application of opposition and anchorage points is correct, and prolonged and unnecessary loading is avoided.

HANGING LIMB

Suspending the limb from an infrastructure or from the ceiling orients the limb in a vertical position. By lowering the surgical table, the animal's own weight distracts the fracture and helps to align the joint surfaces.[9,10] Intraoperative imaging is greatly facilitated because both the frontal and sagittal planes are unobstructed and the C-arm or portable radiograph machine can be freely moved around the patient.

Indications

This technique is mostly indicated for comminuted fractures of the antebrachium and tibia when used alone. The subsequent application of a temporary circular or linear external fixator can greatly improve the stability of the fracture reduction.

Procedure Technique

The animal is positioned for surgery in dorsal recumbency, with the affected limb suspended and draped. The anchorage point should be exactly over the limb to exert a linear traction along the long axis of the fractured bone (**Fig. 4**). The use of a sterile snap-hook system allows the surgeon to disconnect the limb from the anchorage point to evaluate joints' flexion and plane of motion after temporary plate application.[9]

Potential Complications

The weight of the animal restricts the achievement of the fracture reduction. This technique does not provide control over the horizontal plane. It is, therefore, important to verify rotational alignment after temporary fixation by disconnecting the limb from the suspending hook and flexing and extending the adjacent joints. In tibial fractures, traction applied to the pes frequently results in a caudal translation of the distal fragment. This phenomenon must be taken into account before plate positioning.

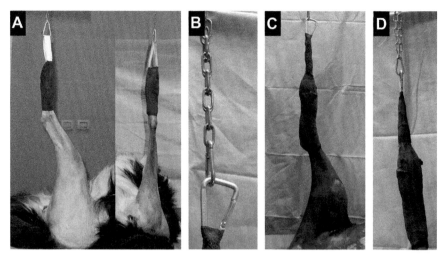

Fig. 4. (*A*) Hanging limb technique for tibial fracture treatment: patient positioning. (*B*) A sterile snap-hook system is secured to the paw. (*C*) The paw and the pulley system are wrapped with sterile self-adherent tape. (*D*) Allowing the surgeon to disconnect the leg during the procedure.

INTRAMEDULLARY PINNING

An IM pin used as a distraction device is an effective method to overcome muscle resistance and gradually restoring length and axial alignment of a fractured bone[9] The IM pin placed near the neutral axis of the bone is very resistant to bending forces and, therefore, capable of maintaining axial alignment.[11] Advantages in using an IM pin for indirect reduction in MIPO include the following.

1. An additional surgical approach is usually not required for normograde pin insertion.
2. Pin progression in the distal fragment allows fracture distraction by overcoming the muscles contraction.
3. The bone surface is free for further plate application.
4. Plate application is easier owing to partial stabilization and alignment of the fracture.
5. Proper limb alignment can be confirmed by observing joint orientation during flexion and extension of the proximal and distal joints.

Indications

All long bone fractures can be treated with indirect reduction achieved by means of an IM pin; however, in the case of a radius fracture, the IM pin is to be inserted in the ulna. Long oblique and comminuted fractures with a large fracture gap are suitable for IM pin reduction. Pin progression in the distal bone segment is especially simple in the case of comminuted fractures, because usually there is no overriding of the main segments.

If the fracture pattern is characterized by a small proximal or distal segment, it will be more challenging to obtain and temporarily maintain a correct axial alignment. This is due to the small bone stock and consequent inadequate pin–bone purchase.

Short oblique or transverse fractures are more demanding. Muscle contraction produces large fracture dislocation and segment overriding is always present. Gradual and progressive traction has to be applied over a period of time to overcome muscle contraction and achieve fracture alignment. Elevating and distracting the fractured bone ends using bone-holding forceps through the surgical approaches reduces segment overriding and allows pin progression in the distal fragment.[9]

Smooth pins with tips at 1 or both ends are used, and their size normally ranges from 1.2 to 4.0 mm in diameter. Correct pin selection is related to bone diameter and determined from preoperative radiographs during surgical planning. The diameter of the pins used should be approximately 30% to 50% of the diameter of the bone's medullary cavity.[4]

Procedure Technique

Surgical proximal and distal approaches, as described for MIPO application in dogs, are to be performed before IM pin insertion.[1,12] The proximal intact bone segment is secured with a bone-holding forceps and the pin is advanced distally. If the pin is properly aligned, it progresses easily in the medullary cavity. In the case of difficult progression, the pin is likely penetrating the cortex and should be redirected. The pin tip is cut and the pin passed carefully through the fragmented area of the bone.

To cut the distal tip of the pin 2 options are available:

1. Withdraw the inserted pin, cut the tip, and reinsert it with the same direction. or
2. Proceed with pin insertion until the tip emerges from the distal approach, then cut the tip.

The pin can be advanced by drill, pushed through using the drill with the motor stopped[10] or by hand using a mallet or Jacob's chuck.

Without the pointed tip, the distal part of the IM pin leans against the metaphyseal bone of the distal segment, distracting the fracture gap while restoring bone length and aligning the main bone segments.[4,13]

Long pins left out from the entrance point help in the intraoperative evaluation of pin direction. A second pin with the same length can be used to evaluate IM pin depth in the distal segment's medullary canal.

Holding the distal segment with point-reduction forceps percutaneously, or with bone-holding forceps applied through the distal approach, helps in maintaining the correct axial alignment during pin progression. To achieve adequate stability, the pin must be seated in the cancellous bone of the distal metaphyseal region.

Once in place, the IM pin assists in maintaining the axial alignment of the bone in both frontal and sagittal planes. However, because it does not effectively counteract torsional forces, it is important to check torsional alignment before plate application, especially in comminuted fractures.

Proper pin positioning and bone alignment can be assessed clinically, but thorough intraoperative diagnostic imaging is recommended, especially in proximal bone segments. Once correct pin placement is confirmed, the IM pin can be left in place to function as a plate-rod construct or removed when the plate has been sufficiently secured to the major bone segments.[4,12] If the pin is left in place, the proximal portion could be cut close to its exit from the bone. More commonly, if the diameter of the pin allows it, the pin is bent at its exit from the proximal segment and cut to allow its removal following fracture healing.

Humerus

Lateral approach The lateral approach is mainly used in proximal and middle-third fractures. The patient is positioned in lateral recumbency with the affected limb uppermost. The proximal approach is performed on the craniolateral aspect of the greater tubercle. The curvature of the bone and the level of the shaft fracture determine the point for insertion of the pin on the cranial crest of the greater tubercle. A point-reduction forceps can be used to hold the proximal segment during pin insertion.

The IM pin is driven from the proximal segment by entering the bone on the lateral slope of the ridge of the greater tubercle near its base.[10,11] Initial drilling is done with the pin held perpendicular to the bone surface. After tip penetration of the outer cortex, the pin is redirected distally into the medullary canal to shift parallel to the caudomedial cortex. The pin must be seated just proximal to the supratrochlear foramen.[10]

Medial approach This approach is mainly used in mid-diaphyseal and distal third fractures. The patient is positioned in lateral recumbency with the affected limb lowermost and the contralateral retracted caudally. The distal approach is performed along the caudal cortex of the medial epicondyle and soft tissue dissection is performed, being mindful of the ulnar nerve, which should be identified and retracted cranially. Bone-holding forceps can be used to secure the distal fragment during pin insertion. The IM pin enters the bone just distally to the square corner of the medial portion of the condyle, directed parallel to its caudal cortex. Proper pin size must be determined on preoperative radiographs so that it can pass along the medullary canal of the medial epicondyle. The pin progresses through the fracture site and advances proximally along the cranial cortex of the proximal segment.[14]

Femur
The patient is positioned in lateral recumbency with the affected limb uppermost. Once the proximal approach has been performed, the pin is inserted through the subcutaneous fat and the gluteal muscles until the top of the great trochanter is felt with the tip of the pin. During pin insertion, the proximal femur is held with a bone-holding forceps at the angle and rotation of the normal standing position.[10] Maintaining the same axis as the femur, the pin is gently moved medially off the trochanter into the trochanteric fossa, where it will center itself with some pressure. To avoid slippage, the tip of the pin is first seated into the metaphyseal bone of the trochanteric fossa in a cranial direction. Once penetration begins, the pin is aligned with the long axis of the proximal femoral segment.

Tibia
The patient is positioned in dorsal recumbency with the stifle flexed at a right angle. The proximal approach is performed on the medial aspect of the proximal tibia over the medial collateral ligament and slightly extended proximally to the medial aspect of the stifle joint (**Fig. 5**). The pin is then inserted along the medial border of the patellar ligament, entering the proximal end of the tibia between the cranial surface of the tibial tuberosity and the medial condyle of the tibia.[10]

Radius and ulna
Fractures affecting the antebrachium can be reduced both with retrograde and normograde IM pinning of the ulna. The size of the pin should be as large as it can fit in the distal medullary canal of the ulna. The patient is positioned in dorsal recumbency, allowing an easy approach to the radius by extending the elbow and to the ulna by flexing the elbow joint. With minimal soft tissue dissection, the deep flexor muscles on the caudal aspect of the ulna are elevated to expose the fractured ends of the ulna. The pin is retrograde inserted in the proximal segment to exit at the olecranon. The ulnar fracture is reduced and the pin normograde driven across the fracture site and ideally seated in the distal metaphysis of the ulna.[15] Normograde pin insertion

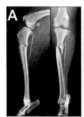
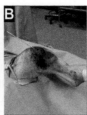
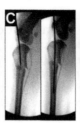
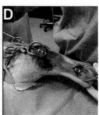
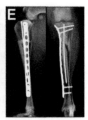

Fig. 5. (*A*) Preoperative radiographs of a mildly comminuted proximal tibia and fibula fracture. (*B*) Normograde IM pinning of the tibia. (*C*) Intraoperative fluoroscopy images showing the indirect reduction of the fracture. (*D*) Plate insertion through the medial proximal and distal incisions using a MIPO technique. (*E*) Immediate postoperative radiographs. (*Courtesy of* A. Pozzi, DVM, MS, DACVS, DECVS, DACVSMR, Zurich, Switzerland.)

is also possible, but more challenging (**Fig. 6**) owing to physiologic procurvatum and the decreasing diameter of the medullary canal.

Potential Complications

If a plate and rod technique is selected to treat the fracture, the IM pin can interfere with bicortical screw insertion, especially in the diaphyseal region. Joint penetration could be possible during pin progression in the distal segment, but is unlikely to occur once the tip has been severed. When a plate and rod construct is applied, pin migration can occur during the postoperative period and pin removal is, therefore, recommended.[4]

LINEAR EXTERNAL FIXATION

Full or half pin frames allow correction of angular deformity and maintenance of bone length. This technique requires shorter setup times, provides complete access to the bone, and allows complete manipulation of the limb, thereby facilitating plate application while avoiding the use of excessive traction because the reduction force is applied solely to the bone and not across the proximal and distal joints.

Indications

Linear external fixation is indicated in fractures of the antebrachium and tibia, because of the relative paucity of soft tissues surrounding them. Similar techniques on the humerus and femur are not recommended because of the large muscle bellies.

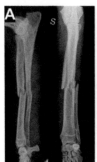
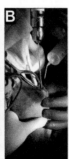
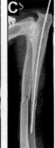
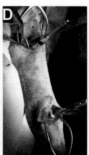
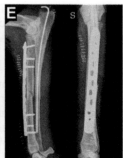

Fig. 6. (*A*) Preoperative radiographs of a comminuted radius and ulna fracture. (*B*) Normograde IM pinning of the ulna. (*C*) Intraoperative radiograph. (*D*) Temporary plate stabilization with push-pull devices. (*E*) Immediate postoperative radiographs.

Procedure Technique

During the surgical positioning of the patient, the affected limb is securely suspended from a ceiling hook and draped. Using a sterile hook system allows the surgeon to disconnect the leg during the procedure.[9] Transfixation full-threaded pins or half-threaded pins are placed in the proximal and distal metaphyses of each bone segment. Their diameter must not exceed 20% to 30% of the width of the medullary canal.[16] The pins are centered in the bone on the sagittal plane and parallel to their respective joint surface. The proximal pin should be placed sufficiently posterior so as not to interfere with plate positioning.[17] It is mandatory to place fixation elements only in safe soft tissues corridors.[18] Care must be taken before pin insertion to avoid multiple attempts that would increase the risk of iatrogenic fracture or bone necrosis. Intraoperative radiographic control or fluoroscopy is used to assess correct pin placement.

The table is then lowered or a pulley system used to raise the limb, suspending the patient by the fractured limb. The weight of the patient distracts the fracture and helps to align the joint surfaces. If necessary, manual distraction on the threaded pin can improve alignment. The connecting bars are placed and limb alignment clinically evaluated. Intraoperative fluoroscopy or radiology is valuable in the assessment of correct alignment.[9]

Only after good reduction and alignment have been achieved the plate can be inserted and secured to the bone.

Potential Complications

Special care is needed to avoid intra-articular pin placement and to ensure that the pins are effectively parallel to the proximal and distal joint surfaces to prevent malalignment. It is important to avoid pin placement into fissures or superficial cortical areas, possibly resulting in fractures. Attention must be paid to avoid nerve or vessel injury during pin insertion, respecting safe corridors.

Leaving empty holes is not ideal, because this can lead to subsequent bone fracture, probably because of the stress riser effect caused by creating a defect in the cortical bone. Placing a hole too close to 1 cortex, eccentrically, rather than penetrating the bone in its middle area could also create a stress riser.

DePuy Synthes (West Chester, PA) markets a unilateral linear fixator system specifically developed to facilitate MIPO applications in human patients. The Minimally Invasive Reduction Instrumentation System (MIRIS) (DePuy Synthes Trauma) has cannulated reduction handles that are slid over and secured to implanted half pins. The handles are used to manipulate the secured major fracture segments. A carbon fiber connecting rod is secured to each of the reduction handles with connecting clamps. When the clamps are tightened, the articulated reduction handle construct maintains alignment and reduction, simplifying MIPO implant placement.[19,20]

A recent canine cadaveric study was performed comparing the use of the MIRIS and a 2-ring circular construct to facilitate alignment and reduction during MIPO applications using a comminuted radius and ulna fracture model. MIRIS allowed for shorter reduction times and simplified plate placement, without compromise to fracture reduction and alignment.[21]

The application of the MIRIS was a relatively efficient process; however, obtaining initial half-pin purchase in the proximal metaphysis of the radius was sometimes difficult owing to the convexity of the radius in this region. Placement of the half pins, which have a 75% larger diameter than the 1.6-mm Kirschner wires used in the circular fixator construct, could potentiate postoperative morbidity, including fracture of the radius through the pin tract. The potential for fracture may increase if the initial pin placement is unsuccessful. The authors reported lower difficulty of plate placement scores associated with use of the MIRIS, attributing it to the construct being situated unilaterally, on the opposite side of the limb to location of the plate insertion incisions. The MIRIS only impeded plate application when the distal half-pin was situated directly subjacent to a screw hole in the plate.

The authors concluded that although both constructs were useful in performing MIPO, the MIRIS was simpler to apply and interfered nominally with plate placement. The authors also published their initial clinical experience using the MIRIS for MIPO application in dogs and concluded that MIRIS was easy to apply and consistently resulted in reductions that were near anatomic, with acceptable restoration of length and alignment. Plate and screw placement was unimpeded by the MIRIS, facilitating implant application and complications observed were not related with the MIRIS use.[22]

CIRCULAR EXTERNAL FIXATION

Tensioned small diameter wires and circular rings can be used with a simple, efficient technique, described by Jackson and colleagues,[17] which allows for precise reduction, length restoration, excellent control of rotation, and easy access for imaging. Once held at the correct length, the frame construct will resist shortening and, perhaps, distraction forces during plate positioning. The application of the frame is straightforward and may be rapidly accomplished and the insertion of fine wires is minimally invasive, causing little tissue trauma.

Indications

Circular external fixation indirect reduction technique is indicated in tibia, radius, and ulna fractures. Humerus and femur fractures are less commonly reduced by this technique because of the large muscle bellies and the impingement given by the thorax and the abdomen. When used for those segments, half rings are used. This method is particularly useful in fragmented or segmental fractures where the reduction is difficult to maintain. It is challenging in proximal and distal third fractures, where the frame can interfere with proper plate positioning and fixation. When this is the case, the reduction can be maintained by a transarticular frame.

Procedure Technique

The frame is preassembled with 2 rings or arches (partial rings) arranged in a single block configuration for the proximal and distal fragment. When arches are used, the proximal one is oriented with the open portion cranially, to avoid interference with elbow or stifle flexion. The distal arch is oriented with the open portion cranially, to avoid interference with the carpus and hock flexion. This frame construct allows for a better limb alignment evaluation during the surgical procedure.

The surgeon must choose a ring or arch size that can be placed around the animal's limb while still having enough space between the skin and the inner margin of the ring to position the plate. The rings or arches are connected using 2 threaded rods, positioned to avoid interference with safe corridors, and subsequent plate application. The transosseous wire size is selected according to established guidelines.[23]

A standard hanging limb preparation is performed with the animal in dorsal recumbency, in a way that to retain the possibility of attaching and detaching the limb from the hanging support. The first transosseous wire is placed in the proximal radius or tibia, parallel to the mediolateral axis of the elbow or stifle joint and perpendicular to the longitudinal axis of the proximal segment. The proximal wire should be placed sufficiently posterior so as not to interfere with plate positioning.[17]

The preassembled frame is passed over the limb and connected to the proximal wire. The distal transosseous wire is inserted in a direction that is parallel to the antebrachiocarpal, or hock joint, and perpendicular to the longitudinal axis of the distal segment. It is recommended to place fixation elements preferably in safe soft tissue corridors. Care must be put before wire insertion to avoid multiple attempts that would increase the risk of iatrogenic fracture or bone necrosis.

Proper placement of the wires is confirmed through intraoperative radiographs or fluoroscopy. The distal wire is then connected to the frame. The wires are tensioned to a maximum of 30 kg to avoid arch deformation.[23]

Fracture reduction is achieved by gentle and progressive distraction of the rings or arches. Distraction is applied by turning the nuts on the threaded rods. By ensuring that the 2 wires are inserted perpendicular to the longitudinal axis and parallel to each other in both frontal and sagittal planes, correction of alignment and rotation is achieved because the bone length is restored (**Fig. 7**). In most trauma cases, the use of conical couples instead of flat nuts is very useful, because they allow rotation and inclination of the rings and the threaded bars to each other, thus allowing multiple planes of correction.

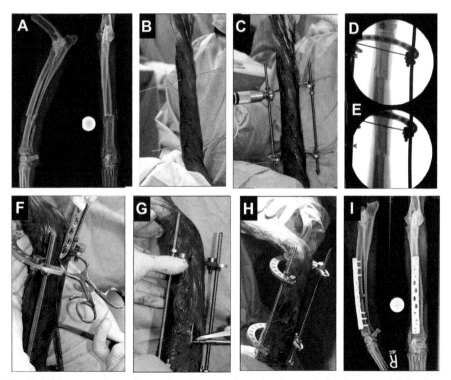

Fig. 7. (*A*) Preoperative radiographs of a comminuted radius and ulna fracture. (*B*) Application of the ring fixator. (*C*) Fracture distraction applied by turning the nut. (*D*) Intraoperative fluoroscopy showing fracture reduction. (*E*) Plate insertion in a MIPO fashion. (*F*) Screw insertion. (*G, H*) Limb alignment evaluation. (*I*) Immediate postoperative radiographs. (*Courtesy of* A. Pozzi, DVM, MS, DACVS, DECVS, DACVSMR, Zurich, Switzerland.)

Reduction and axial alignment can be improved by modifying the frame's spatial alignment, using the following methods.[24]

- The angled bar technique. This technique is used with systems that do not have hemispheric nuts and washers available and consists of changing the angle of a threaded bar between the rings or arches. This bar is connected to the rings or arches, offset by the amount of the deformity to be corrected but in the opposite direction. When the nuts on the previous straight connecting bars are loosened and the nuts on this angled bar are tightened, the angled bar becomes perpendicular to the rings, rotating the bone segment in the direction opposite to that of the deformity.
- Hemispheric nuts and washer technique. This method can be used with systems in which hemispheric nuts and washers are available. The nuts are loosened, the distal ring or arch is rotated in the direction opposite to the deformity, and the nuts are tightened again after deformity correction, leaving the threaded bars at an angle to the rings. Hemispheric nuts and washers can also be used to correct angular deformities. For example, if a valgus deformity is present, the length of the lateral threaded bar connecting the rings may be increased, while the nuts of the threaded bar on the medial side may be released to avoid them holding the rings in the previous position, preventing the frame construct from moving.
- Shifting of the bone along the wire. If a dislocation ad latum is present, it can be corrected by shifting the bone along the wire, thus changing its position on the horizontal plane.
- Rotation of the bone along the fulcrum of the wire. Once distraction of the fracture segments has been achieved, a residual angular deformity may still be present. The bone segment may be aligned using the wire as a fulcrum, thus changing its axis. For this procedure to be performed, it is mandatory that just 1 wire is inserted in each segment. If more than 1 wire is inserted in the bone segment, it will be locked.

Potential Complications

Special care has to be put to avoid intraarticular wire placement[18] and to ensure that the wires are effectively parallel to the proximal or distal joint surfaces respectively to prevent malalignment. It is important to avoid the placing of the transfixation pin into fissures or superficial cortical areas, possibly resulting in fractures. Care must be put to avoid nerve or vessel injury during wire insertion. The use of small-size wires leaves a very small empty hole, diminishing the risk of stress riser effect and secondary fractures.

Pozzi and colleagues[25] compared MIPO and open reduction and internal fixation of radius–ulna fractures in dogs and reported that all fractures obtained radiographic union although infection developed in 1 dog in each stabilization group. No statistical difference was found in operating time, postoperative alignment, gap width, or time to union (MIPO, 51.9 ± 18.4 days; open reduction and internal fixation, 49.5 ± 26.5 days). Although bone segments could easily be slid along the fixator wires, translational malalignment was less effectively corrected than the other types of malalignment; moreover, although not directly compared, simple fractures were more likely to have translational malalignment than comminuted fractures. The authors did not report any rotational or frontal angulation malalignment after MIPO.[25]

Bone-Holding Forceps

Small bone-holding forceps inserted far from the fracture site through the proximal and distal surgical approaches can be used to align the fracture.[26] The most distal and proximal parts of the bone segments are secured with the bone-holding forceps and the segments are distracted and manipulated to reduce the fracture. This method is most successful in the radius–ulna and tibia fractures in which the reduced muscle mass allows more accurate palpation and easier reduction.[1,10]

Nevertheless, a forceps is a space-occupying device and should be applied to the bone in a position that allows subsequent plate application. For example, in a tibial fracture the bone-holding forceps grip the cranial and caudal bone aspects to allow medial plate placement. It should also be noted that bone-holding forceps are passive devices, requiring an assistant to maintain reduction until plate fixation is completed.

In humerus and femur fractures it is often more challenging to achieve and maintain proper fracture reduction with this method because of the large surrounding muscle. Therefore, in such cases, bone-holding forceps are mostly used in combination with other reduction techniques, such as IM pinning. For example, in a femoral fracture the bone-holding forceps could be applied through the proximal surgical approach at the level of the subtrochanteric region to hold and maintain the proximal segment in a levered position during pin insertion (**Fig. 8**). A second bone-holding forceps, applied through the distal surgical approach at the level of the supratrochlear region, can be used to distract and manipulate the distal segment allowing pin insertion and progression.

Bone-holding forceps can also be used as an aid to further improve segment alignment when other indirect reduction techniques are used. Occasionally, a point reduction forceps can be used percutaneously (**Fig. 9**) to approximate a severely displaced fragment or long oblique fractures.[26]

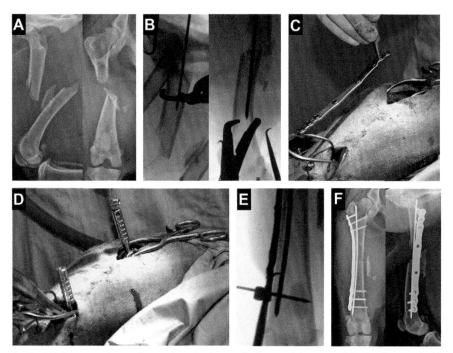

Fig. 8. (*A*) Preoperative radiographs of a butterfly femoral fracture. (*B*) The forceps holds the proximal segment during normograde IM pinning. (*C*) Intraoperative radiograph. (*D*) Temporary plate stabilization with push-pull devices. (*E, F*) Immediate postoperative radiographs.

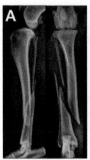
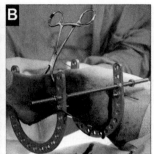
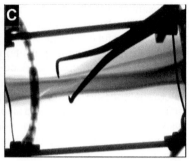

Fig. 9. (*A*) Preoperative radiographs of a long oblique tibia and fibula fracture. (*B*) The point reduction forceps is used percutaneously to approximate the fracture. (*C*) Intraoperative fluoroscopy. (*Courtesy of* A. Pozzi, DVM, MS, DACVS, DECVS, DACVSMR, Zurich, Switzerland.)

FRACTURE DISTRACTOR

The fracture distractor is a mechanical device that applies the forces directly to the bone segments. Some of them are available.

Dynamic 2.0 Distractor

The Dynamic 2.0 distractor is composed of a threaded bar enclosed into 2 stainless steel telescopic cylinders. To function as distractor, the bar is locked at 1 end of 1 cylinder, while the other can be moved proximally or distally by sliding inside the other cylinder (Ad Maiora). The movement is micrometrical, generating a very high force of distraction on the fractured area. Adjacent parts of the body remain unobstructed. The fracture distractor allows easy distraction of the bone segments, even when severe muscle contraction is present.

It works like a temporary fracture distractor if plating is the scheduled procedure, or like a definitive stabilization device if more pins are added once the fracture reduction is achieved. The special clamps allow bone segment movement in all the planes, thus facilitating reduction maneuvers (**Fig. 10**). In very unstable fractures, or when the plate could be potentially weak because of the features of the fracture or the patient's temperament, it can be used like a temporary ancillary stabilization device together with the plate, to be removed after the early bony callus developed.

Titan Distractor

The Titan distractor is composed of 2 threaded bars connected by a knob that carry 2 orthogonal arms. When the knob is rotated, distraction or compression of the arms

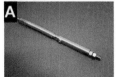
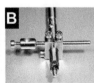
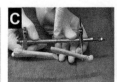
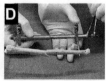

Fig. 10. (*A*) The dynamizable linear fixator. (*B*) A fixator clamp allows multiplanar fracture segment adjustment. (*C*) Application of the dynamizable fixator to a plastic model simulating an overlapped fracture. Note the central part of the fixator body that is almost close. (*D*) After fracture reduction, the central part of the fixator body is larger than before distraction. The clamps can now be set to better adjust the fracture reduction.

can be achieved. The connection with the bone is provided by traction stirrups, the use of which is described elsewhere.[27]

Indications

The fracture distractors are generally reserved for use in large breed dogs, with muscle contraction and fragment overriding or in old fractures where callus and muscle contracture must be overcome. The Dynamic linear distractor can be used in almost all sizes of patients.

Procedure Technique

Dynamic 2.0

Two threaded pins are inserted in the metaphyseal area of both the proximal and distal segments. The distractor is then attached to the pins and the sliding cylinder can then be moved distally, distracting the fracture. The offset position of the distractor allows the surgeon to access the fracture site for implant application. Varus, valgus, or rotational malalignments can be corrected thanks to the special clamp that allows to move the fragments in every plane. When used like an ancillary temporary device, the distance from the bone and the clamp should be decreased to increase the frame stiffness, once the plate is secured to the bone.

Titan distractor

A 1.5-mm diameter K-wire is placed through the proximal fragment and connected to a traction stirrup (Ad Maiora s.r.l.). A second K-wire is inserted through the distal fragment and connected with a second traction stirrup. Then, the distractor (Titan distractor, Ad Maiora s.r.l.) is connected to the stirrups (**Fig. 11**). By rotating the distraction knob to lengthen the distractor, the fracture overlapping is reduced. The distraction should be progressively increased, as usual, to avoid iatrogenic damages to the tissues. Owing to the great adaptability of application of the traction stirrup to many different areas of bones, its application can be extended to virtually all the bones, including vertebral fractures.

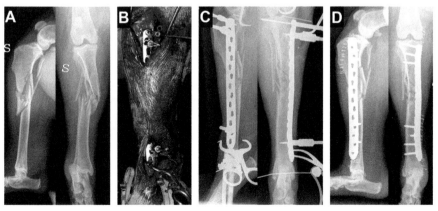

Fig. 11. (A) Preoperative radiographs of a comminuted tibial fracture presented in **Fig. 3**. (B) Temporary plate stabilization with 2 push and pull devices. (C) Intraoperative radiographs showing the indirect reduction of the fracture. (D) Immediate postoperative radiographs.

Potential complications

Although the fracture distractor can be used to indirectly reduce comminuted fractures, it can be difficult to apply bridging plates in an MIPO fashion with the distractor in place.[8] The Dynamic 2.0 distractor should be used with long pins to avoid interference with plate positioning. It should also be placed so that it does not interfere with plate positioning. For example, if a craniomedial plate is scheduled, it should be placed laterally.

Reduction through plate application

The use of anatomically precontoured standard or locking plates in MIPO treatment of diaphyseal fractures helps to ensure proper reduction and correct limb alignment.[28]

Indications

This technique should be combined with one of the previously described methods of indirect reduction to restore the correct bone length before plate application. Only small displacements and angulations on both the frontal and the sagittal planes can be corrected while maintaining stability as the reduction occurs.[1]

Procedure technique

Plate precontouring The orthogonal radiographic views of the contralateral intact limb are used to select the adequate plate whole length and to contour the plate preoperatively.[26] Plate length is evaluated on the mediolateral view and should be close to the length of the whole bone. Schmokel and associates[29] recommend the use of a long plate in MIPO applications to dissipate the stress on the construct. Furthermore, longer plates with a limited number of screws positioned at the plate ends have been shown to sustain greater loads before failing than shorter plates with a screw placed in each plate hole.[30]

Accurate plate precontouring is usually performed on the craniocaudal view to ensure proper axial alignment of the main fragments and correct bone length.[29] Plate bending and twisting are performed to adapt plate ends to the shape of both the proximal and the distal metaphyseal regions of the fractured bone.

Standard plates With standard bone plates, screw tightening produces frictional forces between the plate and the bone and, during weight bearing, the shearing load is transferred directly from the bone to the plate.[31] Therefore, accurate anatomic plate contouring is mandatory to maintain primary fracture reduction during screw tightening.[32]

After plate insertion, the proximal plate end is positioned on the center of the bone and fixed with a cortical screw inserted perpendicular to the cortex. This screw is not fully tightened to allow movement of the distal plate end. Bone-holding forceps can be used to center the plate over the bone or to achieve plate–bone contact. The bone cortex of the distal segment is then exposed and the plate end centered over the bone and fixed with a second cortical screw. Plate position is then checked by means of intraoperative imaging, after which both screws are tightened and fracture reduction is controlled before the final fixation.

If the axial alignment is not satisfactory, another cortical screw should be inserted closer to the fracture site through a separate stab incision to act as a reduction screw. This process allows the displaced segment to be pulled against the plate and reduced in a more anatomically correct position.[33]

Locking plates With locking plates, a rigid connection between the plate hole and the screw is achieved; therefore, no frictional forces are produced between the plate and the bone.[31] The advantage of locking plates is the minimal contouring required for their application in comparison with standard plates. The locking plate acts as an internal fixator and, therefore, does not displace the fracture segments during locking-screw tightening, regardless of the precision of contouring.[32] To provide stable fixation, proper locking of the screw is essential. Temporary stable plate fixation to the bone is recommended before the insertion of the first locking screws.

The push–pull device (Synthes, Solothurn, Switzerland) is a temporary reduction device applied through a plate hole to hold the locking compression plate against the bone (see **Fig. 11**). This device is self-drilling and connects with the quick coupling for power insertion. After monocortical insertion, the flange is turned clockwise until it pulls the plate securely against the bone. Once the plate is secured by the other screws, the push–pull device is removed and a screw can be inserted in the same hole.[34]

Another temporary reduction device is the pin stopper, part of the Fixin system (Traumavet, Rivoli, Italy). The pin stopper is a perforated stainless steel cylinder that can be inserted over a smooth pin and locked with a small screw nut (**Fig. 12**). The pin is inserted in the plate hole through a dedicated conical drill guide. Bicortical pin insertion is recommended to improve torsional stability. Pin insertion progresses until the stainless steel cylinder reaches the top of the conical drill guide and consequently pushes the plate against the bone. The use of a threaded pin can improve this action once the threaded tip enters the bone cortex.[35]

With a properly contoured implant, positioning temporary reduction devices in a hole that is further away from the ends of the plate allows better plate–bone contact and consequently more accurate fracture reduction (see **Fig. 12**).

Potential complications

Inadequate plate contouring may result in loss of primary reduction and axial malalignment during cortical screw tightening or temporary plate fixation. Axial malalignment can also occur if bone length is not completely restored and segment overlapping is still present before plate application. If the proximal and distal screws are not inserted into the center of the bone, because of the plate being offset, or if their direction is not

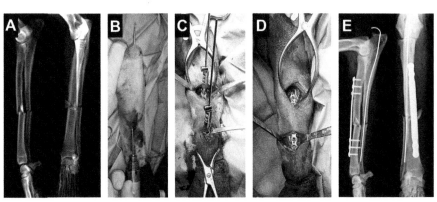

Fig. 12. (*A*) Preoperative radiographs of a radius and ulna fracture. (*B*) Retrograde insertion of the IM pin in the ulna. (*C*) Two pin stoppers are inserted through the plate for temporary plate fixation and indirect fracture reduction. (*D*) Intraoperative aspect after the plate application. (*E*) Postoperative radiographs showing indirect fracture reduction and temporary plate fixation.

perpendicular to the cortical surface, segment rotation and translation may occur at the fracture site.[33]

Care must be taken during tightening of the first screws. The insertion torque applied could still result in dislocation of the bone segments. Therefore, palpation and assessment through visual or intraoperative imaging is recommended to avoid poor fracture reduction.

ASSESSMENT OF ALIGNMENT

After fracture indirect reduction has been achieved, care must be taken to carefully assess limb alignment. Malalignment is the most common complication associated with MIPO, because the fracture site is not exposed and the surgeon cannot rely on direct visualization of correct reduction to restore alignment. It must be underlined that a loss of length or a moderate malalignment on the sagittal plane (procurvatum or recurvatum) does not affect the patient's functional outcome, whereas malalignment on the frontal (varus or valgus) or axial plane can severely compromise limb function. Limb alignment can be assessed both by clinical evaluation and intraoperative fluoroscopy or radiology.

Proper patient positioning and surgical draping are mandatory to allow correct alignment evaluation. The limb should still be completely visible in both sagittal and frontal planes after draping, and the distalmost and proximal-most joints should be evaluated in their range of motion. This setting allows for the identification of anatomic landmarks, which is fundamental for clinical evaluation. Familiarity with the normal relationship between external anatomic landmarks is as essential as in-depth knowledge of bone anatomy in preventing malalignment.[36] The availability of a sterile bone model in the operating room can also help the surgeon to recognize these landmarks on the fractured limb.

Clinical evaluation can easily be performed on the antebrachium and crus, but it can be challenging for the arm and thigh, owing to the presence of large muscle bellies. Therefore, for the proximal bone segments, reliance on intraoperative diagnostic imaging is strongly recommended. Access to a C-arm should be ensured to provide complete visualization of the proximal and distal joints in both frontal and sagittal planes. If fluoroscopy is not available, intraoperative radiographs can be obtained with a portable radiograph machine. Intraoperative radiographs are satisfactory for distal limb segments but suboptimal for proximal ones. Furthermore, the issue of radioprotection for the personnel is raised by the latter technique.

Clinical Evaluation

Tibia
The rotational and frontal alignment are subjectively evaluated with the stifle and hock joints flexed at 90°, by aligning the patella, the tibial crest, and the long axis of the III and IV metatarsal bones, and by reestablishing the sagittal plane of the hind limb. Furthermore, the position of the calcaneus can be assessed during flexion and extension of the stifle. If internal tibial torsion is present, the calcaneus seems to be displaced laterally, whereas, with external tibial torsion, it seems to be displaced medially. Moreover, observing the orientation of the foot with respect to the sagittal plane of the crus while palpating the malleoli is very helpful.[36]

Antebrachium
The same clinical assessment described for the tibia is used to evaluate the alignment of the forearm. The humeral condyle, the radius, and the long axis of the III and IV metacarpal bones are used to reestablish the sagittal plane of the forearm. The

position of the flexed manus is useful to assess axial malalignment. A medial position indicates an external radial torsion, whereas a lateral position suggests an internal radial torsion.

Femur

The anatomic relationship between bone landmarks can also be reestablished in the femur, although it is more difficult. Rotational alignment can be judged by palpation or by direct visualization of the greater trochanter and femoral trochlea through the proximal and distal approaches. The lateral aspect of the femoral trochlea can be palpated or observed through a stifle mini-arthrotomy. The distal part of the femur is then held in a true lateral position. The position of the greater trochanter is then inspected through the proximal approach. If the femur is aligned correctly on the axial plane, the greater trochanter should be slightly caudal compared with the long axis of the bone. According to Dejardin and Guiot,[36] with the femur in a true lateral position, the midpoint of the greater trochanter should be slightly caudal to the coronal plane with the distal aspect of the line of origin of the vastus lateralis muscle aligned with the coronal plane.

Furthermore, in a correctly aligned femur, the surgeon can perform a 90° external and 45° internal rotation of the hip. This method is recommended only if the plate has been temporarily secured to the bone.

Humerus

The anatomic landmarks used for clinical evaluation are the humeral epicondyles, the greater tubercle, and the bicipital groove. These landmarks can be used to roughly evaluate humeral axial alignment. When holding the humeral epicondyles in a true mediolateral position, it should be possible to palpate the greater tubercle cranially and the bicipital groove medially.

Intraoperative diagnostic imaging

As stated elsewhere in this article, reliance on intraoperative diagnostic imaging is mandatory in the case of proximal limb fractures and generally suggested for all bone segments. The anatomic details and relationship with the adjacent bones are evaluated through 2 orthogonal projections. These must include the whole bone segment and the proximal and distal joints. Comparison with the contralateral unaffected limb is also useful if the required projections have been previously obtained.

Intraoperative fluoroscopy enables several quick spot projections of all these structures and is, therefore, the most useful method of assessing bone alignment.

SUMMARY

Indirect fracture reduction is used to align diaphyseal fractures in small animals when using minimally invasive fracture repair. Indirect reduction achieves functional fracture reduction without opening the fracture site. The limb is restored to its previous length and spatial alignment is achieved to ensure proper angular and rotational alignment. Fracture reduction can be accomplished using a variety of techniques and devices, including hanging the limb, manual traction, distraction table, external fixators, and a fracture distractor.

REFERENCES

1. Hudson CC, Pozzi A, Lewis DD. Minimally invasive plate osteosynthesis: applications and techniques in dogs and cats. Vet Comp Orthop Traumatol 2009;22: 175–82.

2. Luenig M, Hertel R, Siebenrock KA, et al. The evolution of indirect reduction techniques for the treatment of fractures. Clin Orthop Relat Res 2000;375:7–14.

3. Bone L. Indirect fracture reduction: a technique for minimizing surgical trauma. J Am Acad Orthop Surg 1994;2:247–54.

4. King KF, Rush J. Closed intramedullary nailing of femoral shaft fractures. A review of one hundred and twelve cases treated by the Kuntscher technique. J Bone Joint Surg Am 1981;63:1319–23.

5. Wu CC. An improved surgical technique to treat femoral shaft malunion: revised reamed intramedullary nailing technique. Arch Orthop Trauma Surg 2001;121: 265–70.

6. Rovesti GL, Margini A, Cappellari G, et al. Intraoperative skeletal traction in the dog. A cadaveric study. Vet Comp Orthop Traumatol 2006;19:9–13.

7. Rovesti GL, Margini A, Cappellari G, et al. Clinical application of intraoperative skeletal traction in the dog. Vet Comp Orthop Traumatol 2006;19:14–9.

8. Johnson AL. Current concepts in fracture reduction. Vet Comp Orthop Traumatol 2003;16:59–66.

9. Piermattei DL, Flo G, DeCamp C. Handbook of small animal orthopedics and fracture repair. 4th edition. Philadelphia: W.B. Saunders Company; 2006. p. 227–660.

10. Rudy RL. Principles of intramedullary pinning. Vet Clin North Am 1975;5:209–28.

11. Reems MR, Beale B, Hulse DA. Use of plate and rod constructs and principles of biological osteosynthesis for repair of diaphyseal fractures in dogs and cats: 47 cases (1994-2001). J Am Vet Med Assoc 2003;223(3):330–5.

12. Pozzi A, Lewis DD. Surgical approaches for minimally invasive plating osteosynthesis in dogs. Vet Comp Orthop Traumatol 2009;22(4):316–20.

13. Johnson AL, Hulse DA. Fracture reduction. In: Fossum TW, editor. Small animal surgery. 2nd edition. St. Louis (MO): Mosby Yearbook Inc; 2002. p. 889–93.

14. Dejardin L, Guiot L. "MIO in diaphyseal humeral fractures". Lectures abstracts booklet, Small Animal MIO Traumatology Course 2011. Las Vegas (NV).

15. Witzberger TH, Hulse DA, Kerwin SC, et al. Minimally invasive application of a radial plate following placement of an ulnar rod in treating antebrachial fractures. Vet Comp Orthop Traumatol 2010;23:459–67.

16. Edgerton BC, An KN, Morrey BF. Torsional strength reduction due to cortical defects in bone. J Orthop Res 1990;8:851–5.

17. Jackson M, Topliss CJ, Atkins RM. Technical tricks: fine wire frame assisted intramedullary nailing of the tibia. J Orthop Trauma 2003;17(3):222–4.

18. Marti JM, Miller A. Delimitation of safe corridors for the insertion of external fixator pins in the dog. J Soc Adm Pharm 1994;35:78–85.

19. Apivatthakakul T, Babst R, Bavonratanavech S, et al. Instruments. In: Babst R, Bavonratanavech S, Pesantez R, editors. 2. Minimally invasive plate osteosynthesis. 2nd edition. New York: Thieme New York; 2012. p. 51–62.

20. Minimally invasive reduction and plate insertion instruments technique guide. West Chester (PA): DePuy Synthes; 2015.

21. Gilbert ED, Lewis DD, Townsend S, et al. Comparison of two external fixator systems for fracture reduction during minimally invasive plate osteosynthesis in simulated antebrachial fractures". Vet Surg 2017;46:971–80.

22. Townsend S, Lewis DD. Use of the Minimally Invasive Reduction Instrumentation System for facilitating alignment and reduction when performing minimally invasive plate osteosynthesis in three dogs. Case Rep Vet Med 2018;2018: 2976795.

23. Ferretti A. The application of the Ilizarov technique to veterinary medicine. In: Maiocchi AB, Aronson J, editors. Operative principles of Ilizarov. Baltimore (MD): Williams & Wilkins; 1991. p. 551–70.

24. Rovesti GL, Bosio A, Marcellin-Little DJ. Management of 49 antebrachial and crural fractures in dogs using circular external fixators. J Soc Adm Pharm 2007;48: 194–200.

25. Pozzi A, Hudson CC, Gauthier CM, et al. Retrospective comparison of minimally invasive plate osteosynthesis and open reduction and internal fixation of radius-ulna fractures in dogs. Vet Surg 2013;42(1):19–27.

26. Guiot LP, Dejardin LM. Prospective evaluation of minimally invasive plate osteo-synthesis in 36 nonarticular tibial fractures in dogs and cats. Vet Surg 2011;40: 171–82.

27. Rovesti GL, Devesa-Garcia V, Urrutia PG, et al. Evaluation of a distractor to increase the joint space of the stifle joint in dogs: a cadaveric study. Vet Comp Orthop Traumatol 2015;28:179–85.

28. Eidelman M, Ghrayeb N, Katzman A, et al. Submuscular plating of femoral frac-tures in children: the importance of anatomic plate precontouring. J Pediatr Or-thop B 2010;19:424–7.

29. Schmokel HG, Hurter K, Schawalder P. Percutaneous plating of tibial fractures in two dogs. Vet Comp Orthop Traumatol 2003;16:191–5.

30. Sanders R, Haidukewych GJ, Milne T, et al. Minimal versus maximal plate fixation techniques of the ulna: the biomechanical effect of number of screws and plate length. J Orthop Trauma 2002;16:166–71.

31. Miller DL, Goswami T. A review of locking compression plate biomechanics and their advantages as internal fixators in fracture healing. Clin Biomech 2007;22: 1049–62.

32. Wagner M. General principles for the clinical use of the LCP. Injury 2003;34(2): B31–42.

33. On Tong G, Bavonratanavech S. AO manual of fracture management - minimally invasive plate osteosynthesis (MIPO). Davos, Switzerland: AO Publishing; 2007. Clavadelerstrasse 8, Davos Platz.

34. Haaland PJ, Sjöström L, Devor M, et al. Appendicular fracture repair in dogs using the locking compression plate system: 47 cases. Vet Comp Orthop Trau-matol 2009;22:309–15.

35. Petazzoni M, Urizzi A, Verdonck B, et al. Fixin internal fixator: concept and tech-nique. Vet Comp Orthop Traumatol 2010;23:250–3.

36. Dejardin L, Guiot L. "Limit and complications of MIO". Lectures abstracts booklet. Las Vegas (NV): Small Animal MIO Traumatology Course; 2011.

Perioperative Imaging in Minimally Invasive Osteosynthesis

Laurent P. Guiot, DVM, MS[a], Loïc M. Déjardin, DVM, MS[b],*

KEYWORDS

- Minimally invasive osteosynthesis • Fluoroscopy • Surgical planning • Imaging

KEY POINTS

- Peri-operative imaging using various appropriate modalities is critical to the successful planning and performance of any orthopedic surgery.
- The use of intra-operative imaging, while not an absolute prerequisite for long bone fractures, considerably facilitates the smooth and effective execution of minimally invasive osteosynthesis of articular fractures.
- One must keep in mind, however, that the risk of overexposure to radiation with fluoroscopy and conventional radiology is real, particularly when considering its insidious effect over time.
- Strict adherence to the "As Low As Reasonably Achievable" (ALARA) principles is critical to mitigate the deleterious effect of radiation exposure while optimizing surgical outcome.

Diagnostic and interventional imaging techniques are an integral part of the surgical planning and execution of any orthopedic procedure. Although this statement is true with conventional osteosynthesis, the reliance on imaging techniques is even more pronounced when minimally invasive surgery is used to achieve fracture repair. In minimally invasive osteosynthesis (MIO), surgical approaches are minimalistic and performed away from the injury sites, which impedes the surgeon's ability to ascertain proper surgical execution. This article reviews the imaging modalities used perioperatively in MIO.

Perioperative imaging begins with the acquisition and interpretation of high-quality preoperative orthogonal radiographs of the affected segment and contralateral side. In some cases additional projections such as oblique or stress views may be added to routine exposures to obviate subtle lesions or ligamentous deficiencies. Advanced imaging techniques, typically in the form of a computed tomography (CT) scan, are

Disclosure: The authors have nothing to disclose.
The article is an update of "Guiot LP, Déjardin LM. Perioperative imaging in minimally invasive osteosynthesis in small animals. Vet Clin North Am Small Anim Pract. 2012;42(5):897-911."
[a] ACCESS Bone & Joint Center, ACCESS Specialty Animal Hospital, 9599 Jefferson Boulevard, Culver City, CA 90232, USA; [b] Orthopaedic Surgery, Collaborative Orthopaedic Investigations Laboratory, Department of Small Animal Clinical Sciences, College of Veterinary Medicine, Michigan State University, 736 Wilson Road, East Lansing, MI 48824, USA
* Corresponding author.
E-mail address: Dejardin@msu.edu

Vet Clin Small Anim 50 (2020) 49–66
https://doi.org/10.1016/j.cvsm.2019.08.003
0195-5616/20/© 2019 Elsevier Inc. All rights reserved.

added to the preoperative workup when standard radiography is insufficient to fully characterize an injury. Completion of preoperative assessment is followed by the establishment of a proper surgical plan, which may or may not include the use of intra-operative imaging.

Although not absolutely necessary, intraoperative imaging using fluoroscopy (C-arm) is often helpful with MIO, particularly in periarticular trauma. In addition, arthroscopy can be used as an aid to fixation for intra-articular injuries as it provides a minimally invasive way to assess fragment apposition and inform on implant position with respect to articular surfaces. One must keep in mind, however, that the use of ionizing radiation may have long-term insidious health effects. Therefore, the benefits of this technology should be carefully weighed against potential health hazards.

Finally, postoperative imaging is used to critically assess repair adequacy, including alignment and implant positioning. This step is essential for the prediction of clinical outcome and decision making for revision should it be necessary. It also helps to build operative skills because postoperative radiographs reveal the quality of surgical execution as a comparison with preoperative planning.

PREOPERATIVE IMAGING

The goals of preoperative imaging include:

1. To identify the nature, location, and extent of injury
2. To determine the ideal mode of fixation, including preselecting surgical implants
3. To establish optimal operating room setup

Passive restraint techniques are recommended over manual restraints for acquisition of radiographs:

1. To improve personnel safety
2. To enhance image quality (suppression of motion artifacts)
3. To allow subtle position adjustments until accurate projections are acquired
4. To standardize images and allow for sequential comparison

With the advent of digital radiography, image calibration has become critical because sizing cannot be inferred from the primary image. Although magnification ratio can be grossly estimated from the manufacturer's specification handbook in most machines, an actual calibration marker is necessary to obtain accurate representation of the actual size of the segments in the radiographs (**Fig. 1**). The marker may be spherical or linear. It must be equidistant from the receptor to the segment evaluated and parallel to it if linear. The marker is then used to calculate a magnification ratio, which in turn permits precise analog (acetate) or digital templating. Positioning of the marker closer to the X-ray beam *or to the cassette* will induce an optical magnification of the marker greater *or smaller* than that of the bone inducing under *or over* estimation of the bone size, respectively.

Imaging of the contralateral segment is necessary in MIO as it is used:

1. To optimize preoperative implant selection (type [plate/interlocking nail], size, and length)
2. To compare with the fractured segment to identify normal versus abnormal structures
3. To accurately evaluate postoperative alignment

The main limitation associated with standard radiography is the inability to reproduce a 3D configuration of structures examined. It is, however, a relatively cost-effective modality that addresses preoperative needs in most instances.

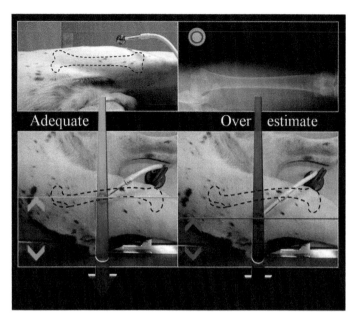

Fig. 1. Illustration of the effect of placement of a magnification marker (spherical or linear) for a horizontal beam projection of the femur (the X-ray beam is directed from the top of the image as shown in by the arrows). To avoid image distortion, the marker must be superimposed with the bone of interest (*left*). Only then will the magnification of the marker and the bone be identical on the radiographic image. Placement of the marker closer to or away from the X-ray generator will lead to misinterpretation of the magnification ratio in excess or default respectively (*right*). Similarly, the bone of interest should be parallel to the radiographic cassette.

Advanced imaging is indicated in cases with comminuted fractures involving the periarticular regions (**Fig. 2**A, B) or for the assessment of complex structures such as the sacroiliac region in the pelvis (see **Fig. 2**A). In orthopedic practice, a CT scan is often preferred over an MRI scan because it offers better and faster rendering of

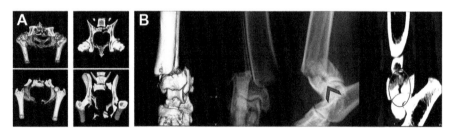

Fig. 2. (*A*) Three-dimensional reconstruction of two dogs with sacral fractures. In the first case (*top*), there is a comminuted fracture of the sacral body and left wing. Such lesion precludes fixation using a compression screw and should be treated conservatively to prevent iatrogenic neurological lesions. Conversely, the simple parasagittal fracture in the second case (*bottom*) maybe treated surgically using MIO techniques with little risk of iatrogenic trauma. (*B*) - Preoperative radiographs (*center*) and CT scan (left and right) of a periarticular distal tibial fracture. The radiographs were suggestive of a fissure extending in the frontal plane towards the talocrural joint. The 3D reconstruction (left) and coronal (*right*) CT images confirmed the presence of a complete fissure extending through the subchondral bone in the frontal plane.

osseous structures. The images acquired are visualized in 2D using multiplanar reconstruction techniques or in 3D by using thresholding to select the bone and hide the soft tissues. Both visualization modes are used in conjunction to gain the most information possible and facilitate the establishment of an accurate surgical plan.

A CT scan is best suited in such cases and provides 2D transverse images and a 3D reconstruction of the affected bones. Transverse images are used for precise assessment of fissure lines, which is essential in optimizing implant placement, particularly with epiphyseal fractures (see **Fig. 2**B). Coronal and parasagittal images also provide invaluable information in cases of sacroiliac luxation associated with comminuted sacral fractures (see **Fig. 2**A).

The use of 3D imaging helps in understanding such complex intra-articular fractures and improves preoperative planning. Furthermore, 3D reconstruction is beneficial in evaluating fragment distribution and can be used to guide reduction maneuvers. The main shortcomings associated with CT imaging are availability and cost. However, because the benefits of accurate planning and subsequent avoidance of intraoperative complications likely overcomes these limitations, CT imaging should be considered an integral part of preoperative planning when using MIO. Alternative modalities, such as MRI and ultrasound are seldom used in veterinary orthopedic trauma, but advanced applications for identifying stress fractures and musculotendinous lesions may prove them to be beneficial in some instances.

The choice of a specific implant is then made based on fracture configuration, as identified with preoperative imaging, patient signalment, and surgeon's preferences. All systems described for conventional osteosynthesis may find MIO applications. Once a fixation system is selected, specific implant dimensions must be determined. Appropriate templating is mainly based on the preoperative radiographs of the contralateral intact side, corrected for magnification. Using premagnified (usually by 4% and 12%) acetate templates superimposed over the radiographs is a cost-effective, however, fairly inaccurate method. In contrast, digital templating can be performed using one of the several dedicated software currently available. Most software will allow the surgeon to plan the entire procedure, including fracture reduction, planning of the location and magnitude of corrective osteotomies in angular limb deformity cases, implant selection and size, implant positioning and contouring (plates), and predetermination of plate screw or interlocking bolt lengths (**Fig. 3**). Considering the cost of this software, interested surgeons are encouraged to become familiar with the system and ascertain that it is compatible with in-house picture archiving and communication systems and that desired templates are available.

Implant position is based on a detailed evaluation of the fractured bone. The fracture pattern, including the presence and extent of fissures, as well as the spread of the fragments, should be carefully evaluated as it may influence the choice and/or position of an implant.

INTRAOPERATIVE IMAGING
Indications

The most obvious limitation of MIO is the inability to directly assess the bone fragments and fracture lines during surgery secondary to the lack of fracture site visualization. Indirectly, this negatively affects the evaluation of (1) fragment apposition, (2) segmental alignment, and (3) identification of structural abnormalities that could be affecting the fractured bone, such as the presence of fissures. Intraoperative imaging such as arthroscopy and fluoroscopy reduce this relative blindness by providing live feedback on the reduction status, alignment restoration, and implant position.

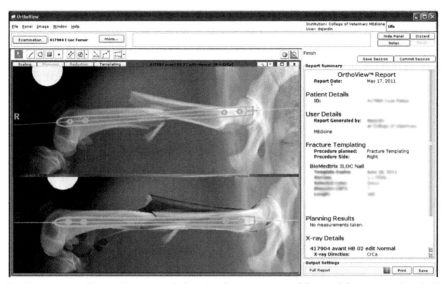

Fig. 3. Montage illustrating surgical planning for treatment of femoral fracture with a dedicated preoperative digital planning software. Digital manipulation of the fragment using the reduction tool provided with the software, allows the surgeon to visualize realignment. In this case, an angle-stable nail was preferred over and LCP as its intramedullary location greatly facilitates realignment. In contrast complex plate countering and use of MIPPO technique make maintenance of alignment during fixation more challenging.

Benefits of these imaging modalities vary based on fracture pattern and location. Whereas it is evident that arthroscopy is only valuable in articular trauma, fluoroscopy has a broader range of application in MIO.

Intraoperative fluoroscopy can provide valuable insights in most MIO procedures but is only truly necessary in periarticular fractures. Importantly, overreliance on fluoroscopy may translate into suboptimal outcomes, a shortcoming that tends to be overlooked by inexperienced surgeons. When considering diaphyseal fractures affecting lower segments (ie, radius-ulna and tibia), readily palpable anatomic landmarks are available and may be used along with joint range of motion to assess fragment location and orientation. This allows for accurate assessment of the alignment, thus reducing the need for intraoperative fluoroscopy. In contrast, upper segments (ie, humerus, femur, and pelvis) are more difficult to assess because of the presence of large soft tissue envelopes and their proximity to the body wall. Fluoroscopy is helpful, and sometimes necessary, in these locations to assist with reduction maneuvers and improve intraoperative assessment of alignment.

Diverging from traditional AO precepts of anatomic reconstruction and rigid fixation, modern AO principles promote the use of bridging osteosynthesis applied using minimally invasive techniques in diaphyseal fracture repair.[1–3] In this mode of fixation, the shaft is no longer reconstructed because fragments are left untouched during surgery to preserve their viability. Implant are selected to span the entire fracture site to create a construct that is semirigid to elastic. With implant extending from joint to joint (adults) or physis to physis (immature animals), intraoperative imaging can be used to ascertain that screws or locking bolts are not violating these essential structures (**Fig. 4**). Diaphyseal fragments are somewhat ignored fluoroscopically and the focus is set on evaluating alignment of adjacent joints. In fractures confined to the diaphysis, the use of a C-arm may facilitate the repair but is not paramount to success. Careful

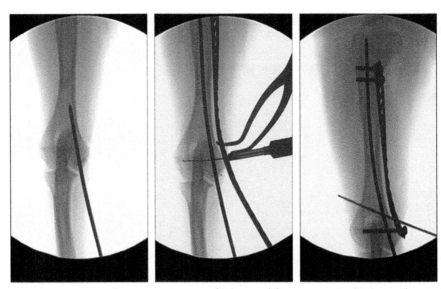

Fig. 4. Intraoperative fluoroscopy images of a humeral fracture repaired using a plate rod combination. The rod is inserted normograde from the medial epicondyle for maximal anchorage (*left*). Following rod insertion, a plate is slid epiperiosteally along the medial cortex. The C-arm is used to ensure proper plate contouring and optimal insertion of the screws (*center* and *right*). Note the orientation of the two distal screws inserted above and below the supracondylar foramen. The distal most screw was placed parallel to the elbow joint to maximize anchorage and prevent inadvertent joint penetration..

evaluation of metaphyseal/epiphyseal anatomic landmarks should provide enough insights to execute the surgery and fluoroscopy is optionally used as a secondary verification tool.

In contrast, all traditional AO principles of intra-articular fracture repair still hold true when using MIO. Fractures involving articular surfaces must be anatomically reduced and stabilized using rigid fixation and interfragmentary compression when possible. In these cases, proper assessment of the reduction status is critical and requires the use of intraoperative imaging. Finally, in nonarticular epiphyseal and metaphyseal fractures, fluoroscopy is systematically used to ensure proper anchorage of the implants in the limited bone stock available for fixation. This guarantees optimal implant insertion and reduces risks of inadvertent joint penetration by the implants (see **Fig. 4**).

Fluoroscopy
Equipment Numerous items are used with intraoperative fluoroscopy. Many choices, ranging from type of machine to supporting accessories, must be made by the surgeon in preparation for use in the context of MIO. Some equipment is optional, but other considerations such as personnel safety equipment are mandatory and regulated by national or regional radiation safety laws. Broadly, these items may be categorized as *required* for those necessary for the safe acquisition of images or *optional* for those that may be used to improve personnel safety and image quality.

Required equipment
1. Intraoperative fluoroscopy unit (full-size or mini C-arm)
2. Lead gowns and thyroid shields (for all personnel in the operating room [OR])

3. Individual radiation dosimeters
4. Warning signs of ionizing radiation use

Optional equipment (recommended)
1. Radiolucent operating table (optional based on procedure and type of C-arm)
2. Attenuating gloves
3. Protective glasses
4. Sandbags and resting devices
5. Radiolucent operating table (optional based on procedure and type of C-arm)

Intraoperative fluoroscopy unit C-arms are mobile fluoroscopic systems that consist of an X-ray generator and an image intensifier mounted on a movable C-shaped arm (**Fig. 5**). They are categorized as full-size or mini based on the dimension of the arm with a free operating space between generator and detector of ~800 mm (31.5″) and ~350 mm (13.8″), respectively. The X-ray tube and image intensifier or detector are mounted coaxially at the opposite ends of the C-arm. Note that image intensifiers are being supplanted by digital detectors, which are more sensitive and require less radiation than older generation systems. The beam is collimated to the size of the detector to reduce radiation exposure and optimize image quality. Further manual collimation can be applied during surgery to minimize scatter and unnecessary radiations. The C-arm is attached via an articulated arm to the control unit or mounted on an independent wheeled base that facilitates maneuverability (mini or full-size C-arms, respectively). Four basic motions of the arm are enabled with various amplitudes based on individual models. These movements are remotely

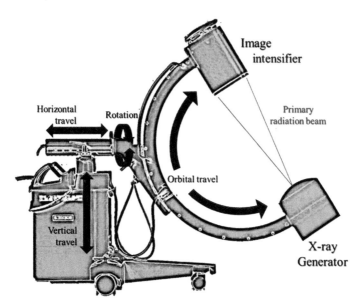

Fig. 5. Full size C-arm diagram showing the four basic motions of the arm. Note the position of the X-ray generator downward compared to the image intensifier. This setting is preferred to selectively reduce scatter radiation towards the surgery crew. Alternatively, the X-ray generator may be placed high above the table with the image intensifier below the table, closer to the patient. While this configuration may improve image definition, it also generates larger amount of harmful scattered radiation back to the surgical team and therefore should be discouraged.

or manually operated depending on the type of motorization of the arm. Motorized arms are available in full-size units only to improve mobility and allow memorization of specific positions to obtain repeatable projections throughout a procedure. Computerized image processing coupled to position recognition is also used to create 3D rendering in advanced applications. The basic arm motions are:

1. Horizontal traveling ($\sim$200 mm)—"in-out"
2. Vertical travel/surge ($\sim$460 mm)—"up-down"
3. Orbital travel ($\sim$115°)—"swing"
4. Rotation about horizontal axis ($\pm$210°)—"rotate"

The arm unit is coupled to a workstation used for image display, processing, and storage. The workstation and C-arm may be independent as in full-size C-arms or part of a single unit as with most mini C-arms. Numerous software have been developed for advanced applications ranging from digital subtractions to 3D image reconstructions. Basic functions allow image manipulation to modify contrast, reorient and recall previous images, which amply covers the needs for MIO applications. Current machines include compatibility programs to integrate the C-arm images to picture archiving and communication systems using DICOM format. Alternatively, images may be stored on the machine (not recommended), printed, or exported to various media including USB flash drives and external hard disks. Compatibility with the other systems in use in an institution should be taken into account before purchase to enhance work flow and minimize data loss.

The choice of a particular machine depends on the primary purpose of the C-arm. The first choice to be considered is between a full-size and a mini C-arm. Although both may be suitable for orthopedic procedures, their functionalities are very different. The final decision will be based on the availability of other equipment (such as a radiographic and fluoroscopy room), and the allocated budget.

Full-size C-arms have a broader spectrum of applications than minis and extending well beyond orthopedic surgery. Newer generations have 3D reconstruction capabilities, which can be useful in periarticular trauma, and advanced *cine mode*, which are necessary for interventional radiography procedures.[4] They are, however, significantly more expensive and less mobile than mini C-arms. Consequently, full-size C-arms are most often used as static units in veterinary applications where the machine remains in the same position throughout a procedure. If necessary, they may be mobilized intraoperatively by a dedicated radiology technician, but maneuvers increase risks of inadvertent contamination of the surgical field. Most commonly the patient will be repositioned to obtain the desired projection(s). Images are generally acquired through the radiolucent surgery table because the broad C allows enough clearance above the surgery site with the generator in the lowermost position. One major drawback associated with this usage may be the additional dose necessary to acquire images when compared with images obtained off the table. The increase in dose is correlated to the amount of attenuation produced by the table which is a function of the tabletop material and thickness. Using a purpose-built fluoroscopy table will optimize image quality while minimizing radiation demand.

Mini C-arms are less costly but offer fewer options than full-size C-arms. Their major advantage is an improved mobility allowing more flexibility than full-size units when working on extremities. They also produce lower levels of ionizing radiation, which helps to reduce personnel exposure during surgical procedures.[5] With mini C-arms, the machine is maneuvered around the patient to produce orthogonal images. The "weaker" X-ray generator limits the use of these machines in *cine mode*, and the *subtraction modes* are typically not available. The portability of the mini C-arm is such that they are mainly operated by the surgeon and the need for an unscrubbed radiology technician is much reduced. The entire C-arm, including the generator and the image intensifier, is sterilely covered to be included in the surgical field, which facilitates manipulations and improve aseptic technique. Owing to the smaller distance between the generator and the amplifier, they are not commonly used through the operating table because they will not provide enough clearance to permit easy access to the surgery site. Their portability may allow easy in and out motion to circumvent this limitation, but the lower output from the generator will restrict this application to smaller patients and/or extremities.

Radiation safety equipment Basic safety steps must be implemented during image acquisition by all personnel within range (typically the entire OR). These include individual lead aprons, thyroid shields, individual dosimeters, mobile shields, protective glasses, and attenuating gloves. In addition, adequate warning and labeling outside the OR must be posted to prevent inadvertent exposure of personnel. Aprons are available in different protective strengths measured in lead equivalence (typically between 0.25 and 0.5 mm lead equivalence). Lower shielding capability is acceptable because the dosage necessary for image acquisition is smaller with image intensifiers when compared with radiographic acquisitions (0.1–0.6 mA compared with 20–60 mA for imaging identical structures, respectively). Light-weight, custom-fitted, and "zero fatigue" aprons are suitable to reduce upper back and extremities fatigue problems associated with extended and repetitive use.

To complement the standard aprons, thyroid shields must be used. Other protective equipment, including leaded glasses and attenuating gloves, should be considered. These specific shields are highly recommended to reduce incidence of thyroid carcinoma, cataracts, and sarcomas associated with chronic, cumulative radiation exposure.[6–10]

Surgery table The use of dedicated operative tables may be extremely valuable. The characteristics of the ideal table vary somewhat with the type of C-arm unit in use and the procedure to be performed. The different properties that should be taken into account include

1. Dimensions
2. Radiolucency
3. Motion amplitude/motorization
4. Position of the stand(s)/wheels
5. Accessories including rails and patient restraints

It is advisable to use radiolucent tables to allow imaging through the table as needed. Whereas this is seldom necessary for the treatment of long bone fractures when using a mini unit, it is required for the treatment of upper segments including sacroiliac luxations. Radiolucent table have variable degrees of attenuation that may be expressed in aluminum equivalence. The attenuation depends on the material in use and on the thickness at the site of exposure. Attenuation coefficients less than 0.5 to 0.7 mm aluminum equivalence are ideal. Carbon fiber and some hard polymers are optimal for such applications, and custom-built boards using these materials may be adapted to a nonradiolucent table if necessary.

Motorized tables that allow progressive motion in all directions are valuable to adjust patient position before and during the procedure. Beside classic vertical motion (surge), surgical tables may feature X/Y tabletop motion (head-to-toe and side-to-side float, respectively), Trendelenburg/reverse Trendelenburg longitudinal tilt (head-down/toes-up and head-up/toes-down pitch, respectively), and lateral roll. The controls are hand or foot activated by an unscrubbed assistant or the surgeon.

The tabletop is either mounted on dual stands or as a cantilever on a single stand. Tables on a cantilever are more "C-arm friendly" because the bottom of the table is clear for most its length. This allows unrestricted horizontal C-arm motion under the table. The maximum weight capacity may be reduced when compared with similar-sized dual stand tables, and table specifications should be verified before use with larger patients.

Accessory rails and restraints are extremely valuable during MIO procedures. They are used to facilitate C-arm access to the area of interest, attach monitoring and anesthesia equipment (ie, endotracheal tube), and secure the patient to the table to prevent inadvertent motion during reduction maneuvers. The presence of accessory rails below (rather than on the edges of) the table is not recommended as it could interfere with proper visualization of the patient.

Intraoperative radioprotection Intraoperative fluoroscopy uses ionizing radiation comparable with that produced by conventional radiography. These emissions are known to produce deleterious effects on living organisms through production of free radicals and direct alteration of DNA sequences. In medical imaging applications, both the patient and the personnel are exposed, and strict regulations must be adhered to when using equipment that produces ionizing radiation. These regulations are grouped under the concept of radiation protection or radiological protection. Radiation protection in medical radiology consists of justification of a practice involving radiation exposure, optimization of radiation protection, and monitoring of individual dose limits. The interested reader should consult the following document: 1990 Recommendations form the International Commission on Radiological Protection (ICRP Publication 60); Ann ICRP, 1991, 21.

The term ALARA (as low as reasonably achievable) or ALARP (as low as reasonably practicable—in the United Kingdom) was introduced in the 1970s and refers to the principle of keeping radiation doses and release of radioactive material to the environment as low as possible, based on technologic and economic considerations.[11] The ALARA concept was integrated into the radiological protection protocols extending its application to personnel at work and the patient who is directly exposed to the radiation for diagnostic and treatment purposes.[12] The 3 pillars of ALARA in radiation safety are:

1. Time (spend less time in radiation fields)
2. Distance (increase distance between radioactive sources and workers or population)
3. Shielding (use proper barriers to block or reduce ionizing radiation)

These mitigation methods are a practical and effective means of minimizing radiation effects. The reduction in time of exposure directly reduces acute and cumulative dose exposure; increasing distance reduces doses following the *inverse square law*; and shielding refers to a mass of absorbing material placed around a reactor, or other radioactive source, to reduce the radiation to a level safe for humans. The Sievert (Sv) is a unit of dose equivalent radiation used to quantify the biological effect of ionizing radiation.

Exposure time Practically, in the OR setup, the first principle translates into complete avoidance of *cine mode* if possible and reducing the number of images to the minimum necessary for accurate diagnosis. In that regard, a recent study compared the exposure time and dose between senior (experienced) and junior (inexperienced) surgeons performing minimally invasive nail osteosynthesis. Senior surgeons used significantly less fluoroscopic time and as a result were exposed to markedly lower doses per operation than junior surgeons (4.43 vs 6.95 min, respectively).[13] This observation should prompt mentoring surgeons to sensitize their trainees to remain mindful of their time spent on fluoroscopy and review radiation exposure routinely.

Operating room personnel/radiation source distance The surgeon and assistants should maintain the largest possible distance from the C-arm during image acquisition (**Fig. 6**). This can be achieved by using extended tools and instruments to hold the limb if necessary and avoiding facing the primary radiation beam. The *inverse square law* stipulates that the dose of radiation is reduced by the power of 2 of the distance to the X-ray source, making distance from the source of radiation the best protection. For example, when the distance between source and surgeon is doubled, the dose of radiation is reduced to a quarter of the initial dose.

$$I_2 = I_1 \frac{(D_1)^2}{(D_2)^2},$$

where I_1 and I_2 are radiation intensity at distances D_1 and D_2, respectively, and D_1 and D_2 are initial and final distance from the X-ray source.

Note that the inverse square law applies to primary beam electromagnetic radiation from X-rays, but that the primary beam is rarely the source of personnel exposure. Instead, the surgical team is most likely to be affected by scatter radiation. Scattered radiation is radiation that arises from interactions of the primary radiation beam with the atoms in the object being imaged. Scatter radiation has random direction and poses the greatest radiation risk to occupational workers. Backscatter refers to those

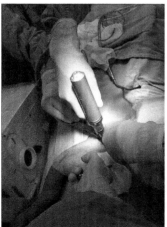 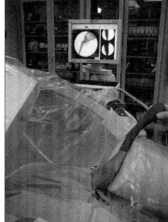

Fig. 6. Intraoperative photographs of MIO procedures. In the left picture, the main surgeon along with the assistant has his hands in the primary beam. In this situation configuration, C-arm images *should not be taken* as it would result in high exposure levels. In the right image, all personnel are off the primary beam and the patient leg is held as far away as possible. This is an acceptable position to acquire images safely. Further improvement could include the use of a forceps placed at the leg extremity to further increase distance from the exposition field.

photons that return in the direction from which they came, that is backward toward the tube.[14] Forward scatter continues in the general direction of the original photon with a few degrees of directional change; these photons are generally projected toward the image receptor and are the cause of image fog. It is that scatter that is propagated at various angles that can reach the surgery crew and poses a hazard. In particular, with the lower kVp settings used by C-arms, scatter is the greatest between 90° and 180°. In addition, scatter is proportional to the amount of matter exposed to the primary beam. Therefore, when using full-size C-arms through the table for larger patients, the generator should be placed under the table to direct most of the scatter downward, toward the OR floor, rather than upward, toward the surgery crew.

Shielding The exposure level also varies considerably with the type of fluoroscopically assisted procedure and the radiation protection used by the OR personnel. As an example, a recent study showed that the total effective dose to the surgeon during a routine hip replacement or a routine kyphoplasty was ~5 and 250 μSv, respectively, when a 0.5-mm lead equivalent apron was used alone. This dose was significantly reduced to ~2.5 and 95 μSv, respectively, when an additional thyroid shield was worn.[15]

The use of shielding as a cardinal principle of radiation protection is required by both the National Council on Radiation Protection and Measurement (NCRP), the Nuclear Regulatory Commission, and various federal and state regulations. Shielding applies to the room in which ionizing radiation is in use, the personnel, and the patient.[16] Different materials are used for shielding including lead and barium in aprons and attenuating gloves, respectively. The thickness of a shielding material ultimately determines how much radiation will be attenuated. Most shields are made of 0.25, 0.5, or 1.0 mm lead equivalent. Lead aprons of 0.5 mm lead equivalent will attenuate approximately 75% of a 100-kVp beam. However, most radiology, surgery, and orthopedic departments purchase 0.25- and 0.5-mm lead equivalent aprons, meaning that the exit radiation reaching the wearer can approach 50% to 25%. *This is an important reason why, to optimize protection, shielding must be coupled to the other two cardinal principles of radiation protection, limited time of exposure to ionizing radiation and distance from the source.* Assuming that these principles are followed, exposure to radiation can remain very low, particularly when compared with other sources of radiation. The use of proper protective gear over a 6-month period has been shown to reduce cumulative radiation exposure of surgeons by up to 45% (eg, thyroid, 0.51 and 0.79 mSv with or without shield, respectively; waist, 0.48 and 0.86 mSv with or without an apron, respectively). These values were well within the NCRP safety guidelines.[17] In comparison, a chest radiograph or chest CT generates approximately 0.1 or 12 mSv of dose equivalent radiation, respectively; passengers on a transatlantic flight receive doses ranging from 0.001 to 0.01 mSv/h. It is currently recommended that the maximum dose to OR personnel does not exceed 10 mSv/y.[18]

Operative technique The layout of the OR is essential and should facilitate C-arm maneuvers and prevent interference with the surgical procedure. The importance of this step is, however, often underestimated. Similarly, it should be emphasized that adequate patient positioning is critical to the smooth execution of the surgical procedure, from fracture reduction, to restoration of alignment, to suitable implant location. In particular, proper patient positioning will allow better, full visualization of the joints adjacent to the fracture in 2 orthogonal planes. In turn this will considerably limit the number of intraoperative images required to evaluate intraoperative realignment and therefore exposure of the surgical team to harmful radiation (**Table 1**).

	Static Full-Size C-Arm/Through Table	Mobile Mini C-Arm/Table Top
Humerus	Dorsal recumbency Leg extended caudally (CC view) Leg abducted (Lat view)	Lateral approach (interlocking nail) Lateral recumbency/surgery leg up Medial approach (plate or plate rod) Dorsal recumbency/surgery leg abducted
Radius-ulna	Dorsal recumbency Leg extended caudally (CC view) Leg abducted (Lat view)	Dorsal recumbency Leg extended caudally (CC view) Leg abducted (Lat view)
Pelvis (SI luxation)	Lateral recumbency/surgery leg up Perfect lateral spine projection required	Optional, in conjunction with full-size C-arm to provide VD image (horizontal beam projection)
Femur	Lateral recumbency/surgery leg up Leg extended and abducted (CC view) Leg held horizontally (Lat view)	Lateral recumbency/surgery leg up Pelvis elevated to allow CC view
Tibia	Dorsal recumbency Leg extended caudally (CC view) Leg abducted (Lat view)	Lateral recumbency/surgery leg down

Table 1
Recommended position for optimal use of a C-arm based on fractured segment and C-arm size

Abbreviations: CC, craniocaudal; Lat, lateral; SI, sacroiliac; VD, ventrodorsal.

Patient position should be evaluated in each case by both the anesthesiologist and the surgeon to prevent anesthetic complications and facilitate the surgical procedure. First and foremost, the position must not compromise patient safety. From an anesthesia standpoint, the final patient position should allow easy access to airways, prevent ventilation compromise, permit adequate monitoring and allow use of an extracorporal warming devices. From a surgical standpoint, the patient should be positioned so as to facilitate all surgical phases including approach and reduction maneuvers, as well as implant insertion and fixation. It must also permit unrestricted C-arm mobility around the patient so that intraoperative views of adjacent joints, in both sagittal and frontal planes, can be easily obtained throughout the surgical procedure (**Fig. 7**). One should bear in mind that poor positioning may result in circulatory compromise, perioperative pressure ulcers, and neurologic injury, even in routine surgical procedures. In addition, poor positioning will impair image accuracy, which in turn may lead to inadequate restoration of alignment and/or improper fracture fixation. Once positioning is deemed adequate, the patient should be secured on the table using resting devices, sandbags or tape to prevent inadvertent displacement during the surgery. Following completion of patient positioning, C-arm mobility is reassessed to ensure that orthogonal views of the joints proximal and distal to the fracture can be obtained (see **Fig. 7**). This ultimate preoperative assessment is made before final preparation to allow iteration of the patient position as necessary.

In-depth knowledge of the loco-regional anatomy is critical to a successful surgical outcome. Although this statement holds true in all surgical fields, this prerequisite is even more critical with MIO because direct visualization of the fracture site is not available to the surgeon. Although mini open approaches remote from the fracture site are most often used in MIO, in advanced applications, implants may be fed

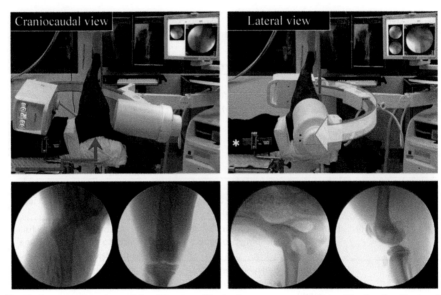

Fig. 7. Preoperative view of the OR set up illustrating proper patient positioning for the treatment of a femoral fracture. The pelvis has been elevated to allow unrestricted C-arm motion around the limb. This provides intraoperative views of the joints adjacent to the fracture in two orthogonal planes, facilitates restoration of alignment and in turn reduces exposure to radiation.

transcutaneously through large gauge needles used as cannulas. In such cases, the surgeon relies exclusively on percutaneous landmarks and on intraoperative fluoroscopy to achieve fracture reduction, to restore alignment and to complete fixation. Because a comprehensive 3D understanding of the bone's anatomy is necessary to enable adequate implant contouring and fixation, using dry specimens in the OR in addition to CT reconstruction, is highly recommended.

Assessment of reduction status and implant position using the C-arm may be critical in MIO procedures. Similar to that recommended with conventional radiographs, orthogonal views of the joints adjacent to the fracture site should be obtained. Furthermore, the X-ray beam should consistently be perpendicular to the long axis of the bone and centered over the area of interest to minimize image distortion. Alignment is verified before final fixation using adequate landmarks in the frontal and sagittal planes for the joint proximal and distal to the fracture site. If both joints cannot be seen within 1 C-arm image, a first image is obtained from the proximal joint and then the C-arm is translated to take an image of the distal joint without changing the plan of imaging or the leg's position. The same procedure is repeated for the orthogonal projection.

Arthroscopy Although not standard in small animal fracture repair, arthroscopy may be used to enhance the surgeon's ability to monitor intra-articular fracture reduction minimally invasively (**Fig. 8**). Standard arthroscopic equipment and instrumentation including light source and camera heads are used in a routine fashion with appropriately sized 30° arthroscopes. Scope and instrument portals are similar to those used for elective arthroscopic procedures in most instances. Fracture configuration may occasionally dictate the need for alternate portals or modifications of standard ones.

Arthroscopy can be used in combination with intraoperative fluoroscopy because both technologies are complementary to ascertain optimal articular fragment

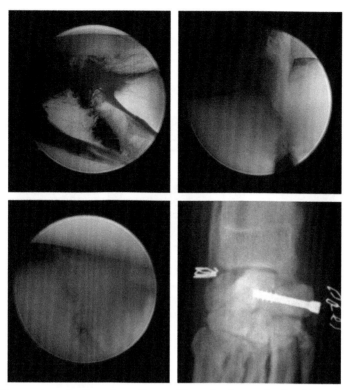

Fig. 8. Arthroscopic evaluation of a radiocarpal bone fracture reduction. Upon joint entry, a blood clot is seen over the fracture edges (*top left*). Joint lavage improves visualization (*top right*). A double point bone holding forceps was used to compress the fracture and achieve interfragmentary compression (*bottom left*) and a headless compression screw was used for stabilization (*bottom right*).

apposition and implant placement, respectively (**Fig. 9**). Arthroscopic evaluation of articular fracture poses some obstacles when compared with exploration of nontraumatized joints. Joint capsule tears are commonly associated with articular fractures, which can prevent the proper distension of joint space necessary to allow intra-articular work. The presence of blood clots may obstruct joint inspection and irrigation fluid extravasation can progressively cause significant impediment to surgical execution. Judicious use of ingress/egress flow is necessary to minimize these deleterious effects and optimize fracture reduction and fixation. In the case of unsuccessful arthroscopic exploration, conversion to a standard, open approach should be considered before inflicting iatrogenic damage to the articular surfaces.

POSTOPERATIVE IMAGING

Critical assessment of postoperative images is performed immediately postoperatively. The 4 "A" rules are applied to perform a comprehensive radiographic reading and produce an accurate radiographic diagnosis.[19] The 4 "A"s of radiographic evaluations are:

1. Alignment: Refers to the anatomic relationship between the joints adjacent to the fracture site. It includes axial alignment (ie, length) and alignment in the frontal (varus-

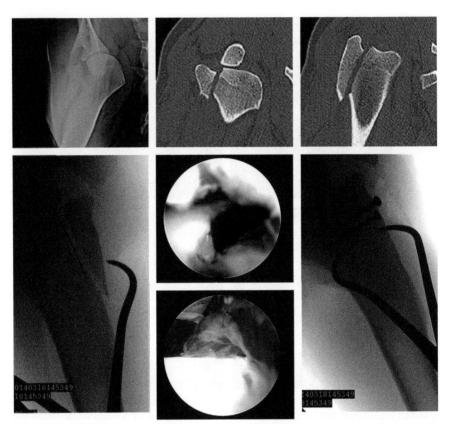

Fig. 9. Proximal articular humeral fracture involving the bicipital groove and deltoid tuberosity. Radiographic evaluation (*top left*) was insufficient to fully characterize the lesion and CT images were obtained (*top center* and *right*). Intraoperative fluoroscopy (*bottom left* and *right*) was used in combination with arthroscopy (*bottom center*) to allow for minimally invasive fracture reduction and stabilization. A double point bone holding forceps was applied percutaneously under C-arm guidance. Note the use of a needle to mark the fracture orientation (*bottom left*). Arthroscopy was used concurrently to monitor the apposition at the level of the articular surface (*bottom center*). Lag screw fixation was used to compress the fracture (*bottom right*).

valgus) and sagittal (procurvatum-retrocurvatum) planes. Ideally, postoperative alignment is directly compared with the intact contralateral limb. Severe malalignment should be immediately identified and corrected to avoid long-term consequences of aberrant transarticular forces that would result from such deformities.

2. Apposition/adjacency: This is the relationship between fracture fragments. In bridging osteosynthesis, apposition is seldom used as an outcome measure because reconstruction of the bony columns is not intended, nor desired. Instead, adjacency of fragments can be used as a measure of fragment dispersion compared with the normal shaft diameter.

3. Apparatus: Includes primary and secondary fixation devices. Assessment of apparatus aims at determining adequacy of the repair in terms of strength and stiffness. It also aims at identifying inadvertent misplacement of implants (ie, joint penetration).

4. Activity: Refers to biological activity as evaluated on follow-up images. These will be compared with the immediate postoperative images to identify progression of healing in terms of callus formation and remodeling. Reevaluation of alignment, apposition, and apparatus is also performed on each follow-up radiograph. Implant and/or bone failure should be addressed as needed.

In conclusion, perioperative imaging using various appropriate modalities is critical to the successful planning and performance of any orthopedic surgery. Although not an absolute prerequisite, the use of intraoperative imaging considerably facilitates the smooth and effective execution of MIO. One must keep in mind, however, that the risk of overexposure to radiation with fluoroscopy and conventional radiology is real, particularly when considering its insidious effects over time. Therefore, the primary concern of the surgeon must be safety of the surgical team. If properly implemented, basic, simple steps will be effective in reducing radiation exposure, which in turn will make MIO a safe alternative to traditional open reduction and internal fixation. One should also remember that intraoperative imaging is in no way a substitute to fine surgical skills and in-depth knowledge of surgical anatomy.

REFERENCES

1. Johnson AL, Houlton JEF, Vannini R. AO principles of fracture management in the dog and cat. Stuttgart (Germany): Georg Thieme Verlag; 2005.
2. Perren SM. Evolution of the internal fixation of long bone fractures. The scientific basis of biological internal fixation: choosing a new balance between stability and biology. J Bone Joint Surg Br 2002;84:1093–110.
3. Tong GO, Bavonratanavech S. Minimally invasive plate osteosynthesis (MIPO). 1st edition. Davos (Switzerland): AO Publishing; 2007.
4. Stubig T, Kendoff D, Citak M, et al. Comparative study of different intraoperative 3-D image intensifiers in orthopedic trauma care. J Trauma 2009;66:821–30.
5. Athwal GS, Bueno RA Jr, Wolfe SW. Radiation exposure in hand surgery: mini versus standard C-arm. J Hand Surg Am 2005;30:1310–6.
6. Mrena S, Kivela T, Kurttio P, et al. Lens opacities among physicians occupationally exposed to ionizing radiation—a pilot study in Finland. Scand J Work Environ Health 2011;37:237–43.
7. Vano E, Kleiman NJ, Duran A, et al. Radiation cataract risk in interventional cardiology personnel. Radiat Res 2010;174:490–5.
8. Venneri L, Foffa I, Sicari R. Papillary thyroid carcinoma of an interventional cardiologist. A case report. Recenti Prog Med 2009;100:80–3 [in Italian].
9. Ainsbury EA, Bouffler SD, Dorr W, et al. Radiation cataractogenesis: a review of recent studies. Radiat Res 2009;172:1–9.
10. Furlan JC, Rosen IB. Prognostic relevance of previous exposure to ionizing radiation in well-differentiated thyroid cancer. Langenbecks Arch Surg 2004;389:198–203.
11. Risk management: ALARP at a glance, in Executive LHaS (ed) Health and Safety at Work etc. Act 1974. 2011. Available at: http://www.hse.gov.uk/risk/theory/alarpglance.htm. Accessed October 7, 2019.
12. Willis CE, Slovis TL. The ALARA concept in radiographic dose reduction. Radiol Technol 2004;76:150–2.
13. Blattert TR, Fill UA, Kunz E, et al. Skill dependence of radiation exposure for the orthopaedic surgeon during interlocking nailing of long-bone shaft fractures: a clinical study. Arch Orthop Trauma Surg 2004;124:659–64.

14. North D. Pattern of scattered exposure from portable radiographs. Health Phys 1985;49:92–3.

15. Theocharopoulos N, Perisinakis K, Damilakis J, et al. Occupational exposure from common fluoroscopic projections used in orthopaedic surgery. J Bone Joint Surg Am 2003;85-A:1698–703.

16. Christodoulou EG, Goodsitt MM, Larson SC, et al. Evaluation of the transmitted exposure through lead equivalent aprons used in a radiology department, including the contribution from backscatter. Med Phys 2003;30:1033–8.

17. Lo NN, Goh PS, Khong KS. Radiation dosage from use of the image intensifier in orthopaedic surgery. Singapore Med J 1996;37:69–71.

18. Kirousis G, Delis H, Megas P, et al. Dosimetry during intramedullary nailing of the tibia. Acta Orthop 2009;80:568–72.

19. Piermattei DL, Flo GL, DeCamp CE. Fractures: classification, diagnosis, and treatment. In: Farthman L, editor. Handbook of small animal orthopedics and fracture repair, vol. 1. St. Louis (MO): Saunders Elsevier; 2006. p. 25–159.

Interlocking Nails and Minimally Invasive Osteosynthesis

Loïc M. Déjardin, DVM, MS[a],*, Karen L. Perry, BVM&S, CertSAS, MRCVS[a],
Dirsko J.F. von Pfeil, DVM[b], Laurent P. Guiot, DVM, MS[c]

KEYWORDS

- Interlocking nail • Angle-stable interlocking nail • Bone healing • Traumatology
- Minimally invasive osteosynthesis • Minimally invasive nail osteosynthesis

KEY POINTS

- Ongoing reviews of osteosynthesis clinical outcomes led to a radical paradigm shift towards emphasizing the biological component of fracture healing; this became the foundation of a new approach in fracture management known as biological osteosynthesis.
- Interlocking nails are solid intramedullary rods featuring transverse cannulations and locking devices at both extremities. As such, interlocking nails are by design well suited for bridging osteosynthesis.
- As intramedullary devices, interlocking nails have unique biological and mechanical benefits that make them ideal implants for minimally invasive nail osteosynthesis, a technique known as MINO. Interlocking nailing has emerged as an attractive alternative to bone plating, and to some surgeons, the method of choice for osteosynthesis of diaphyseal and epi-metaphyseal fractures as well as for revisions of failed plate osteosynthesis.
- Thanks to a new angle-stable locking design, indications for interlocking nailing have been expanded to comprise treatment of metaphyseal and epiphyseal fractures including those with articular involvement and angular limb deformities such as distal femoral varus or and associated patellar luxations.
- To reduce the risk of implant yield or fatigue as well as iatrogenic cranial cruciate ligament injury, tibial nails should be bent to follow the natural tibial recurvatum.

Disclosure: Some of the work presented here was supported by the Michigan State University Companion Animal Fund (grants: CAF nos. 81-2156-D, 81-2625-D, 31-1086-D, and 81-1086) as well as by implant donations from BioMedtrix. L.M. Dejardin is the inventor of the I-Loc interlocking nail described in this article. L. M. Dejardin holds a US patent for the I-Loc nail and receives royalties from Michigan State University as well as honoraria from BioMedtrix for teaching interlocking nailing techniques. None of the other authors have anything to disclose. The article is an update of Déjardin LM, Guiot LP, von Pfeil DJ. Interlocking nails and minimally invasive osteosynthesis. Vet Clin North Am Small Anim Pract 2012;42(5):935-62.
[a] Department of Small Animal Clinical Sciences, College of Veterinary Medicine, Michigan State University, 736 Wilson Road, East Lansing, MI 48824, USA; [b] Sirius Veterinary Orthopedic Center, 3125 South 61st Avenue, Omaha, NE 68106, USA; [c] ACCESS Bone & Joint Center, ACCESS Specialty Animal Hospital, 9599 Jefferson Boulevard, Culver City, CA 90232, USA
* Corresponding author.
E-mail address: dejardin@cvm.msu.edu

INTRODUCTION

In an effort to improve on the poor functional outcomes associated with external fixation or coaptation, and/or long-term patient immobilization, starting in the late 1950s, open reduction and internal fixation (ORIF) became the modus operandi recommended by the AO (Arbeitsgemeinschaft für Osteosynthesefragen) Foundation for the treatment of long bone fractures.[1] Although strict adhesion to ORIF principles of anatomic reduction and rigid fixation allowed restoration of absolute mechanical stability, it came with a hefty biological price inherent to extensive iatrogenic surgical trauma, including disturbance of the fracture hematoma and inevitable damage to the local soft tissues and blood supply. As a result, despite improved outcomes compared with earlier techniques, ORIF precipitated the development of a new set of complications, including delayed or nonunion, implant failure, and osteomyelitis. As an example, humeral and tibial fractures in dogs treated with conventional techniques carry complication rates of up to 40% and 18%, respectively.[2,3] Such observations led to the reiteration of the early AO principles of preservation of blood supply, gentle soft tissue handling, and early mobilization, and practically to a biologically friendlier "Open But Do Not Touch" (OBDNT) approach to osteosynthesis. Nonetheless, OBDNT techniques, which still favor manipulation of the bone fragments (albeit remotely), continued to put an emphasis on mechanical rigidity of the repaired bone, as illustrated by the extensive use of the plate-rod combination (PRC) in the treatment of comminuted fractures.[1]

Over the past 2 decades, the ongoing review of clinical outcomes by the AO led to a radical paradigm shift toward further emphasizing the biological component of fracture healing.[1] This became the foundation of a new philosophic approach known as minimally invasive osteosynthesis (MIO).[4–8] With MIO, the fracture site is not exposed, which in turn preserves the fracture hematoma and promotes earlier fracture healing. Rather, indirect reduction techniques through gentle manipulation of the main bone fragments and small approaches remote to the fracture site are used to introduce the implant epiperiosteally (plate) or in an intramedullary manner (interlocking nail [ILN]). In addition, quasi abandonment of interfragmentary screws, cerclage wires, or bone grafts, as well as anatomic reduction, became hallmarks of MIO.[9] This evolution favors the preservation of a biological environment essential to bone healing. From a mechanical perspective, emphasis is put on restoration of alignment rather than anatomy and on achieving optimal construct stability rather than rigid interfragmentary stability. This is accomplished through several iterations of traditional osteosynthesis techniques, such as increased reliance on longer more compliant bridging implants that bypass the fracture site altogether. Today, biological osteosynthesis principles and MIO are readily implemented in human orthopedics and are slowly gaining momentum and acceptance in veterinary medicine.[5,6,10] Although numerous acronyms have been used to describe specific implant-related minimally invasive surgical techniques, adherence to these new principles is collectively known as MIO. This article will address the use of minimally invasive nail osteosynthesis (MINO) in the treatment of long bone fractures in companion animals.

HISTORY OF INTERLOCKING NAILING

The interlocking nail concept in the treatment of long bone fractures evolved from the original intramedullary nail and later "detensor" nail designed by Küntscher[11] (Germany) in the 1940s and late 1960s. The first true interlocking nail was developed in the 1970s by Huckstep[12] (Australia) to treat femoral fractures in humans. Following the successful experimental and clinical use of modified Huckstep nails in animals by

Johnson and Huckstep[13] and Muir and colleagues,[14–16] several dedicated veterinary systems were independently designed in the early 1990s by Dueland and Johnson[17] (United States), Duhautois and van Tilburg[18] (France), Durall and Diaz[19] (Spain), and Nagaoka and colleagues[20] (Japan). These systems are not compatible with each other. In an effort to address some of the limitations of currently available designs, a new angle-stable ILN (AS-ILN) was developed at Michigan State University.[21–24] Currently, 2 systems are available in the United States. The Original Interlocking Nail System is a standard nail system commercialized by Innovative Animal Products (IAP), Rochester, MN, and the I-Loc is an AS-ILN commercialized by BioMedtrix, Booton, NJ. Throughout the remainder of the text, IAP and I-Loc may be used to refer to standard and angle-stable nails, respectively.

INTERLOCKING NAIL DESIGNS

Regardless of their designs, ILNs have common characteristics. They are solid intramedullary rods featuring transverse cannulations at both extremities and sometimes along the whole length of the nail (Durall system). The nail is locked in place via bone screws or partially threaded bolts that engage the cis- and trans-cortices as well as the nail. The proximal nail extremity features keying flanges for rigid coupling between the nail and an alignment guide via extension rods. The distal end of the nail presents a dull or trocar point to facilitate insertion.

Standard Nail Design and Instrumentation

Implants

To accommodate dogs and cats of various sizes, nails are available in several diameters (4, 4.7, 6, 8, and 10 mm) and lengths (68–230 mm). Each nail extremity features 1 or 2 smooth cannulations that accommodate locking screws or bolts of different size (2.0, 2.7, 3.5, and 4.5 mm) depending on nail diameter (**Fig. 1**). To improve the versatility of the device, particularly with regard to its use in the treatment of metaphyseal fractures, cannulations are either 11 or 22 mm apart. The smaller spacing is more suitable for metaphyseal fractures when limited bone stock is available for the placement of 2 interlocking bolts.

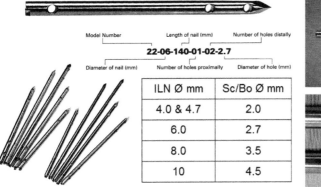
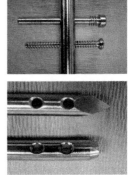

Model Number · Length of nail (mm) · Number of holes distally

22-06-140-01-02-2.7

Diameter of nail (mm) · Number of holes proximally · Diameter of hole (mm)

ILN Ø mm	Sc/Bo Ø mm
4.0 & 4.7	2.0
6.0	2.7
8.0	3.5
10	4.5

Fig. 1. Standard nails from Innovative Animal Products come in various sizes (diameter and length) to accommodate dogs and cats. The nails can be locked using partially threaded solid bolts (preferred) or standard cortical bone screws. The nail extremities feature proximal keying flanges for coupling of the nail to an insertion handle or an alignment guide and a trocar or dull tip distally. *Courtesy* of Medical Innovations, Inc., Rochester, MN.

Instrumentation

The use of the standard nails from IAP requires dedicated instrumentation comprising (1) an insertion handle, (2) a drill jig featuring a series of holes whose location matches that of the nail cannulations, (3) extension rods for attachment of the nail to the insertion handle or to a drill jig, (4) a set of drilling (and tapping) sleeves and size matched drill bits and taps, and (5) a dedicated depth gage (**Fig. 2**). Once the drill guide is rigidly secured to the nail via the extension rod, accurate transcortical insertion of the locking devices is possible.

Angle-Stable Nail Design and Instrumentation (BioMedtrix)

Implants

In an effort to improve construct stability, facilitate surgical procedures and adherence to MIO principles of bridging osteosynthesis, the I-Loc nail was designed as an angle-stable, compliant implant. Compared with standard nails, the main differences relate to the design of the locking mechanism, the profile of the nail, and the implantation technique.[21,25]

Locking mechanism Each nail cannulation (2 at each extremity) features a self-centering and self-locking mechanism consisting of a threaded Morse taper. The main characteristic of the locking bolt is its threaded conical central section that matches both taper and thread of the nail cannulations. This creates an angle-stable rigid linkage between bolt and nail. The bolts also feature a solid triangular end-section designed to drive the bolt through the cis-cortex into the nail and a thinner

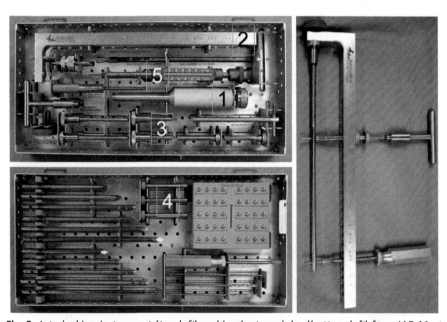

Fig. 2. Interlocking instrument (*top left*) and implant modules (*bottom left*) from IAP. Most currently available interlocking nail systems rely on specific instrumentation for their implantation including 1) an insertion handle, 2) a drill jig, 3) extensions linking nail and drill jig, 4) drilling and tapping sleeves and 5) a dedicated depth gage. Assembled nail (*right*) illustrating the matching locations of the nail and alignment guide cannulations (Medical Innovations, Inc., Rochester, MN.)

cylindrical end-section conceived to engage the trans-cortex. Both end-sections are free of threads (**Fig. 3**). Although the diameters of the locking bolt sections are nail specific, the length of each end-section is common to all bolts and can be cut to size as appropriate.

Nail profile The AS-ILN features an hourglass profile designed to limit iatrogenic damage to the endocortices and medullary blood supply and also to increase overall construct compliance (compliance is the inverse of stiffness). Furthermore, the thinner core diameter of the nail facilitates its insertion and virtually eliminates the need for reaming of the medullary cavity (see **Fig. 3**). Because of the conical geometry of the nail cannulations and matching central bolt section, proximal asymmetrical keying flanges are used to guarantee appropriate nail orientation as well as accurate connection of the nail to a customized alignment guide via a single dedicated extension. Finally, an oblong bullet-shaped distal tip was designed to optimize fracture reduction, particularly with regard to restoration of bone length, while limiting the risk of joint violation (see **Fig. 3**). Currently, the I-Loc AS-ILN is available in 6 diameters ranging from 3 to 8 mm in 1-mm increments. The small nails (3, 4, and 5 mm) are intended for use in cats and small dogs and are available in lengths ranging from 62 to 158 mm in 8-mm increments. The lengths of the larger nails (6, 7, and 8 mm) range from 122 to 235 mm.

Implantation technique An important modification of the surgical technique is the use of temporary smooth locking posts to create a rigid frame between the nail and alignment guide. These posts are systematically inserted in a proximal to distal sequence, rather than alternating from distal to proximal as with standard nails. This step progressively reduces the alignment guide lever arm and therefore its potential deviation from the nail axis, which in turn further limits the risk of off-site distal bolt insertion.

Instrumentation
As with most veterinary nail systems, an alignment guide is necessary for accurate bolt insertion. In addition to typical nailing equipment, instrumentation specific to this

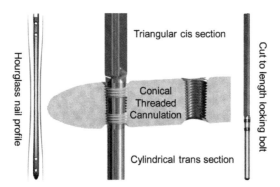

Fig. 3. Schematic of the I-Loc® AS-ILN locking mechanism from BioMedtrix (*center*). Each nail cannulation features a threaded cone the dimensions of which match those of the central section of the locking bolt. The locking bolt central section features two threads (green highlight) which purpose is to engage the cannulation. Once tightened, the bolt is rigidly locked into the nail thus creating an angle-stable link between nail and bolt. The nail hourglass profile is intended to reduce iatrogenic endosteal damage, optimize revascularization of the medullary cavity and increase overall construct compliance (*left*). Because of the fixed nail/bolt relationship, cortical threads on the end-sections of the bolt are unnecessary (*right*). *Courtesy* of BioMedtrix LLC., Whippany, NJ.

system includes (1) a cutting awl and a trial nail used to open the medullary cavity proximally and the distal metaphysis, respectively, (2) smooth locking posts used to temporarily link nail and alignment guide, (3) a dedicated depth gage for simultaneous measurement of the cis- and trans-bolt end-sections, and (4) a dedicated bolt shearing tool (**Fig. 4**). To simplify surgical steps throughout the procedure, system components are linked using cam-based quick couplings.

BIOMECHANICAL PROPERTIES OF INTERLOCKING NAILS

With the recent paradigm shift toward biological osteosynthesis, interlocking nails have emerged as an attractive alternative to bone plating, and to some surgeons, have become the method of choice for the repair of most comminuted diaphyseal fractures in human and veterinary patients. With the development of the I-Loc angle-stable nail, the range of indications for nail osteosynthesis has been expanded to address epi-metaphyseal fractures, including those with articular components.[26,27]

General Considerations

The efficacy of ILNs rests on several mechanical and biological advantages inherent to the fixation method. Like any intramedullary device, ILNs are placed near the neutral axis of the fractured bone and consequently are shielded against deleterious cyclic bending. Throughout physiologic activity, bones are subject to various forces that create tensile and compressive loads on opposite cortices and, as a net result, bending moments along the entire bone. The neutral axis of a bone is a concept that describes the location where tensile and compressive loads are virtually

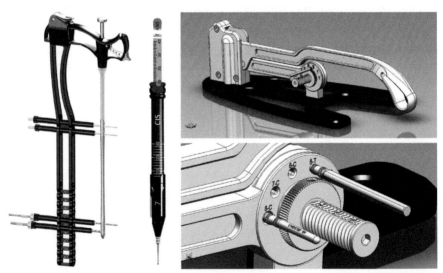

Fig. 4. Schematic representation of an assembled I-Loc® nail and dedicated instrumentation used for implantation (*left*). The position of the alignment guide can be adjusted along the insertion handle to accommodate patients of various sizes. Temporary smooth locking bolts (proximal two holes) are used to rigidify the frame during fixation, thus reducing the risk of distal off-site bolt insertion. Cam shaped quick couplings are used to consecutively link the insertion handle to an awl and a trial nail (not shown) as well as to the nail and alignment guide. A dedicated depth gage (*center*) is used to concomitantly measure the lengths of the bolt end-sections which are then cut using a custom shearing bolt (*right*). *Courtesy* of Bio-Medtrix LLC., Whippany, NJ; with permission.

eliminated along with their resulting bending moment.[28] As a consequence, the further away an implant is positioned from the bone neutral axis, the more susceptible it is to fatigue failure from cyclic bending.[29,30] Although the exact position of the neutral axis is unknown, and likely varies during activity, it is assumed that it is located near or within the medullary cavity. From a mechanical standpoint, this makes an interlocking nail superior to a bone plate or an external fixator, particularly when anatomic reconstruction is not pursued, as is the case with MIO. In addition, most ILNs are made of cold worked 316L stainless steel[21,31] and have a relatively larger and more homogenous area moment of inertia (AMI) than comparable bone plates.[32,33] Both features account for their intrinsic high resistance to bending. The AMI of an implant characterizes material distribution with respect to the plane or axis of deformation and is proportional to the implant bending or torsional stiffness. The AMI is proportional to the 4th power of the ILN diameter and to the 3rd power of a plate thickness. Consequently, although the AMI of the solid section of a plate varies considerably based on the plate orientation, it is constant regardless of the direction of applied load in nails. As an example, the AMI of the solid section of a 3.5-mm broad dynamic compression plate (DCP) bent along its flat surface is only 25% that of an 8-mm ILN but approximately 3 times greater if the same plate is bent on edge.[33]

Finally, unlike solid intramedullary pins, ILNs can resist torsional, compressive, and shear forces by using screws or bolts passing through both bone cortices and nail cannulations (locking effect).[21,31] However, standard nail holes act as stress concentrators promoting nail failure through the holes.[34,35] Because screws or bolts do not rigidly interact with the nail, filling the standard nail holes, as found with bone plates, does not reduce local stresses. Furthermore, assuming that in most cases the locking devices are oriented perpendicular to the sagittal plan of the limb, ILNs are structurally weaker in medio-lateral bending because the nail AMI is smaller in a bending plane parallel to the nail hole.[32,36]

Interlocking nails also have biological advantages.[5,37,38] Following fracture, severe disruption of the intramedullary vascularization occurs. As a result, the extra-osseous blood supply becomes a critical component of bone healing. When applied remotely to the fracture site via limited approaches, ILNs preserve the soft tissues and thereby the extra-osseous blood supply. Indeed, to reduce disruption of the fracture environment, ILNs can be placed in a normograde fashion. This less-invasive approach reduces postoperative morbidity and promotes fracture healing and functional recovery.

Standard Nail Biomechanics

Early generations of standard nails featured relatively large cannulations, which weakened the nail making them prone to fatigue failure through the nail hole.[31,34] To address this drawback, the 6- and 8-mm IAP nail hole diameters were reduced in current designs to accommodate 2.7- and 3.5-mm locking screws or bolts, instead of the previous 3.5- and 4.5-mm screws. Although such changes resulted in a 52- and 8-fold increase in the nail fatigue life, respectively, screw failure became predominant over nail failure.[34] Indeed, screw size reduction results in an approximately 40% decrease in the screw AMI, which translates to a similar decrease in bending yield strength. To limit the incidence of screw failure, partially threaded solid bolts featuring a self-tapping thread at the level of the cis-cortex, have been devised and are currently recommended (**Fig. 5**).[39,40] A recent study demonstrated that, under axial loads, metaphyseal insertion of the bolts further extends their fatigue life and decreases the incidence of catastrophic failure. Yet another theoretic advantage of metaphyseal, rather than diaphyseal, bolt location is the subsequent increase in construct working length and therefore compliance.

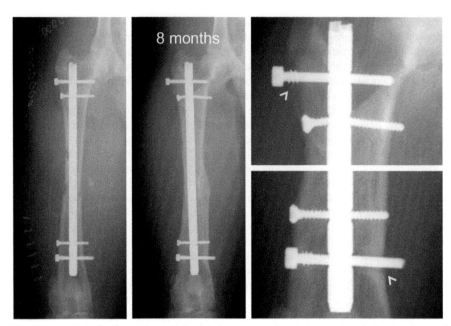

Fig. 5. Immediate (*left*) and 8 month (*center*) postoperative radiographs of a healed femoral fracture. The femur was treated using MIO with an 8 mm standard nail locked with two 3.5 mm solid bolts and two 3.5 mm cortical screws. The relative strength of the locking devices is illustrated by the plastic deformation of the proximal screw (*top right*). Delayed healing was observed in this case, presumably as a result of post-operative instability as suggested by the backing out of the proximal bolt as well as by the osteolysis around the distal bolt (*arrows*).

Despite overall favorable clinical outcomes, the reliability of standard ILN designs in assuring fracture repair stability has been challenged in human and veterinary orthopedics. In an original mechanical study, torsional and bending angular deformations were significantly greater with standard nail constructs than in those treated with a PRC; a fixation method often used in the treatment of comminuted fractures.[41] Importantly, IAP nail constructs experienced up to 28° of acute rotational instability, or slack, and showed an overall angular deformation (AD) of up to 40°. In contrast, the PRC maximum AD was 11° and occurred without slack. Construct instability was attributed to the inherent mismatch between locking screws and nail cannulations, which precludes rigid locking, as well as to structural damage to the screw threads and nail holes.[41]

Although veterinary clinical studies have reported that 12% to 14% of diaphyseal fractures treated with standard ILNs required additional fixation to overcome perioperative instability,[42,43] other studies showed that torsional and bending instability significantly reduced bone healing and functional recovery,[44,45] when a standard ILN was compared with an external fixator. These studies suggest that standard human and veterinary ILN systems do not counteract torsional and bending forces as much as initially anticipated. This, in turn, could contribute to complications such as delayed or nonunion. To improve construct stability and reduce the risk of bolt failure, reaming, which allows for implantation of larger nails and locking devices, has been recommended. Although potentially beneficial from a mechanical stand point, reaming severely impairs the medullary blood supply and has been associated with a higher incidence of infection as well as fat embolism, and therefore should be avoided.[46] In contrast, the use of smaller unreamed ILNs better preserves the endosteal and medullary blood supply, which from a biological standpoint, may be preferable. From a mechanical standpoint, however, postoperative stability of unreamed ILNs relies primarily on the efficacy of the locking mechanism.[22]

Angle-Stable Nail Biomechanics

The main impetus behind an AS-ILN design was the realization that the lack of rigid interaction between nail and locking devices in standard nails resulted in acute angular instability (slack). Over the past few years, several *in vitro* studies, using a tibial diaphyseal gap fracture model, have compared the mechanical behavior of 6- and 8-mm screwed or bolted standard nails to that of an AS-ILN prototype (8-mm extremities—6-mm midshaft core diameter).[21–23,36] These studies showed that constructs treated with an AS-ILN sustained significantly less AD in bending and torsion than those treated with IAP nails. More importantly, although AD of the AS-ILN constructs occurred without slack, constructs treated with screwed standard nails sustained nearly 10° and 20° of bending and torsional acute instability, respectively.[21–23,36] The use of locking bolts rather than screws reduced but did not eliminate construct slack in standard nails. Assuming continuous construct deformation, ILNs effectively resist torsional, and presumably bending, moments, through a recoil mechanism known as "spring back" effect.[47] In standard nails, construct slack has been misinterpreted as a spring back effect.[48] One must keep in mind, however, that these 2 mechanisms are very different and may have opposite effects on bone healing. Optimization of the spring back mechanism requires that construct AD occurs without slack and that the nail be somewhat compliant. This was achieved in early human models by the use of slotted nails. Although ideal construct compliance for optimal bone healing is unknown, one can speculate that overly compliant or stiff systems may promote either deleterious local shear stresses or stress shielding. Construct compliance of the AS-ILN was between that of the 6- and 8-mm standard nails.[22]

The high 25% complication rate seen in human tibial metaphyseal fractures treated with standard ILNs has been attributed to increased (up to 20°) construct slack caused by the lack of interference between nail and endocortices in relatively wider metaphyseal regions.[6,49–51] These clinical reports underscore the shortcoming of the current locking mechanism and agree with the authors' experience that approximately 40% of canine tibial fractures treated with standard ILNs require additional fixation to control intraoperative or acute postoperative instability, particularly in comminuted metaphyseal and submetaphyseal fractures. In a subsequent mechanical study, our group demonstrated that an AS-ILN maintained construct bending stability (~4° of AD) regardless of the fracture configuration. In contrast, standard nail AD doubled from up to 11° to up to 22° between transverse and metaphyseal fractures patterns. This strongly suggests that contrary to AS-ILNs, the intrinsic slack of standard ILNs jeopardized construct stability, particularly in a fracture configuration involving the metaphyses.[23] In contrast, the angular stability of the I-Loc nail system has allowed surgeons to expand the indications for interlocking nailing to epi-metaphyseal fractures and/or osteotomies aiming at correcting angular limb deformities such as distal femoral varus associated with medial patellar luxation.[26,27,52]

In a subsequent in vivo study,[24] a 7- × 5.25-mm (extremities and core diameters, respectively) AS-ILN was compared with a 6-mm bolted standard nail using a canine mid-diaphyseal tibial gap fracture model. Dogs treated with standard nails showed tibial rotational slack up to 2 weeks postoperatively and, from 4 to 8 weeks after surgery, were significantly more lame than dogs treated with an AS-ILN. Radiographic clinical union started at 8 weeks and was complete in all AS-ILN dogs at 10 weeks postoperatively. In contrast, bone healing was significantly slower in the dogs treated with the IAP nails, as only 50% of them reached clinical union by 18 weeks (**Fig. 6**). Mechanical testing of the calluses at 18 weeks showed that failure torque and energy were significantly greater in the AS-ILN than standard nail specimens. In addition, contralateral intact tibiae (controls) and AS-ILN-treated tibiae consistently failed via acute spiral fractures along the tibial diaphysis, and tibiae treated with a standard IAP nail failed progressively via transverse fracture through the initial gap (**Fig. 7**).[24]

From a mechanical standpoint, these studies suggest that through re-engineering of the locking mechanism and nail profile, the new hourglass AS-ILN system can eliminate bending and torsional instability associated with the use of current ILNs. Considering the deleterious effect of acute deformation on bone healing, compared with current ILNs, an AS-ILN may represent a mechanically more effective fixation method for the treatment of diaphyseal and metaphyseal fractures.[21–23,36] Similarly, from a biological standpoint, the use of an AS-ILN, rather than a standard nail, yields faster functional recovery and bone healing, as demonstrated by the presence of a stronger and more mature callus.[24]

INDICATIONS FOR INTERLOCKING NAILING
General Considerations

As intramedullary devices, ILNs can only be used in long bones that provide a nonarticular entry point for the nail (which excludes the radius). Although conventional ILNs

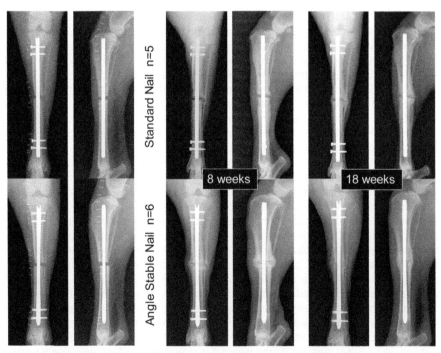

Fig. 6. Radiographic follow-up showing callus progression in a tibial gap fracture model stabilized with either a 6 mm bolted IAP standard nail (top row) or a 7 x 5.25 mm AS-ILN (bottom row). Clinical union, defined as bridging of 3 of 4 cortices, was completed in all AS-ILN dogs by 10 weeks post-operatively. In contrast, at 18 weeks, only 3 of the 5 dogs treated with an IAP nail had reached clinical union. By then, callus remodeling had occurred in the AS-ILN group.

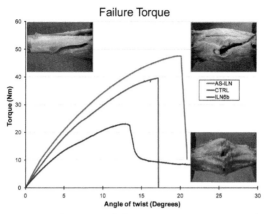

Fig. 7. Representative 18 weeks torque/deformation curves generated during mechanical testing of the bony callus of angle-stable (AS-ILN) and standard 6 mm bolted nail (ILN6b) groups as well as intact contralateral tibia (CTRL). Failure torque was greatest in the AS-ILN group (p<0.05). Calluses were significantly weaker in the standard ILN6b than both control and AS-ILN groups. Failure occurred as an acute spiral fracture in the control and AS-ILN specimens (*top* inserts) and a progressive transverse fracture through the original gap in the standard nail specimens (*bottom* insert).

have traditionally been used to treat diaphyseal fractures of the humerus, femur, and tibia, in recent years, their range of application has been considerably and successfully expanded thanks in part to the use of MINO techniques and to the introduction of an angle-stable locking design. The combined effect of MINO and elimination of perioperative slack with subsequent improvement in construct stability likely contribute to enhancing bone healing even in more challenging cases, including epi-metaphyseal fractures with or without articular involvement, as well as transverse fractures, corrective osteotomies, and revision surgeries. Furthermore, the added strength of the locking mechanism in AS-ILNs in addition to the nail intramedullary location has allowed the authors to stabilize pathologic humeral and femoral fractures rather than resort to amputation.

Common Indications

Thanks to established unique biomechanical advantages, interlocking nail osteosynthesis is the treatment of choice for most long bone diaphyseal fractures in people. Over the past 20 years, thanks to the work of such pioneer surgeons as Johnson and Huckstep,[13] Dueland and Johnson,[17] Duhautois and van Tilburg,[18] Durall and colleagues,[53] Basinger and Suber,[54] Nagaoka and colleagues,[20] and others, interlocking nailing has gained increasing acceptance in veterinary orthopedics as a reliable osteosynthesis method. Although ILNs are often placed through open approaches, the recent use of minimally invasive techniques further amplifies the biological benefits of interlocking nailing (**Fig. 8**).

Early on, ILNs were mostly used for the treatment of closed diaphyseal canine fractures of the femur, tibia, and to a lesser extent, the humerus. Current indications, particularly since the recent availability of an AS-ILN, include open contaminated fractures, particularly from gunshot injuries (see **Fig. 8**) as well as infected and nonunion fractures. A recent case report described the successful use of an ulnar nail in the treatment of a severely comminuted proximal radioulnar gunshot fracture in a dog.[55] This single ulnar nailing technique has been used successfully by our

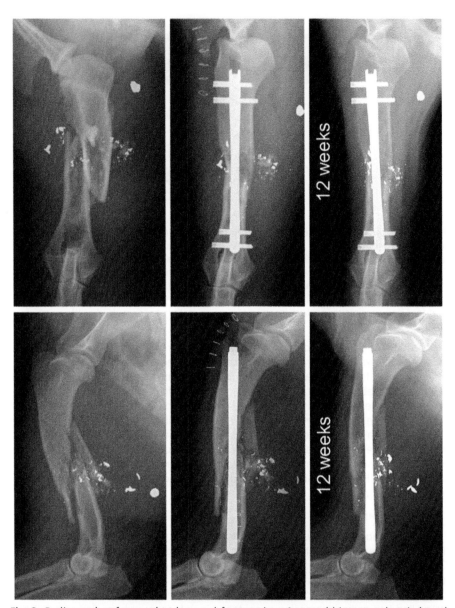

Fig. 8. Radiographs of a gunshot humeral fracture in a 4-year-old intact male mix-breed dog (pre-operative [*left*], immediate post-operative [*center*]). The fracture was treated with a 7 mm AS-ILN using MINO. The fracture site was not approached surgically in an attempt to limit further soft tissue trauma. The dog was weight bearing immediately after surgery, recovery was uneventful. Clinical union was achieved by 12 weeks post-operative (*right*).

team at Michigan State University (MSU) to treat Monteggia and mid-diaphyseal radio-ulnar fractures (**Figs. 9** and **10**). Once reserved to midsize and large dogs, thanks to the introduction of smaller nail models, interlocking nailing is now suitable for the treatment of feline diaphyseal fractures, regardless of fracture pattern.

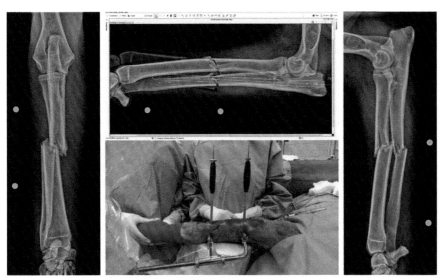

Fig. 9. Pre-operative radiographs as well as digital planning (*center - top*) of a transverse RU fracture in an 18-month, male neutered (70 kg [154 lbs]) Great Dane. Intra-operative photographs (*center - bottom*) illustrating the use of a linear distractor applied to the radius as well as toothed cannulated reduction handles affixed to the ulna (DePuy Synthes Vet, a division of DePuy Orthopaedics, Inc.). Alternative and/or synchronized manipulation of the RU fragments allowed for anatomical realignment of the fracture prior to nail insertion and subsequent fixation.

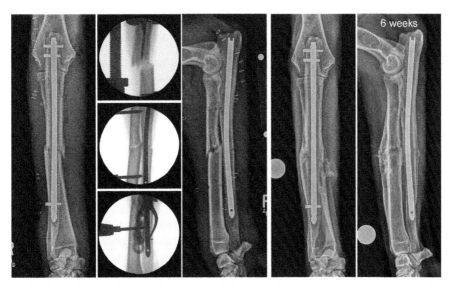

Fig. 10. Immediate post-operative as well as intra-operative fluoroscopic images illustrating fracture reduction which was facilitated by fragment distraction followed by compression once the nail was inserted in the distal fragment (*Left panel*). Follow up post-operative radiographs at 26 weeks show restoration of alignment as well as ongoing bone healing and remodeling.

Extended Indications

Alternative to plate-rod combination

Although the acceptance of MIO is gaining momentum, the treatment of long bone diaphyseal fractures using ORIF with a PRC technique remains widespread among veterinary orthopedic surgeons. The popularity of this technique likely stems from the perception that the intramedullary rod (IMR) facilitates fracture reduction and that it provides added strength to the repair compared with plate fixation alone. From a mechanical standpoint, a PRC is conceptually analogous to an ILN, although the technique requires at least 2 implants, rather than 1, to effectively control all fracture forces. From a surgical perspective, the PRC may be challenging owing to the difficulty of screw placement around the IMR. This technical difficulty is further accentuated should a fixed-angle locking plate be selected for fixation. Consequently, despite the plate-sparing effect of the IMR, the eccentric location of the plate remains a concern when surgical constraints preclude the use of an appropriately sized IMR (**Fig. 11**). Finally, from a biological standpoint, PRC inherently induces more extensive damage to the main blood supplies to the fractured bone, namely its endosteal/medullary, and, to a greater extent, periosteal blood supplies, than an ILN. Presumably, the hourglass profile of the AS-ILN also contributes to limiting iatrogenic damage to the endosteal and medullary blood supply because reaming is unnecessary. Furthermore, the narrow central core diameter of the AS-ILN likely facilitates revascularization of the medullary cavity, which in turn may enhance bone healing and functional recovery. Based on the above observations, the authors surmise that everything else being equal, from both biological and surgical standpoints, an AS-ILN implant is superior to a PRC (**Fig. 12**). From a mechanical standpoint, although direct comparison between PRC and AS-ILN is not available, a recent study showed that an AS-ILN sustains less AD than a size-matched DCP.[22]

Angular limb deformities—patellar luxation

Yet another theoretic argument in favor of ILNs over PRC is that restoration of axial alignment is technically facilitated by the use of an intramedullary device. Indeed, using an epiperiosteal plate often requires complex contouring, particularly in the presence of a callus in cases of revision surgery. This argument holds true in the treatment of angular limb deformities, specifically for those involving multiple corrections. Similarly, correction of distal femoral varus or valgus associated with medial or lateral patellar luxation, respectively, can be facilitated by the use of an ILN rather than a plate (**Fig. 13**). In brief, a medial opening, rather than lateral closing wedge osteotomy, is performed at the level of the CORA. A bone tunnel oriented parallel to the trochlea is created in the distal femoral segment. The tunnel is oriented caudo-distally to prevent exposure of the nail tip should a sulcoplasty be required. The nail is then impacted in the distal epi-metaphyseal tunnel, which ensures realignment of the proximal anatomic axis of the femur with that of the trochlea. Additional benefits of the technique over lateral plate fixation include (1) the opening wedge osteotomy does not need to be located at the CORA, (2) cortical continuity does not need to be restored, and (3) limited surgical approaches may be used because the distal locking bolts are located alongside the trochlea.

Revision surgery—nonunion

In the authors' experience, MINO is of particular interest in the revision of failed pin, plate, and/or PRC osteosyntheses of diaphyseal fractures (see **Fig. 11**). In such cases, implant removal can be performed through periarticular incisions remote to the fracture site. The same approaches can be used for nail insertion and stabilization, often

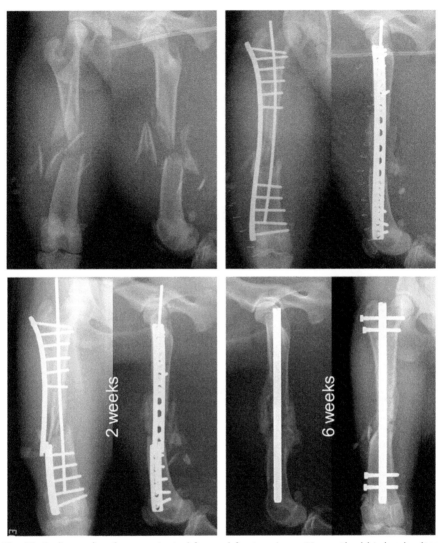

Fig. 11. Radiographs of a comminuted femoral fracture in an 11-month-old Labrador (*top left*). The initial repair consisted of a PRC applied using ORIF technique (*top right*). Although the IMR filled ~30% of the medullary cavity, plate failure occurred 2 weeks post-operatively, presumably due to the relatively small size of the IMR (*bottom left*). Successful revision was achieved using minimally invasive techniques to remove the implants followed by MINO with a standard ILN. One can speculate that primary repair with an ILN is a valid alternative to PRC.

without the need to further disturb the fracture site. Similarly, the treatment of non-unions using MINO has proved beneficial (**Fig. 14**). Following implant removal as appropriate, a reamer is used to reopen the medullary cavity. Furthermore, because the fracture is not exposed, the bone fragments generated during reaming remain in the vicinity of the nonunion site, acting as an autogenous graft. Further grafting may be performed as appropriate under fluoroscopic guidance using a Michel trephine to inject a mixture of marrow and corticocancellous material percutaneously.

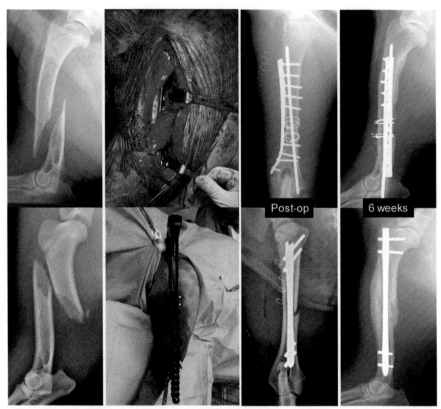

Fig. 12. Radiographs and intra-operative photographs of two similar humeral fractures in a 12 and a 9-month mid-size dog (*top* and *bottom* row, respectively). Note the presence of a long distal fissure in the second case. Anatomical reduction and traditional ORIF with cerclage wires and a PRC was achieved in the first case. In contrast, minimally invasive nail osteosynthesis, or MINO, with an AS-ILN was performed in the second case to achieve realignment without attempting anatomical reduction. While both cases eventually healed, delayed union was observed when osteosynthesis consisted of ORIF with a PRC. Note that, the limited callus formation and presence of discernible fracture line remains at 6 weeks in the PRC case. In contrast, callus remodeling is well underway in the fracture treated with MINO and an AS-ILN.

Metaphyseal and epiphyseal fractures

Presumably because of the limited bone stock available for locking and the inherent instability of current locking mechanisms, a traditionally reported limitation of interlocking nailing is the treatment of metaphyseal and epiphyseal fractures. In humans, up to 58% of valgus malalignment[51] and up to 20° of acute, uncontrolled motion at the fracture site have been documented in ILN-treated tibial metaphyseal fractures.[49] These reports agree with the authors' experience that approximately 40% of canine comminuted metaphyseal and submetaphyseal tibial fractures treated with standard ILNs require additional fixation to control perioperative instability. Various supplemental fixation techniques, including external skeletal fixators, stack pins, and additional plating, have been advocated to circumvent construct instability.[42,54,56] However, these methods may not conclusively achieve optimal stability without additional surgical trauma, which off-sets the biomechanical benefits of MINO.

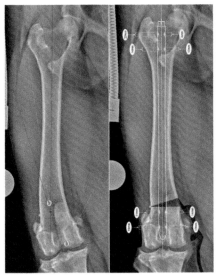
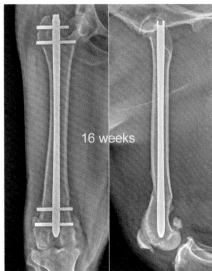

Fig. 13. A distal femoral corrective osteotomy was used for the treatment of a medially lux-ating patella (Grade III/IV). The procedure was planned with a dedicated digital planning software (*Left*) and consisted of a 18° medial opening wedge and a block sulcoplasty. The use of an I-Loc® AS-ILN (BioMedtrix LLC., Whippany, NJ) simplified realignment without need for extensive soft tissue dissection and complex implant contouring required with plate fixation. Post-operative radiographs at 16 weeks show bone remodeling of the ostet-omy site. Note that an approximately 16° recurvatum was created to 1) facilitate the execu-tion of a block sulcoplasty without interference with the nail and 2) induce a slight distalization of the patella to improve tracking in the center of the trochlea.

In contrast, reliance on the rigid locking mechanism of the AS-ILN proved effective in eliminating construct slack in a submetaphyseal comminuted fracture model.[23] Several clinical cases recently performed at MSU have thus far confirmed that an AS-ILN can be used effectively and reliably in the treatment of metaphyseal and epiph-yseal fractures including those with articular involvement. In these cases, the distal nail tip may be custom-lathed to optimize deep nail seating against the subchondral bone plate. In turn, this allows for the safe use of the locking bolts despite the limited avail-able bone stock and the presence of metaphyseal fissures (**Fig. 15**). The surgeon should keep in mind that, although in most cases, the locking bolts are inserted in the frontal plane, this plane can be reoriented to avoid fissures. This property, unique to ILNs, considerably increases the versatility of this fixation method in metaphyseal and epiphyseal fractures.

CLINICAL USE OF INTERLOCKING NAILS
Preoperative Planning

Orthogonal radiographs of the fractured and contralateral intact bone of interest are essential to accurate planning. Imaging of the affected bone is used for evaluation of the fracture location, configuration and for identification of fissures that could extend in the metaphyses. In such cases, a computed tomographic scan with 3D reconstruction may prove beneficial. Radiographs of the intact contralateral bone should take into account magnification and distortion. Therefore the proper use of a

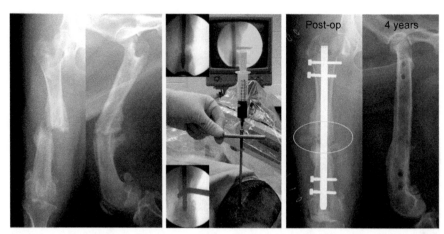

Fig. 14. Three consecutive surgical attempts at repairing a femoral fracture with a single IMR resulted in a chronic, 4 months, highly unstable nonunion. Several biomechanical factors were carefully evaluated during pre-operative planning: 1) multiple previous surgical traumas, 2) extensive muscle atrophy and fibrous adhesions, 3) challenging plate contouring in the presence of a bony callus and 4) poor bone quality due to extensive disuse osteopenia. Accordingly, MINO with a standard nail as well as percutaneous injection of a bone marrow/cancellous autograft mixture (*center*) was selected over plate fixation as the optimal option for revision. Oversize reaming was performed to open the medullary cavity and locally release bone material (central inserts). The graft is clearly visible on the immediate post-operative AP radiograph (*right*). Clinical union was obtained at 12 weeks (not shown). Bone remodeling can be appreciated after implant removal due to the presence of a distal seroma, 4 years post-operatively.

linear or spherical calibration marker placed over the bone of interest is critical. Similarly, to avoid image distortion, the bone diaphysis should be parallel to the plane of the film. Horizontal beam projections are particularly helpful for that purpose.

Selection of the appropriate nail can be performed using premagnified (usually by 4% and 12%) acetate templates superimposed over the radiographs. This cost-effective method is, however, fairly inaccurate. In contrast, digital templating can be performed using one of the dedicated software options currently available. Most software will allow the surgeon to plan the entire procedure (**Fig. 16**). Valuable steps include fracture reduction, planning of the location and magnitude of corrective osteotomies in angular limb deformity cases, implant selection, and positioning, as well as predetermination of the locking bolt lengths. Considering the cost of such software, interested surgeons are encouraged to become familiar with the system and ascertain that it is compatible with their in-house picture archiving and communication system and that desired templates are available before purchase.

Traditionally, selection of the largest possible nail fitting the isthmus of the medullary canal has been recommended.[1] To achieve this, however, reaming is often necessary. The rationale for this recommendation is 2-fold: (1) larger nails can accommodate relatively larger, hence stronger, locking bolts, and (2) the inherent slack of standard nails may be attenuated (in bending) by direct nail bone impingement. Although this may be true for standard nails, it becomes obsolete with the AS-ILN. Considering the biological disadvantages of reaming and mechanical advantages of compliant systems, we recommend that, when using an AS-ILN, the nail largest diameter (extremities) be approximately 75% of the medullary cavity at its narrowest point. Likewise, the longest possible nail should be selected to optimize construct compliance. Seating the nail

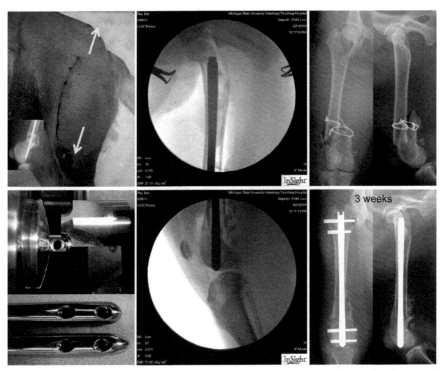

Fig. 15. Proximal and distal rod migration (*top left - arrows*), occurred 2 weeks after repair of a distal metaphyseal femoral fracture with two IMRs and cerclage wires (*top left - insert*). The choice of a plate for revision seemed ill-advised due to the presence of iatrogenic fissures extending toward the lateral fabella, which considerably limited bone stock availability for reliable screw fixation (*top right*). In contrast, based on a previous study from our laboratory, the use of an AS-ILN appeared a valid alternative. The nail tip was custom-lathed to allow deeper seating in the distal epiphysis thus avoiding the distal fissures (*bottom left*). Care was taken to ensure that the subtle protrusion of the rounded nail tip, immediately proximal to the origin of the caudal cruciate ligament, did not interfere with patellar tracking. Robust callus formation was noticed 3 weeks following revision.

distal extremity deep in the epiphysis, flush with the subchondral plates (or physes in immature dogs) provides added benefits including (1) improved bending stability and (2) increased fatigue life of the locking bolts now encased in cancellous bone. Finally, the coupling flanges of the nail should always protrude from its proximal insertion point, namely the greater tubercle, the olecranon, the greater trochanter, and the tibial plateau. In addition to further optimization of construct compliance, this critical location will facilitate nail capture should explantation become necessary.

General Techniques

Although interlocking nails can be applied using an OBDNT approach, MINO implies that the nail is inserted through small incisions remote from the fracture site. The size of the incisions varies with the bone of interest and the skills of the surgeon. A common mistake early on is not to open wide enough to allow for easy fracture realignment and to ensure that placement of the alignment guide and drill sleeves will not be hindered by soft tissues. As an example, the approach to the proximal femur may expand from the level of the acetabulum to the subtrochanteric region initially. This will facilitate

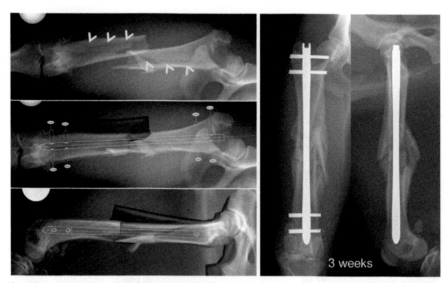

Fig. 16. Preoperative planning using a dedicated digital planning software (*Left*). Selection of an appropriately sized nail is based on digital templating of the intact contralateral bone (*top left*). In this young animal care is taken to ensure that the locking bolts are not bridging the growth plates. Note that the presence of extensive fissures (*arrows*) is not a contraindication for interlocking nailing and does not require further stabilization (*center left*) as long as one locking bolt is placed in healthy bone (*bottom left*). Through an increase in construct compliance, bridging osteosynthesis combined with the use of an hourglass AS-ILN provide beneficial controlled micromotion at the fracture site. Along with adherence to MINO principles, these techniques enhance bone healing as demonstrated by robust callus formation and clinical union by 3 weeks post-operatively (*right*). The hourglass profile of the AS-ILN also promotes revascularization of the medullary cavity and reduces the need for over reduction. Please note 1) the deep seating of the nail in the distal epiphysis as well as the location of the nail flanges flush with the tip of the greater trochanter. This location offers several benefits including, 1) optimization of bending resistance, 2) optimization of construct compliance and 3) ease of nail capture if implant removal were required.

normograde nail insertion through the intertrochanteric fossa and provide access to the trochanter for interlocking bolt placement. With experience the nail is inserted blindly through a proximal stab incision and blunt dissection through the superficial gluteal; the trochanter is exposed through a smaller distal and lateral incision followed by caudal and cranial retraction of the biceps and vastus lateralis muscles, respectively.

Although not absolutely necessary, intraoperative fluoroscopy may be beneficial with MINO to ascertain proper restoration of rotational alignment. One of the benefits of interlocking nailing is that alignment in the sagittal and frontal planes is easily restored by the mere intramedullary location of the implant. Should intraoperative imaging be part of the preoperative planning, the surgeon should verify, before initiating surgery, that complete, unobstructed visualization of the adjacent joints in both cranio-caudal and latero-medial planes are obtainable throughout the procedure.

Preservation of the fracture site during reduction is a hallmark of MINO. However, the use of hanging leg techniques or traction tables is inappropriate for MINO because the resulting extension of the limb precludes nail insertion in any bone segment. In contrast, the use of small bone reduction forceps applied at the level of the epi/metaphyses is acceptable. Alternatively, the application of cannulated toothed reduction handles (DePuy Synthes, Paoli, PA), specially designed for MIO may be preferred particularly for realignment of tibial fractures (**Fig. 17**). Successful reduction should lead to restoration of alignment in the sagittal, frontal, and transverse planes. Multiple unsuccessful attempts should be discouraged as they will induce iatrogenic trauma. Conversion to an open approach must be considered when atraumatic restoration of alignment cannot be completed using MINO techniques. The use of small portals over the fracture, as well as the use of bone graft during primary osteosynthesis, should be regarded as invasive surgical acts unsuited for MINO and therefore be avoided.

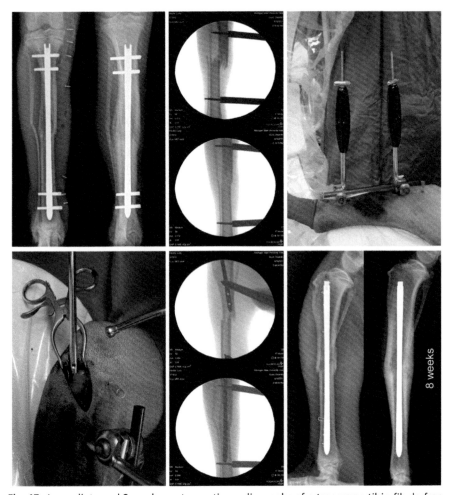

Fig. 17. Immediate and 8 weeks postoperative radiographs of a transverse tibia-fibula fracture in a 7-month-old Labrador treated using MINO with an AS-ILN (*top left* and *bottom right*). Note the continuous bone growth without loss of alignment. Cannulated toothed reduction handles (DePuy Synthes Vet, a division of DePuy Orthopaedics, Inc.) were used to realign the bone fragments. Following reduction, a temporary dedicated Snap-On external fixator was used to connect the so-called joy sticks and maintain stability during normograde nail insertion (*top right* and *bottom left*). The procedure was conducted under fluoroscopic guidance (*center* column).

In MINO, the only acceptable nail insertion technique is normograde. The medullary cavity is first opened using intramedullary pins of increasing diameter or a dedicated awl. The nail is coupled to an insertion handle via an extension, then carefully impacted intramedullary with a hammer until deeply seated in the distal epiphysis. Leverage on the nail during insertion must be avoided because it may result in structural damage to the couplings and will lead to loss of alignment between the nail and drill guide and thus off-site placement of the locking bolts. For these same reasons, the nail must not be used for fracture reduction.

Following proper nail insertion, placement of the locking bolts is achieved through the use of an alignment guide coupled to the nail. System-specific instruments (sleeves, drill bits, temporary locking bolts, depth gages, and so forth) are used for that purpose. Depending on the distribution of the locking bolts on either side of the fracture, ILNs can be used in a static (bolts above and below the fracture) or dynamic mode (bolts on one side of the fracture only). Although dynamic locking is occasionally performed in people,[57] full ILN biomechanical potential is only achieved in static mode, which remains the sole viable option when bridging osteosynthesis is desirable. Dynamic nailing can be achieved at a later date to stimulate bone remodeling once sufficient continuity and strength of the bone column have been restored (**Fig. 18**).[58] Accurate placement of the distal bolts has been challenging with off-site insertion reported in up to 28% of the cases treated with standard nails.[43,53,59] Resting the leg on a Mayo stand, which adds stability, and use of proper drilling techniques are simple surgical steps that may be used to limit this drawback. Light and steady drill pressure, pulse drilling without leaning on the alignment guide, and use of well-balanced high-end drills without recoil are very effective techniques to prevent off-site bolt insertion. Likewise, the use of light, finger-held battery-powered small drills is critical when using small 3- and 4-mm I-Loc nails. Similarly, the use of sharp Stick-Tite-like drill bits helps prevent skidding of the drill bit. Accurate bolt insertion is further facilitated by the use

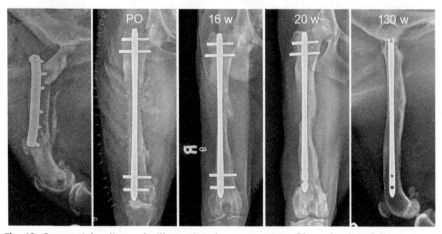

Fig. 18. Sequential radiographs illustrating the progression of bone healing following revision of an infected femoral non-union in an 8 months old, MN, Rottweiler. Failure of the initial plate osteosynthesis, 2 months prior, led to the formation of an approximately 8 cm sequestrum. Revision was performed using a 7-160 mm I-Loc nail and extensive autogenous cancellous bone grafting. While bone healing progressed without complication, graft resorption was noticed over the lateral cortex at 16 weeks. Conversion from a static to a dynamic mode via percutaneous removal of the distal bolts stimulated bone formation over time as seen at 20 weeks and 130 weeks (2.5 years) postoperatively.

of (1) an adjustable alignment guide that can be moved closer to the bone, (2) extended smooth locking bolts that temporarily link the nail to the alignment guide, and (3) self-centering conical bolts. Using these techniques and devices, the rate of off-site placement of the AS-ILN locking bolts was reduced to 1.3% in a series of 100 consecutive trauma cases.[26]

Specific Application

It is beyond the scope of this article to describe specific techniques, which are the objects of specialized courses. The interested reader is encouraged to visit the following Web sites: http://www.innovativeanimalproducts.com/ and http://www.biomedtrix.com/ as well as the AO Foundation http://www.aovet.org/ for course availability on specific nail systems and MIO techniques.

Humeral fractures

Because approximately 55% of all humeral fractures affect the center and/or the distal one-third of the diaphysis, nailing of humeral fractures may be challenging. Preoperative planning is critical to ensure that there is enough bone stock available for distal locking. In particular, fracture pattern (eg, distal fissures) as well as location in relation to the supratrochlear foramen, may limit, even preclude, deep seating of the nail. The use of a single distal bolt has been recommended in such cases. Alternatively, to circumvent this potential limitation, the tip of the nail may be lathed down and allowed to slightly protrude through the roof of the foramen (see **Fig. 8**).

  With the affected leg up and the animal in lateral recumbency, normograde nail insertion is performed via a limited cranio-lateral approach centered over the crest of the greater tubercle. A distal incision immediately above the lateral epicondyle and cranial retraction of the brachialis muscle allow exposure of the distal 25% of the diaphysis, while avoiding the radial nerve.[60] We found that orienting the locking plane ~45° away from the frontal plane in a slightly more cranio-caudal direction facilitates bolt insertion and improves anchorage in the medial epicondylar ridge (see **Fig. 12**).

Radioulnar fractures

Although only 1 case report describes the successful use of an ulnar standard nail to treat a highly comminuted fracture of the proximal radius and ulna[55] our team at MSU has used ulnar nailing on several occasions including Monteggia as well as radio-ulnar fractures in large-breed dogs (see **Figs. 9** and **10**). The relative size of the nail and ulnar medullary cavity, however, remains a limiting factor in the treatment of such fractures.

Femoral fractures

The approaches and nail insertion techniques have been described in the General techniques section. Because of the natural femoral procurvatum, over-reduction, particularly in distal femoral fractures, is necessary when using bridge interlocking nailing (**Fig. 19**). The subsequent subtle loss of anatomic alignment in the sagittal plane, however, is clinically irrelevant. Conversely, this technique allows deep nail penetration in the distal epiphysis without jeopardizing the integrity of the femoral trochlea. By moving the bolts away caudal to the edges of the trochlea, the technique also improves distal bone purchase by the bolts while limiting soft tissue irritation during flexion/extension. Distal normograde nail insertion has been described in distal metaphyseal fractures. This technique, which destroys the articular surface of the distal trochlea, is, however, more invasive and may be avoided by using lathed down nails and over-reduction of the fracture as shown in **Fig. 15**.

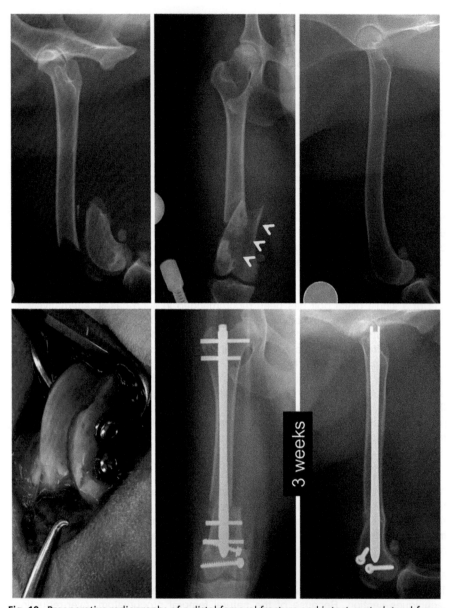

Fig. 19. Preoperative radiographs of a distal femoral fracture and intact contralateral femur in a middle age Labrador (*top row*). Note the presence of distal fissures through the trochlea (*arrow* heads) and the natural procurvatum of the distal femur. The trochlear fracture was stabilized with two lag screws (*bottom left*) while the distal femoral fracture was reduced with a slight retrocurvatum then stabilized with an AS-ILN (*bottom right*). As noted previously, fissures do not preclude interlocking nailing as long as one locking bolt is placed in healthy bone. The hourglass profile of the AS-ILN facilitates nail insertion in curvilinear bones such as the femur and tibia.

Tibial fractures

The limited soft tissue coverage of the tibia makes this bone well suited for closed interlocking nailing even without fluoroscopic assistance. Through a small medial parapatellar incision, standard nails have been traditionally inserted cranial to the footprint of the cranial cruciate ligament insertion.[61] The nail is directed toward the talocrural joint between the malleoli to avoid premature exit through the caudal or lateral tibial cortices. Conventionally, unless reaming is performed, relatively smaller nails are used in the tibia to account for the sigmoid shape of its diaphysis (**Fig. 20**). Because of its hourglass profile, the AS-ILN can be used without reaming. However, using this technique presents several disadvantages, which include (1) possible damage to the cranial cruciate and intermeniscal ligaments, (2) risk of iatrogenic increase

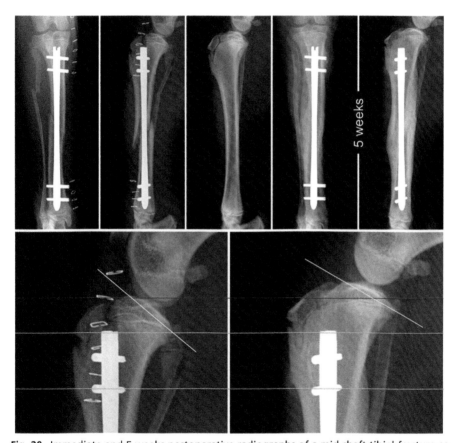

Fig. 20. Immediate and 5 weeks postoperative radiographs of a mid-shaft tibial fracture as well as intact contralateral tibia in a 6 months old German shepherd (top row). The postoperative tibial plateau angle (TPA) was similar to that of the contralateral tibia. Bridging osteosynthesis was achieved by selecting the longest possible nail extending within the constraints of the tibial physes. Observed at 5 weeks, bony union was associated with a mild reduction in TPA (yellow lines) likely due to partial closure of the cranial aspect of the proximal tibial physis. The reduced TPA may have a sparing effect on the cranial cruciate ligament later in life. Conversely, there was no growth disturbance in this case (red line). Note that the magnification between pre and post-operative radiographs (bottom row green lines) is identical.

of the tibial plateau angle and thus subsequent failure of the cranial cruciate ligament, and (3) increased risk of nail yield or fatigue failure in procurvatum and valgus because of the asymmetrical muscle distribution around the tibial diaphysis (**Fig. 21**). To circumvent these shortcomings, tibial nails should be bent to espouse the natural tibial recurvatum of approximately 170°. This simple technique offers several advantages. Firstly, the nail can be inserted more cranially to avoid the cranial cruciate ligament footprint. Secondly, restoration of the anatomic profile of the tibia, mitigates the risk of cranial cruciate ligament failure by maintaining the tibial plateau angle. As importantly, if not more so, this approach also provides mechanical advantages. Indeed, it virtually eliminates the risk of implant yield or fatigue failure by effectively counteracting the bending moments imparted to the nail by the gastrocnemius and tibial cranialis muscles. From a biological perspective, an indirect beneficial effect of bending tibial nails is that fracture fragments tend to realign along the nail shaft, which in most cases renders cortical reconstruction unnecessary and undesirable. This technique is therefore better suited for tibial MINO. Although a perceived drawback of this novel method is the need for free-hand insertion of the distal bolts, simple technical steps can be used to ensure accurate penetration of bolts in their respective cannulations (**Fig. 22**). This technique has been successfully implemented by the authors and is currently recommended in all tibial MINO as well as during ORIF (**Fig. 23**).

Clinical Outcome and Complications

Although postoperative recommendations may vary based on the specifics of a case, our patients are usually sent home within 48 hours after surgery without bandages,

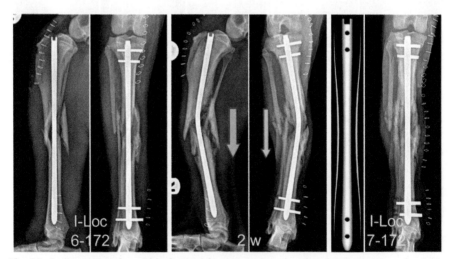

Fig. 21. Radiographs of a midshaft tibial fractures treated with a 6-172 I-Loc® angle-stable interlocking nail applied using MIO techniques (BioMedtrix LLC., Whippany, NJ). Nail yield at 2 weeks occurred as a result of 1) the asymmetrical muscle distribution around the tibia which created bending moments in a cranio-medial to caudo-lateral plane and 2) the location of the fracture vis-à-vis the thinnest section of the hourglass shaped I-Loc® nail. The larger gastrocnemius muscle (*green arrow*) induced tibial procurvatum while the relatively smaller tibial cranialis muscle (*blue arrow*) generated tibial valgus. Successful revision consisted of 1) nail section with a high-speed burr at the point of maximum curvature followed by 2) extraction from the stifle joint and fracture site (proximal and distal nail sections, respectively) then 3) nail replacement by a larger 7-172 nail.

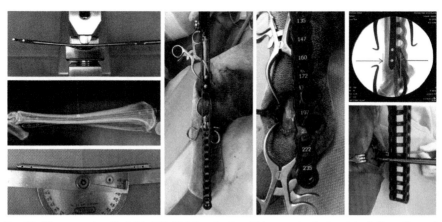

Fig. 22. *To prevent nail yield, ALL tibial nails should be gradually bent to follow the natural procurvatum of the bone. Left panel* - Using a table bending press, the nail is progressively curved from proximal to distal based on preoperative planning. In the vast majority of the cases, the overall nail bending angle is ~170° with a smooth apex at the center on that nail. *Central panel* - Following fracture reduction and nail insertion from the stifle, the proximal bolts are placed using the alignment guide. However, because nail bending will preserve tibial procurvatum, the alignment guide will lie caudal to the distal metaphysis. *Right panel* - The distal bolts are inserted using free hand technique. Briefly, the alignment guide is used to determine the location of the cannulations in a proximal to distal direction while the cranio-caudal location is identified along the bisector of the cranial and caudal tibial cortices as illustrated on the fluoroscopic image. Finally, the cis cortex is drilled along the axis of the cannulation at the intersection between the proximo-distal and cranio-caudal cortical marks as described above. That axis is parallel to the drill sleeve as illustrated on the intraoperative photo. Note: while intraoperative imaging was used for demonstration purpose in the case illustrated here, it seldom used in clinical cases.

other than superficial dressings over the skin incisions. Low-impact activity is recommended until radiographic evidence of adequate (subjective assessment) callus formation (typically 3 weeks).

Standard nails

The success rate of interlocking nailing using traditional nailing techniques and standard nails varies from 83% to 96% with healing times ranging from 13 to 17 weeks.[19,43,59,62] Complications have been reported in up to 17% of cases treated with standard nails.[59] Although most are related to poor indications (eg, metaphyseal fractures with insufficient bone for screw insertion) or technical errors (eg, empty screw hole near a fracture site), some may be attributed to the limitation of the nail designs, including implant fracture, missed screw holes, and delayed or nonunions. Catastrophic nail fractures in early designs are now rare occurrences. Complications, such as delayed or nonunions may be related to torsional and bending slack in standard nails, which may be accentuated by structural failure and/or off-site placement of the locking screws. Although the use of solid bolts may limit the incidence of implant failure it has little to no effect on construct stability.[22] The use of additional implants, such as type I external fixators, has been reported to provide adequate construct rigidity in 12% of cases.[42] Other nonspecific complications include infection, sciatic neuropraxia, coxofemoral luxation (immature dogs), and joint violation.[42,59,63]

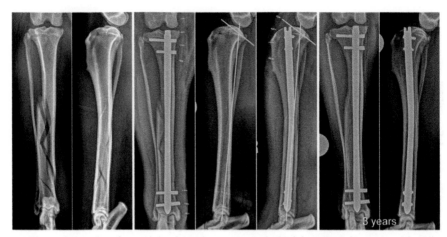

Fig. 23. Radiographs of a mid-diaphyseal comminuted tibial fracture in a 2-year old, 49 kg, female spayed Labrador retriever. Note the extend of the fissures from the mid diaphyseal region down to the distal epi-metaphysis (*left panel*). Using MINO techniques, the fracture was reduced and stabilized with an 8-210 mm I-Loc interlocking nail bent at ~170° (*central panel*). Note the realignment of the fragments and spontaneous closure of the fissure along the nail as well as the restoration of the natural tibial recurvatum and of the normal tibial plateau angle as compared to the intact contralateral tibia (blue lines). Tibial nail bending also allows for preservation of the cranial cruciate ligament footprint through nail insertion in a more cranial location than typically recommended. Bone remodeling can be seen on the 3-year postoperative radiographs. Tibial nail bending has been implemented by the authors since the onset of using the hourglass shaped I-Loc nail as illustrated in the case shown here. Our group believes that this is the reason why we have not seen cases of tibial nail yield as anecdotally reported by some of our colleagues. Accordingly, we strongly recommend that this technique be used systematically when using MINO (as well as ORIF) of tibial fractures.

I-Loc angle-stable nails

The clinical outcome of nail osteosynthesis has been recently reported in 2 prospective case series involving 100 and 25 consecutive traumatic fractures of the femur, tibia and humerus in dogs (I-Loc 6, 7, and 8 mm)[26] and cats (I-Loc 3 and 4 mm).[27]

In the canine study, femoral fractures were seen in 64% of the cases, and tibial and humeral fractures accounted for 28% and 8% of cases, respectively. I-Loc nails of 6, 7, and 8 mm were used in dogs with a mean body weight (±SD) of approximately 25 ± 6, 30 ± 7, and 38 ± 9 kg, respectively, and fractures in dogs weighing as little as 17 kg (I-Loc 6) and as much as 59 kg (I-Loc 8) were successfully treated. MIO was performed in most (61%) of the fractures. Although all nails were applied using a static configuration, as surgeons' experience improved the bolt distribution progressively evolved from a 2-2 distribution (81% of the cases) to simpler 1-2, 2-1, and eventually 1-1 distribution (14% of the cases). Missed cannulations occurred in 6% of the cases and were retrieved during the same anesthetic event in all but 1 case. Overall, the postoperative rate of missed cannulations was 1.3%, which favorably compares to the 14% rate reported with standard nails. Complications requiring additional surgery occurred in 3 cases involving tibial fractures. These consisted of (1) subacute infection in a grade II open fracture, (2) fatigue failure of an undersized nail at 7 weeks, and (3) proximal and medial cortical tearing along the bolts resulting in "biological slack" in a nail inserted immediately adjacent to the medial cortex. All cases were successfully revised with (1) nail removal after clinical union at 15 weeks, (2) replacement of the failed 7-mm nail with an 8-mm nail, and (3) temporary application of a type IA medially applied external fixator frame. All cases healed and fully recovered without further intervention. Minor complications also occurred in 4 tibial fractures in which delayed (up to 3 years) seromas over the distal bolts medially prompted bolt removal under local anesthesia. That complication has not been seen since our recommendation to shorten the cis section of the tibial bolts so that it does not protrude by more than 1 mm over the medial tibial cortex.

In the feline study, femoral, tibial, and humeral fractures, respectively, occurred in 48%, 32%, and 20% of the 25 consecutive cases. Most (62%) of the fractures were comminuted and diaphyseal (76%). In the remaining cases (24%) one or both epimetaphyseal regions were affected. Most femora received a 4-mm I-Loc, whereas the humerus was treated exclusively with 3-mm nails regardless of body weight. Unlike that reported in dogs, MINO was only performed on a third of the cases. In both studies, all patients were weight bearing within 2 days after surgery and full recovery was achieved in all cases.

Nail explantation
Stress shielding has not been a clinical issue with standard nails and is even more unlikely with the compliant AS-ILN design (**Fig. 24**). Accordingly, unless motivated by a

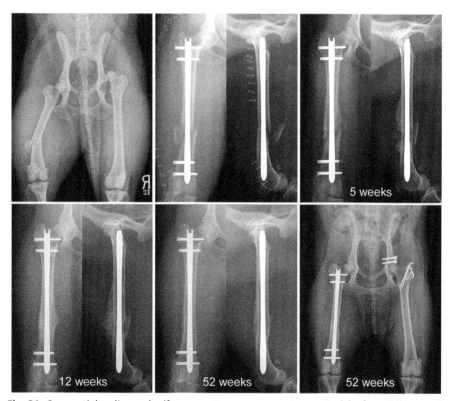

Fig. 24. Sequential radiographs (from pre- to one year postoperatively) of a mildly comminuted diaphyseal femoral fracture and concurrent contralateral hip luxation in a 1-year old Labrador. The fracture was treated using MINO with an AS-ILN. Note the large callus at 12 weeks, as well as its complete resorption with restoration of the normal femoral shape at one year. This suggests that this compliant nail does not shield the repaired bone from physiologic loads and allows normal bone remodeling to occur unhindered. Also note the absence of OA in the reduced hip at one year.

complication, nail removal is unnecessary. Nonetheless, a perceived problem is that explantation may be challenging as a result of difficulties in recapturing the nail. Simple effective strategies may be used to circumvent this potential drawback. Bone wax capping the nail flanges may be used to prevent bone ingrowth. Choosing the longest possible implant, as recommended for semirigid fixation, also places the nail flanges near the proximal aspect of the greater tubercle, greater trochanter, or within the fat pat slightly proud of the tibial subchondral plate. In turn, this facilitates nail identification, coupling to the extension and handle, and finally extraction after removal of the locking devices. The hourglass shape of the AS-ILN has not been a factor preventing nail explantation. In a recent in vivo study,[24] using a twisting and pulling motion, all nails were extracted in less than 30 seconds at loads smaller than 300 N, even though explantation was performed 18 weeks postoperatively, before callus remodeling.

Although no objective clinical data are currently available on the efficacy of MINO and new nail designs, the comparative outcome of standard versus angle-stable nails in an experimental in vivo study demonstrated the biomechanical superiority of the AS-ILN over standard nails.[24] Similarly an internal (Laurent P. Guiot and Loic M. Dejardin, unpublished, 2012) review of 13 femoral and tibial fractures treated with an AS-ILN using MINO showed a mean healing time of 36 ± 9.3 days (21–45 days). This was shorter than that previously reported with standard nails (90–120 days).[59] At present, the AS-ILN has been successfully used in approximately 175 consecutive trauma cases of the femur, tibia, humerus, and ulna, as well as in approximately 30 angular deformity cases. Complications requiring some form of revision surgery were documented in 3 tibial fractures (1.7% of all trauma cases), which compares favorably with 17% of complications requiring revision surgery reported in a series of 134 cases treated with ORIF using standard nails.[59] Atraumatic reduction, preservation of the soft tissue envelope surrounding the fracture site, and MIO techniques, as well as the use of an AS-ILN, may explain both findings.

SUMMARY

Interlocking nailing of long bone fractures has long been considered the gold standard osteosynthesis technique in humans. Thanks to improvements in the locking mechanism design and nail profile, a recently developed veterinary angle-stable nail has become the first true intramedullary fixator providing accurate and consistent repair stability while allowing semirigid fixation. As a result, indications for interlocking nailing have expanded to include treatment of peri-articular fractures, corrections on angular deformities, and revisions of failed plate osteosyntheses. Perfectly suited for MIO, interlocking nailing is an attractive and effective alternative to plate and plate-rod osteosynthesis.

REFERENCES

1. Johnson AL, Houlton JEF, Vannini R. AO principles of fracture management in the dog and cat. 1st edition. New York: AO Publishing & Thieme; 2005.

2. Kirkby KA, Lewis DD, Lafuente MP, et al. Management of humeral and femoral fractures in dogs and cats with linear-circular hybrid external skeletal fixators. J Am Vet Med Assoc 2008;44(4):180–97.

3. Dudley M, Johnson AL, Olmstead M, et al. Open reduction and bone plate stabilization, compared with closed reduction and external fixation, for treatment of comminuted tibial fractures: 47 cases (1980–1995) in dogs. J Am Vet Med Assoc 1997;211(8):1008–12.

4. Tong GO, Bavonratanavech S. Minimally invasive plate osteosynthesis (MIPO). Davos (Switzerland): AO Publishing; 2007.
5. Gerber C, Mast JW, Ganz R. Biological internal fixation of fractures. Arch Orthop Trauma Surg 1990;109(6):295–303.
6. Gerber A, Ganz R. Combined internal and external osteosynthesis a biological approach to the treatment of complex fractures of the proximal tibia. Injury 1998;29(Suppl 3):C22–8.
7. Gautier E, Sommer C. Guidelines for the clinical application of the LCP. Injury 2003;34(Suppl 2):B63–76.
8. Perren SM. Evolution of the internal fixation of long bone fractures. The scientific basis of biological internal fixation: choosing a new balance between stability and biology. J Bone Joint Surg Br 2002;84(8):1093–110.
9. Rozbruch SR, Muller U, Gautier E, et al. The evolution of femoral shaft plating technique. Clin Orthop Relat Res 1998;(354):195–208.
10. Guiot LP, Dejardin LM. Prospective evaluation of minimally invasive plate osteosynthesis in 36 nonarticular tibial fractures in dogs and cats. Vet Surg 2011; 40(2):171–82.
11. Küntscher G. Die Behandlung von Knochenbrüchen bei Tieren durch Marknagelung. Archiv für Wissensch Prakt Tierheil 1940;75:262.
12. Huckstep RL. Proceedings: an intramedullary nail for rigid fixation and compression of fractures of the femur. J Bone Joint Surg Br 1975;57(2):253.
13. Johnson KA, Huckstep RL. Bone remodeling in canine femora after internal-fixation with the huckstep nail. Vet Radiology 1986;27(1):20.
14. Muir P, Johnson KA. Tibial intercalary allograft incorporation: comparison of fixation with locked intramedullary nail and dynamic compression plate. J Orthop Res 1995;13(1):132–7.
15. Muir P, Johnson KA. Interlocking intramedullary nail stabilization of a femoral fracture in a dog with osteomyelitis. J Am Vet Med Assoc 1996;209(7):1262–4.
16. Muir P, Parker RB, Goldsmid SE, et al. Interlocking intramedullary nail stabilisation of a diaphyseal tibial fracture. J Small Anim Pract 1993;34(1):26–30.
17. Dueland RT, Johnson KA. Interlocking nail fixation of diaphyseal fractures in the dog: a multi-center study of 1991–1992 cases. Vet Surg 1993;22(5):377.
18. Duhautois B, vanTilburg J. Veterinary bolted pinning or interlocking nail: clinical study of 45 cases. Vet Q 1996;18:S21.
19. Durall I, Diaz MC. Early experience with the use of an interlocking nail for the repair of canine femoral shaft fractures. Vet Surg 1996;25(5):397–406.
20. Endo K, Nakamura K, Maeda H, et al. Interlocking intramedullary nail method for the treatment of femoral and tibial fractures in cats and small dogs. J Vet Med Sci 1998;60(1):119–22.
21. Dejardin LM, Lansdowne JL, Sinnott MT, et al. In vitro mechanical evaluation of torsional loading in simulated canine tibiae for a novel hourglass-shaped interlocking nail with a self-tapping tapered locking design. Am J Vet Res 2006; 67(4):678–85.
22. Lansdowne JL, Sinnott MT, Dejardin LM, et al. In vitro mechanical comparison of screwed, bolted, and novel interlocking nail systems to buttress plate fixation in torsion and mediolateral bending. Vet Surg 2007;36(4):368–77.
23. Ting D, Cabassu JB, Guillou RP, et al. In vitro evaluation of the effect of fracture configuration on the mechanical properties of standard and novel interlocking nail systems in bending. Vet Surg 2009;38(7):881–7.

24. Cabassu JB, Villwock M, Guillou RP, et al. In vivo biomechanical evaluation of a novel angle-stable interlocking nail design in a canine tibial gap fracture model. Breckenridge (CO): Veterinary Orthopaedic Society; 2010.

25. Dejardin LM, Cabassu J, Guillou RP, et al. In vivo biomechanical evaluation of a novel angle-stable interlocking nail design in a canine tibial gap fracture model. World Veterinary Orthopaedic Congress. Bologna, Italy, September 15–18, 2010.

26. Fauron AH, Gazzola KM, Perry KL, et al. Clinical Application of the I-Loc Angle-Stable Interlocking Nail In 100 traumatic fractures of the humerus, femur and tibia. Abstract presented at the VOS Conference. Snowmass, CO, March 10–17, 2018.

27. Marturello DM, Perry KL, Déjardin LM. Clinical Application of the Small I-Loc Nail in Cats. Abstract presented at the ECVS conference. Budapest, Hungary, July 4–6 2019.

28. Hulse D, Hyman B. Biomechanics of fracture fixation failure. Vet Clin North Am Small Anim Pract 1991;21(4):647–67.

29. Hulse D, Hyman W, Nori M, et al. Reduction in plate strain by addition of an intramedullary pin. Vet Surg 1997;26(6):451–9.

30. Hulse D, Ferry K, Fawcett A, et al. Effect of intramedullary pin size on reducing bone plate strain. Vet Comp Orthop Traumatol 2000;13(4):185–90.

31. Dueland RT, Berglund L, Vanderby R, et al. Structural properties of interlocking nails, canine femora, and femur-interlocking nail constructs. Vet Surg 1996; 25(5):386–96.

32. Muir P, Johnson KA, Markel MD. Area moment of inertia for comparison of implant cross-sectional geometry and bending stiffness. Vet Comp Orthop Traumatol 1995;8:146–52.

33. Roe SC. Biomechanics principles of interlocking nails fixation. 8th Annual American College of Veterinary Surgeons Symposium. Chicago, October 8–11, 1998.

34. Dueland RT, Vanderby R Jr, McCabe RP. Fatigue study of six and eight mm diameter interlocking nails with screw holes of variable size and number. Vet Comp Orthop Traumatol 1997;10:194–9.

35. Bucholz RW, Ross SE, Lawrence KL. Fatigue fracture of the interlocking nail in the treatment of fractures of the distal part of the femoral shaft. J Bone Joint Surg Am 1987;69(9):1391–9.

36. Dejardin LM, Guillou RP, Ting D, et al. Effect of bending direction on the mechanical behaviour of interlocking nail systems. Vet Comp Orthop Traumatol 2009; 22(4):264–9.

37. Broos PL, Sermon A. From unstable internal fixation to biological osteosynthesis. A historical overview of operative fracture treatment. Acta Chir Belg 2004;104(4): 396–400.

38. Wheeler JL, Lewis DD, Cross AR, et al. Intramedullary interlocking nail fixation in dogs and cats: clinical applications. Comp Cont Educ Pract 2004;26(7): 531–43.

39. Aper RL, Litsky AS, Roe SC, et al. Fatigue life and push-out strength of a 2.7mm locking bolt for use in a 6mm interlocking nails. 13th Annual American College of Veterinary Surgeons Symposium. Washington, DC, October, 2003.

40. Dueland RT, Vanderby R, McCabe RP. Comparison of interlocking nail screws and bolts: insertion torque, push-out strength, and mode of failure. 13th Annual American College of Veterinary Surgeons Symposium. Washington, DC, October, 2003.

41. von Pfeil DJF, Déjardin LM, DeCamp CE, et al. In vitro biomechanical comparison of plate-rod combination-construct and an interlocking nail-constructs for experimentally induced gap fractures in canine tibiae. Am J Vet Res 2005;66(9): 1536–43.

42. Basinger RR, Suber JT. Two techniques for supplementing interlocking nail repair of fractures of the humerus, femur, and tibia: results in 12 dogs and cats. Vet Surg 2004;33(6):673–80.

43. Duhautois B. Use of veterinary interlocking nails for diaphyseal fractures in dogs and cats: 121 cases. Vet Surg 2003;32(1):8–20.

44. Schandelmaier P, Krettek C, Tscherne H. Biomechanical study of nine different tibia locking nails. J Orthop Trauma 1996;10(1):37–44.

45. Kaspar K, Schell H, Seebeck P, et al. Angle stable locking reduces interfragmentary movements and promotes healing after unreamed nailing. Study of a displaced osteotomy model in sheep tibiae. J Bone Joint Surg Am 2005;87(9): 2028–37.

46. Klein MPM, Rahn BA, Frigg R, et al. Reaming versus non-reaming in medullary nailing—interference with cortical circulation of the canine tibia. Arch Orthop Trauma Surg 1990;109(6):314–6.

47. Wheeler JL, Stubbs PW, Lewis DD, et al. Intramedullary interlocking nail fixation in dogs and cats: biomechanics and instrumentation. Compend Contin Educ Pract Vet 2004;26(7):519–29.

48. Tarr RR, Wiss DA. The mechanics and biology of intramedullary fracture fixation. Clin Orthop Relat Res 1986;(212):10–7.

49. Lang GJ, Cohen BE, Bosse MJ, et al. Proximal third tibial shaft fractures. Should they be nailed? Clin Orthop Relat Res 1995;315:64–74.

50. Freedman EL, Johnson EE. Radiographic analysis of tibial fracture malalignment following intramedullary nailing. Clin Orthop Relat Res 1995;315:25–33.

51. Buehler KC, Green J, Woll TS, et al. A technique for intramedullary nailing of proximal third tibia fractures. J Orthop Trauma 1997;11(3):218–23.

52. Guillou RP, Guiot LP, Déjardin LM. Angle-Stable Interlocking Nail Fixation for Distal Femoral Corrective Osteotomy Associated with Medial Patellar Luxation. Abstract presented at the VOS Conference, Park City, UT, March 9–16, 2013.

53. Durall I, Diaz-Bertrana MC, Morales I. Interlocking nail stabilization of humeral fractures: initial experiences in seven clinical cases. Vet Comp Orthop Traumatol 1994;7:3–8.

54. Basinger RR, Suber JT. Supplemental fixation of fractures repaired with interlocking nails: 14 cases. 29th Annual Veterinary Orthopedic Society Conference. The Canyons, UT, March, 2002.

55. Gatineau M, Plante J. Ulnar interlocking intramedullary nail stabilization of a proximal radio-ulnar fracture in a dog. Vet Surg 2010;39(8):1025–9.

56. Goett SD, Sinnott MT, Ting D, et al. Mechanical comparison of an interlocking nail locked with conventional bolts to extended bolts connected with a type-IA external skeletal fixator in a tibial fracture model. Vet Surg 2007;36(3): 279–86.

57. Tigani D, Fravisini M, Stagni C, et al. Interlocking nail for femoral shaft fractures: is dynamization always necessary? Int Orthop 2005;29(2):101–4.

58. Durall I, Falcon C, Diaz-Bertrana MC, et al. Effects of static fixation and dynamization after interlocking femoral nailing locked with an external fixator: an experimental study in dogs. Vet Surg 2004;33(4):323–32.

59. Dueland RT, Johnson KA, Roe SC, et al. Interlocking nail treatment of diaphyseal long-bone fractures in dogs. J Am Vet Med Assoc 1999;214(1):59–66.

60. Piermattei DL, Johnson KA. An atlas of surgical approaches to the bones and joints of the dog and cat. 4th edition. Philadelphia: Saunders; 2004.
61. Pardo AD. Relationship of tibial intramedullary pins to canine stifle joint structures—a comparison of normograde and retrograde insertion. J Am Anim Hosp Assoc 1994;30(4):369–74.
62. Diaz-Bertrana MC, Durall I, Puchol JL, et al. Interlocking nail treatment of long-bone fractures in cats: 33 cases (1995–2004). Vet Comp Orthop Traumatol 2005;18(3):119–26.
63. Durall I, Diaz MC, Puchol JL, et al. Radiographic findings related to interlocking nailing: windshield-wiper effect, and locking screw failure. Vet Comp Orthop Traumatol 2003;16(4):217–22.

Percutaneous Pinning for Fracture Repair in Dogs and Cats

Caleb C. Hudson, DVM, MS[a],*, Stanley E. Kim, BVSc, MS[b],
Antonio Pozzi, DMV, MS[c]

KEYWORDS

- Growth plate fracture • Pinning • Percutaneous • Minimally invasive

KEY POINTS

- Pinning is the treatment of choice for the surgical repair of simple physeal fractures.
- All traditional principles of intramedullary or cross-pinning apply when considering the use of percutaneous pinning.
- Fractures should ideally be minimally displaced with a significant portion of bridging periosteum remaining intact.
- A thorough physical and orthopedic examination should be performed to identify any serious concomitant injury.
- For closed reduction of physeal fractures, the precise technique depends on the direction and degree of displacement of the epiphysis.

INTRODUCTION

Steinman pins or Kirschner wires (herein referred to as pins) can be used to stabilize a variety of different physeal fracture configurations in the dog and cat.[1–7] Traditionally, pinning of physeal fractures has been described using an open surgical approach to achieve direct, anatomic reduction and facilitate accurate placement of implants.[3,4,6,8,9] When physeal fracture stabilization using pins is performed in a minimally invasive fashion, the procedure is known as percutaneous pinning.[1,2] Insertion of pins in a minimally invasive fashion through small stab incisions in the skin may offer significant advantages when compared with traditional open pinning, such as

Disclosure: The authors have nothing to disclose.
The article is an update of "Kim SE, Hudson CC, Pozzi A. Percutaneous pinning for fracture repair in dogs and cats. Vet Clin North Am Small Anim Pract 2012;42(5):963-74."
[a] Gulf Coast Veterinary Specialists, 8042 Katy Fwy, Houston, TX 77024, USA; [b] Department of Small Animal Clinical Sciences, College of Veterinary Medicine, University of Florida, 2015 Southwest 16th Avenue, PO Box 100126, Gainesville, FL 32610-0126, USA; [c] Clinic for Small Animal Surgery, Vetsuisse Faculty, University of Zurich, Zurich CH-8057, Switzerland
* Corresponding author.
E-mail address: caleb.hudson@me.com

reduced postoperative pain, accelerated healing, and less iatrogenic trauma to important structures such as the physes and joint capsule.[10] Juxta-articular pediatric fractures in humans are frequently treated in a similar minimally invasive manner.[10–13] Percutaneous pinning is routinely used at the authors' institutions with a high success rate; however, appropriate case selection, fluoroscopic guidance, and surgeon experience are required to achieve consistent, successful outcomes. The purpose of this article is to describe case selection, surgical technique, and anticipated outcomes for percutaneous pinning in the dog and cat.

CASE SELECTION

Traditional principles of case selection for intramedullary or cross-pinning stabilization of fractures apply when considering patients as candidates for percutaneous pinning. Salter-Harris type I and II physeal fractures are the most amenable to percutaneous pinning stabilization, for several reasons. Pins mainly serve to counteract bending forces, whereas rotational and compressive forces are poorly neutralized, even when multiple pins are used. Therefore, juxta-articular, noncomminuted fracture configurations with some inherent stability after reduction are the optimal fracture configurations for stabilization by use of pins alone. Because pins have limited ability to provide long-term stability in all 3 planes when compared with other forms of fixation, pinning alone is generally used in young animals with a rapid capacity for bone healing. As pins cannot provide significant interfragmentary compression, intra-articular fractures should not be treated with pins alone.

Candidates for percutaneous pinning must meet additional criteria to those already described. Fractures should ideally be minimally displaced with a significant portion of bridging periosteum remaining intact on one side. Intact periosteum has the potential to contribute to fracture site stability by acting as a tension band if combined with appropriately positioned pins.[14] In addition, the intact periosteum facilitates closed reduction as it guides correct interdigitation of the fragments. This technique is similar to ligamentotaxis because the soft tissue envelope is used to restore alignment of the fragments. Percutaneous pinning is often still possible in moderately displaced fractures, as long as the interval between trauma and surgical intervention is short. Closed reduction is difficult or impossible in fractures that are not immediately treated (more than 24–48 hours after trauma), owing to muscular contraction and adhesions from early callus formation. Very small fracture fragments can be difficult to palpate and manipulate percutaneously, or identify with intraoperative fluoroscopy; hence an open approach is more suitable in these cases. For example, distal femur fractures in cats require very accurate pin placement to avoid damaging the long digital extensor tendon, which, in some cases, might only be possible with an open approach. Fracture fragments that are covered by large amounts of soft tissue may be difficult to align with indirect methods, which may preclude the use of percutaneous pinning. Finally, Salter-Harris type II fractures with large metaphyseal fragments (Thurstan Holland fragments) should be reduced with an open approach.

The authors currently perform percutaneous pinning for Salter-Harris types I and II fractures of the distal femoral, femoral capital, proximal tibial, tibial apophyseal, distal tibial, distal radial, and proximal humeral physes.

PREOPERATIVE MANAGEMENT AND PLANNING

Preoperative planning for percutaneous pinning fracture stabilization must begin with appropriate case selection, as already described. A thorough physical and orthopedic examination should be performed to identify any significant concomitant injury. At a minimum, thoracic radiographs and orthogonal projection radiographs of the affected bone are acquired. Radiographs typically require moderate sedation or anesthesia to achieve optimal positioning and projections. It is strongly recommended that radiographs of the contralateral intact bone be obtained. Comparing radiographic projections of the injured bone with the contralateral normal bone can help accurately differentiate minimally displaced physeal fractures from normal physeal anatomy. Contralateral intact bone radiographs can also be very useful for comparison intraoperatively to assist in achieving anatomic fracture reduction. Rarely, stressed view radiographic projections are necessary to demonstrate location and degree of instability of a physeal fracture. All radiographic projections should be obtained with a magnification marker in place at the level of the fracture site to allow radiographic images to be accurately size calibrated for planning measurements. Radiographic tracings of the fracture fragments in normal alignment, or digital templating software, can be used to preoperatively select pin size, and choose anticipated pin insertion sites and trajectory. Preemptive selection of pin size and positioning is often more accurate when planned from the normal contralateral bone radiographs, because it is not uncommon for fracture segments to be rotated out of plane of the radiographic projection on the images of the fractured bone.

As manipulation of the affected limb may not be well tolerated during initial orthopedic examination, sedation for radiographs presents an opportunity to carefully palpate the fracture site. Thorough palpation of the fracture is particularly crucial when considering patients as candidates for percutaneous pinning. Preoperative palpation should be performed carefully to avoid additional iatrogenic damage to the fracture site. Occasionally, minimally displaced fractures that retain extensive soft tissue integrity may be stable enough to treat conservatively with cage rest with or without adjunctive external coaptation. At the other end of the spectrum, physeal fractures that are several days old may have already developed soft tissue callus formation and muscle contraction that precludes indirect reduction. Reduction may be attempted at the time radiographs are obtained, but this requires heavy sedation or anesthesia. Radial and tibial physeal fractures should be temporarily immobilized with a Robert Jones bandage (nonreduced fractures) or a soft padded bandage and an appropriate splint (reduced fractures) to prevent further displacement of the fracture segments and decrease discomfort associated with motion at the fracture site. As limb immobilization for humeral and femoral fractures is difficult to attain with external coaptation, the main goal of initial manipulation of these fractures is to assess fracture site stability rather than to obtain reduction at the fracture site. The authors routinely administer parenteral opioids with or without an oral or parenteral nonsteroidal anti-inflammatory drug for analgesia before surgery.

PREPARATION AND PATIENT POSITIONING

At the time of surgery, the entire affected limb must be aseptically prepared to enable adequate intraoperative maneuvering required for closed reduction and percutaneous insertion of pins. A full limb preparation is also required to allow conversion to a traditional open approach if needed. The hanging limb preparation is useful to fatigue contracted muscles and facilitate closed reduction. Femoral capital physeal fractures are approached with the patient in lateral recumbency, affected limb uppermost. For hindlimb fractures at the level of the distal femur and below, patients are positioned in dorsal recumbency, optimally with the leg projecting off of the end of the surgical table. Humeral proximal physeal fractures are approached with the patients in lateral recumbency, affected leg uppermost or dorsal recumbency using a hanging limb technique with a vacuum bag positioned to elevate the chest off of the operating table. Distal radial physeal fractures can be approached with the patient in dorsal recumbency (preferred) or lateral recumbency with the affected leg uppermost. Before final aseptic limb preparation, trial images with the fluoroscopy unit should be acquired to ensure that the fracture site can be imaged appropriately. Use of towel clamps may hinder optimal visualization of the fracture segments during intraoperative imaging. Drapes can be sutured or stapled into place in lieu of using towel clamps. Adhesive dressings (Ioban, Opsite) can become wrapped up by pins during insertion, and are thus generally avoided. If using large-gauge needles as a guide for percutaneous pin insertion then adhesive dressings may be applied. A radiolucent operating table is advantageous but not essential.

FRACTURE REDUCTION AND SURGICAL APPROACH

For closed reduction of physeal fractures, the precise technique depends on the bone, the involved physis, and the direction and degree of displacement of the epiphysis. The first principle in reduction is to minimize harm to the physis. To achieve this, the maneuver should generally be 90% traction and 10% leverage.[14] Initial traction may slightly increase the displacement and angular malalignment at the fracture site. The epiphysis is then translated into alignment while maintaining traction. Reduction is completed by realignment of any angular malalignment. Audible or palpable grinding of the physeal cartilage should be avoided. Assessment of reduction is performed with intraoperative fluoroscopy.

Although rarely used in the authors' institutions, reduction can be facilitated by use of a traction device, temporary external skeletal fixation, or a traction table. Temporary pins for skeletal traction should not be placed directly through the epiphysis because of the risk of iatrogenic fracture and interference with definitive pin placement. The insertion sites for the traction and countertraction pins should be placed well proximal and distal to the epiphysis, in the diaphysis of the affected bone and in the diaphysis or metaphysis of the bone on the opposite side of the joint of the displaced epiphysis. Traction instruments can be cumbersome and bulky, so these devices are not recommended for routine use with percutaneous pinning. Manual reduction is sufficient in most cases. Alternatively, temporary half pins can be safely placed in the diaphysis of the affected bone and used to facilitate manual control of the larger fracture segment, while the epiphyseal segment is indirectly controlled by manipulating the long bone proximal or distal to the joint closest to the physeal fracture site.

Following fracture reduction, small stab approaches are made over the proposed pin insertion sites. The stab incisions should extend down to the periosteum to provide a tract for the pin to pass through. Alternatively, large-gauge hypodermic needles can be inserted percutaneously through the skin and soft tissues until the tip of the needle lodges against the periosteal surface of the bone at the proposed pin insertion site. The needles serve as a guide for pin insertion as well as a tissue guard to prevent soft tissues from being damaged by the pin during insertion.[15] The skin incisions or needle insertion sites should be located slightly distal to the proposed pin insertion site for distal physeal fractures, and slightly proximal to the proposed pin insertion site for proximal physeal fractures, to account for anticipated pin trajectory through the soft tissues. Pins are placed from the epiphyseal or apophyseal segment toward the metaphyseal/diaphyseal segment to maximize purchase as well as to help maintain reduction of the fracture site during pin insertion. The exception to this rule on pin insertion direction is for capital physeal fractures, in which the pins are inserted from the lateral aspect of the femur and the tips are directed into the femoral capital epiphysis.

Comments on surgical approach relevant to specific physeal fractures are included below.

Capital Physeal Fracture

The femoral capital physis has a natural "L" shape, which assists closed reduction of capital physeal fractures. To reduce capital physeal fractures, the thigh over the mid-diaphyseal region of the femur is grasped and manually manipulated while the coxofemoral joint region is assessed using fluoroscopy. The femoral neck is typically displaced dorsally and cranially, so a caudally and distally directed force is applied to reduce the capital physeal fracture site. As an alternative to manipulating the femoral shaft from the thigh, a pointed reduction forceps can be applied to the greater trochanter and used to apply traction to the femur and reduce the fracture. Care must be taken not to avulse the greater trochanter with the reduction forceps. Once the capital physeal fracture is reduced, manual compression force is applied directed along the long axis of the femoral neck to maintain fracture reduction. The coxofemoral joint is then put through a range-of-motion and several orthogonal images are obtained with the fluoroscopy unit to confirm fracture reduction.

Distal Femoral Physeal Fracture

The distal femoral epiphysis is usually displaced caudally and proximally. To reduce the distal femoral epiphysis, distally directed traction force is applied to the tibia. The stifle joint is then hyperextended while a caudally directed force is applied to the mid-thigh region over the femoral diaphysis. Once reduced, the caudally directed force on the mid-thigh is maintained, but the stifle can be carefully flexed by manipulating the tibia. As the stifle is flexed, a cranial/proximally directed force is applied along the shaft of the tibia from distal to proximal to counteract the caudally directed force applied to the mid-thigh and maintain the distal femoral epiphysis in reduction. Orthogonal fluoroscopic images are obtained to verify physeal fracture reduction. A gap or a step at the cranial aspect of the physis indicates an incomplete reduction. Alignment in the frontal plane should be carefully evaluated in Salter-Harris type II fractures with Thurstan Holland fragments.

Tibial Apophyseal Fracture (Tibial Tuberosity Avulsion)

The tibial apophysis typically displaces predominantly proximally owing to the pull of the quadriceps muscle group exerted through the patellar tendon. To reduce tibial apophyseal fractures, the stifle joint is initially hyperextended by applying a caudally directed force over the femoral diaphysis in the mid-thigh region while a cranially directed force is applied over the caudal aspect of the distal tibia. While the stifle is hyperextended, a pointed reduction forceps is applied percutaneously to the middle of the apophyseal segment with the tips inserted from the medial and lateral sides. The pointed reduction forceps is then used to apply a distally and caudally directed force to the tibial apophysis to bring the apophysis into reduction. Alternatively, a technique known as the "spiking" technique may be used to reduce the apophysis.[2] The spiking technique involves inserting a pin percutaneously through the skin over the tibial apophysis while the apophysis is still in a displaced position. The pin is oriented over the desired insertion point of a stabilizing pin through the apophysis and the trajectory of the pin is directed to be as perpendicular as possible to the apophyseal physis. The pin is then inserted although the apophysis until the tip is just protruding through the caudal aspect of the apophyseal segment. The pin inserted in the apophysis is then used as a handle to reduce the apophyseal segment.[2]

Proximal Tibial Physeal Fracture

The proximal tibial physis typically displaces caudally and may also displace in a caudolateral or caudomedial direction with Salter-Harris type II fractures. Proximal tibial physeal fractures can usually be reduced by hyperextending the stifle joint. A caudally directed force is applied over the femoral diaphysis in the mid-thigh region while a cranially directed force is applied over the caudal aspect of the distal tibia. Varus or valgus stress can also be applied as needed if the epiphysis is laterally or medially displaced, respectively. Orthogonal fluoroscopic images are obtained as needed during the reduction process to verify accuracy of fracture reduction.

Distal Tibial Physeal Fracture

The distal tibial epiphysis often displaces caudally and proximally owing to the contraction of the tarsal extensors, but can displace cranially, medially, or laterally as well. To reduce a caudally displaced epiphyseal segment, the distal limb is first distracted using a distally directed force applied to the paw, to overcome the contraction of the crus musculature. The tarsal joint is hyperflexed by applying a cranially and proximally directed force to the metatarsals and paw, while at the same time applying a caudally directed force to the cranial aspect of the mid-crus region over the mid-tibial diaphysis. Physeal fracture reduction is confirmed with orthogonal projection fluoroscopy images.

Proximal Humeral Physeal Fracture

The proximal humeral epiphysis typically displaces caudally, but may also displace medially or laterally, particularly with Salter-Harris type II fractures. To reduce the proximal humeral epiphysis the shoulder is hyperextended by applying a cranially and proximally directed manual force to the mid-brachium over the caudal aspect of the humeral diaphysis. Varus or valgus stress can also be applied to the brachium if the epiphysis is laterally or medially displaced, respectively. Fluoroscopy is then used to confirm adequate reduction of the proximal humeral epiphysis.

Distal Radial Physeal Fracture

The distal radial epiphysis usually displaces caudally if the distal ulnar physis is also fractured. If the distal ulnar physis is intact, the distal radial epiphysis will often be minimally laterally displaced. For a caudally displaced epiphysis, a distal distraction force is first manually applied to the paw, followed by a cranially directed force manually applied to the metacarpals with a simultaneous caudally directed force applied over the mid-antebrachium to hyperextend the carpal joint. For a laterally displaced radial epiphysis, a laterally directed force is applied over the medial aspect of the distal radial diaphysis/metaphysis at the same time that a medially directed (varus) force is applied to the metacarpals. Appropriate physeal fracture reduction is confirmed with fluoroscopy before pin insertion.

SURGICAL PROCEDURE

General principles of traditional open physeal fracture repair with pins must be adhered to with percutaneous pinning. To decrease the risk of premature physeal closure, pins must be placed as perpendicular to the physeal plate as possible. Angulation of pins greater than 45° to the physis predisposes to epiphysiodesis.[16] Threaded pins are not routinely used by the authors for percutaneous pinning because of the inherent weakness at the thread-shaft interface, risk of hindering longitudinal bone growth, and difficulty with pin removal if required. Trocar-tipped pins facilitate precise entry in the epiphysis without "walking" or migration of the pin tip across the bone surface, which is important with percutaneous pinning because the pin insertion site is not directly visualized during pin insertion.

Although immature bone may be soft enough to allow pins to be placed by hand, battery-driven or air-driven drills should be used for optimal accuracy. An oscillating drill function is useful to minimize soft tissue entanglement around the pin during insertion. The use of large-gauge needles as pin guides and soft tissue guards as previously mentioned also minimizes soft tissue entrapment around the pins during insertion. Intraoperative fluoroscopy should be used before, during, and after inserting the pins to ensure optimal pin positioning. Without fluoroscopy, it is often extremely difficult to place pins accurately, owing to the limited exposure performed for percutaneous pinning. It is important to bear in mind that the number of pins and size of pins should be kept to a minimum to decrease iatrogenic physeal damage, yet the selected pins should be large enough to provide adequate stability. When using cross pins, the implants should cross away from the fracture site to achieve optimal stability. The pins should be inserted until the pin tip is seated into the trans-cortex. The pin length should then be carefully measured, the pin backed out partially, excess pin length cut off accurately, and finally the pin should be countersunk to beneath the surface of the bone to prevent damage to a joint surface or to prevent protrusion into the surrounding soft tissues. If the measurements and cut are performed correctly, the pin tip will once again be seated in the trans-cortex when the cut end of the pin is countersunk. If the pin insertion site is extra-articular, the pin may be bent over to decrease risk of pin migration rather than being countersunk. Bending the pin also improves the ability to fully seat the pin to the bone surface through the limited exposure site. Pins ends should never be bent over or left protruding from the bone when they are inserted inside a joint through an articular cartilage surface. Pins placed outside of a joint may be cut long and left protruding out into the soft tissues or even through the skin to facilitate pin removal once the fracture site is healed. The authors prefer not to leave the cut pin ends long, as the high degree of soft tissue motion around the joint tends to result in soft tissue irritation and subsequent seroma formation or premature pin migration.

Comments on surgical technique relevant to specific physeal fractures are included below.

Capital Physeal Fracture

The pin insertion site is located in the region of the third trochanter, just distal to the greater trochanter on the lateral aspect of the femur. Because of the relatively thick soft tissue coverage over this portion of the femur, the use of large-gauge needles inserted percutaneously to serve as pin drill guides and soft tissue guards during pin insertion is recommended. The pins should be directed from lateral to medial as well as being directed in a slightly caudodistal to cranioproximal direction, following the course of the femoral neck. Two or 3 pins should be inserted and the trajectory of the pins should be parallel to optimize biomechanical performance. As the pins are inserted across the capital physis, orthogonal projection fluoroscopy images or continuous video fluoroscopy monitoring in orthogonal planes should be used to ensure that the pins do not penetrate the cortex of the femoral head. If a pin tip does penetrate the cortex, the pin should be carefully backed out until the tip is below the level of the cortex. For any pin where the tip penetrates the cortex of the femoral head during insertion, consideration should be given to bending over the end of the pin that protrudes through the lateral femoral cortex to prevent the pin from inadvertently migrating into the coxofemoral joint. The authors do not recommend countersinking the pins used to stabilize capital physeal fractures because it increases the chances of inadvertent penetration of the coxofemoral joint. The pins should be bent over and cut short or cut short without bending (to facilitate future removal).

Distal Femoral Physeal Fracture

Two pins are typically inserted to stabilize distal femoral physeal fractures. Pin insertion location is at the level of the distal end of the trochlear ridges, just medial and lateral to the middle of the trochlear ridges in the frontal plane. On the lateral side the pin insertion site is next to the origin of the long digital extensor muscle. The pins can be inserted through stab incisions or through large-gauge needles. Pin trajectory is proximal and slightly cranial to prevent the pins from prematurely exiting through the caudal cortex of the femur. The more lateral pin also angles slightly medially relative to the insertion point, while the medial pin angles slightly lateral relative to the insertion point. The pins may cross in the diaphysis before seating in the transcortex of the femur. Alternatively, the pins may reflect off the endosteal surface of the femur, in which case the pins can be inserted until seated in the proximal femoral metaphysis. Because the pins used to stabilize distal femoral physeal fractures are placed intra-articularly, the pin ends should be cut short and countersunk as described above. **Figs. 1–5** depict preoperative and postoperative radiographs, as well as intraoperative images demonstrating percutaneous pinning of a distal femoral physeal fracture in a dog.

Tibial Apophyseal Fracture (Tibial Tuberosity Avulsion)

One or 2 pins are typically inserted to stabilize tibial apophyseal fractures. Two pins are preferred if the size of the apophyseal segment will accommodate insertion of 2 pins, because a single pin offers little resistance to rotation. The pins can be inserted through a stab incision or through large-gauge needles. The pin insertion sites are just proximal and distal to the middle of the cranioproximal surface of the apophyseal segment if 2 pins are being inserted, and right in the center of the apophyseal segment if a single pin is being inserted. Pin trajectory is directed through the tibial apophysis into the proximal tibial metaphysis in a cranioproximal to caudodistal direction as well as a slightly lateral to medial direction to ensure optimal bone purchase in the tibial metaphysis. Pin tips should be seated in the caudomedial tibial cortex. If the previously described spiking technique is used for apophyseal reduction, then once the apophysis is reduced, the pin which has already been inserted through the tibial apophysis can be immediately driven into the proximal tibial metaphysis to stabilize the apophyseal physis. Pin ends can be cut short and countersunk, bent over, or left protruding for easy removal once the fracture is healed.

Proximal Tibial Physeal Fracture

In many patients with proximal tibial physeal fractures, the tibial apophysis remains attached to the proximal tibial epiphysis. Once the proximal tibial epiphysis and tibial apophysis are reduced, the fracture can be stabilized by inserting 2 pins through the tibial apophysis into the proximal tibial metaphysis in a cranioproximal to caudodistal direction as well as a slightly lateral to medial direction to ensure optimal bone purchase in the tibial metaphysis, similar to the technique described above for tibial apophyseal fracture stabilization. This 2-pin technique results in the least disruption of the proximal tibial physis but likely does not offer as much resistance to rotational

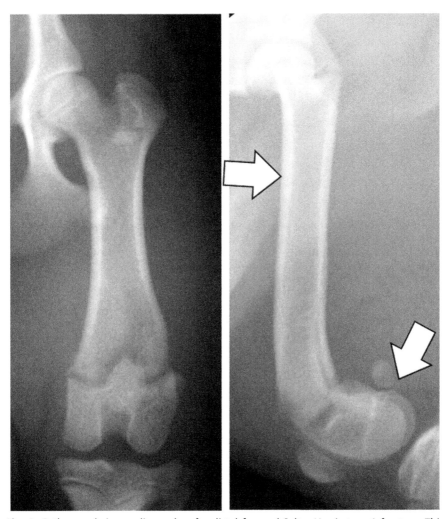

Fig. 1. Orthogonal-view radiographs of a distal femoral Salter-Harris type 1 fracture. This injury is amenable to repair by percutaneous pinning, because the fracture segments are minimally displaced. Arrows indicate the direction of force applied on the fracture segments for closed reduction.

forces as the cross-pinning technique using 3 pins. For the cross-pinning technique, the first pin is inserted through the tibial apophysis as described above. A second pin is inserted near the caudomedial border of the proximal tibial epiphysis just cranial to the medial collateral ligament and is directed distally, laterally, and slightly cranially until the tip is seated in the lateral tibial cortex. A third pin is inserted near the caudolateral border of the proximal tibial epiphysis, just cranial to the fibular head. This pin is directed distally, medially, and slightly cranially until the tip is seated in the medial tibial cortex. The pin ends can be cut short and countersunk or bent over and cut off. **Figs. 6–9** depict preoperative and postoperative radiographs, as well as intraoperative fluoroscopy images demonstrating reduction and percutaneous pinning of a proximal tibial physeal fracture in a dog.

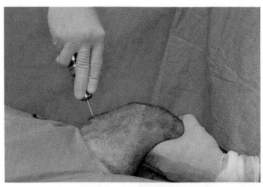

Fig. 2. Closed reduction of a distal femoral physeal fracture can be achieved with manual traction and leverage. For the left hind limb, the surgeon's left palm is placed under the stifle and the distal tibia is firmly grasped. In this case, a temporary half pin is used to assist manipulation of the proximal fragment. Distal traction and cranial leverage is applied to the distal segment with the stifle partially flexed, while the proximal segment is pushed caudally.

Distal Tibial Physeal Fracture

Two pins are typically used to stabilize distal tibial physeal fractures. The pins are often inserted through stab incisions without the use of needles because minimal soft tissue coverage is present over the distal tibial region. The medial pin insertion site is located near the distomedial tip of the medial malleolus. The pin is directed from distomedial to proximolateral. Care is taken to ensure that the pin does not impinge on the articular surface of the distal tibia. The tip of the pin is seated in the lateral cortex of the distal tibial diaphysis/metaphysis. The lateral pin insertion site is near the distolateral end of the lateral malleolus. The pin is directed from distolateral to proximomedial and crosses from the fibula into the epiphysis of the distal tibia and then through the distal tibial physis and metaphysis to seat in the medial cortex of the distal tibial diaphysis/metaphysis. In some cases, the authors have inserted a third pin from the craniolateral aspect of the distal tibial epiphysis, directed in a craniodistal to caudoproximal direction, as well as a slight lateral to medial direction, until the tip of the pin seats in the caudomedial tibial cortex. The decision to use

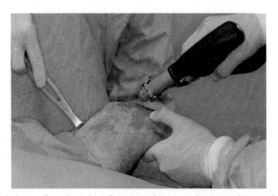

Fig. 3. Pins should always be placed with an air-driven or battery-driven drill. An oscillating function is useful to decrease the risk of entangling surrounding soft tissue structures.

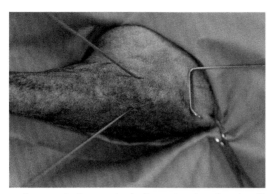

Fig. 4. Percutaneous placement of cross pins before trimming the pins. Note that the precise trajectory of the pins can be difficult because of the very limited approaches; intraoperative fluoroscopy is highly recommended when performing percutaneous pinning.

a third pin is made intraoperatively if the pin inserted through the lateral malleolus of the fibula does not seem to be adequately stabilizing the lateral aspect of the distal tibial epiphysis. The pin ends can be cut short and countersunk or bent over. The authors do not typically leave the pin ends long owing to the limited soft tissue coverage over the distal tibia. **Figs. 10–15** depict intraoperative fluoroscopic images and postoperative radiographs of a distal tibial physeal fracture in a cat treated with percutaneous pinning.

Proximal Humeral Physeal Fracture

Two pins are typically used to stabilize Salter-Harris type I proximal humeral physeal fractures. The pin insertion site is on the most superficial portion of the greater tubercle of the humerus. Pins can be inserted through a stab incision or through large-gauge needles. The pins are directed from cranioproximally to caudodistally and also in a slight lateral to medial direction. The pins are typically inserted parallel with each other. Pins can be cut short and countersunk or bent over and cut short. For some Salter-Harris type II fractures of the proximal humeral physis, 2 pins through the greater tubercle may not provide appropriate stabilization. A cross-pinning technique can be used for proximal humeral physeal fractures that need additional stability. The authors recommend that the pins be inserted through large-gauge needles when the cross-pinning technique is used owing to the significant amount of musculature present medial and lateral to the shoulder joint. A pin can be inserted from the lateral aspect of the proximal humeral epiphysis and is directed distally, medially, and cranially until the tip is seated in the medial humeral cortex. The lateral pin insertion site should be kept as lateral as possible, as this pin will typically be placed through the lateral articular surface of the humeral head. This lateral pin should be cut short and countersunk to below the articular surface. The medial aspect of the shoulder has significant soft tissue coverage and the proximity of the thorax limits the ability to drive a pin at the correct trajectory to stabilize the proximal humeral epiphysis from the medial side. For these reasons, the authors advocate insertion of the third pin with a distolateral to proximomedial trajectory when the percutaneous cross-pinning technique is used for the proximal humeral epiphysis. The insertion site is the lateral aspect of the proximal humeral diaphysis/metaphysis. The pin is directed proximally, medially, and slightly caudally until the tip is seated in the proximal humeral epiphysis. The

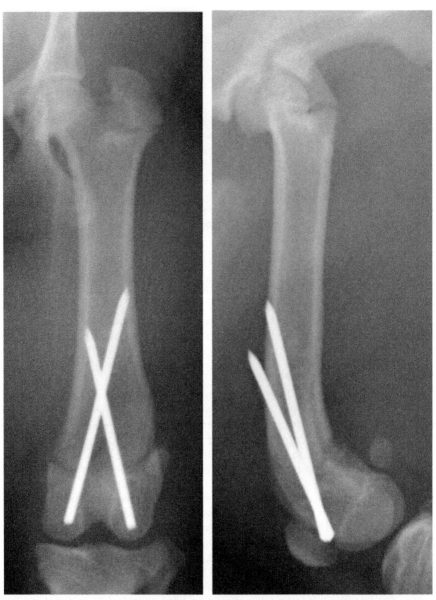

Fig. 5. Orthogonal-view postoperative radiographs of a distal femoral Salter-Harris type I fracture treated with percutaneous pinning. Note that the pins cross proximal to the fracture; pin entry sites are cranial to the weight-bearing surfaces, and seated to the level of the subchondral bone.

tip of the pin should not be allowed to exit through the articular surface of the humeral head. Orthogonal projection fluoroscopy images should be used to guide insertion depth of the third pin and to ensure the pin does not penetrate the articular surface. This third pin can be cut short and countersunk (not recommended owing to the possibility of inadvertent penetration of the articular surface) or bent over and cut short.

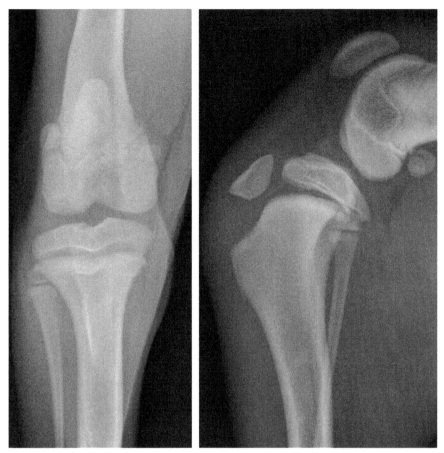

Fig. 6. Orthogonal-view radiographs of a proximal tibial Salter-Harris type 1 fracture in a 5-month-old male Labrador retriever. This injury is amenable to repair by percutaneous pinning, as the fracture segments are minimally displaced.

Distal Radial Physeal Fracture

Two pins are typically used to stabilize distal radial physeal fractures. Pin insertion sites are the medial and lateral aspects of the distal radial epiphysis. The medial pin insertion site is located just proximal to the tip of the medial styloid process. This pin is directed from distomedially to proximolaterally and the pin tip is seated in the lateral cortex of the distal radial metaphysis/diaphysis. The lateral pin insertion point should be located just cranial to the lateral styloid process of the ulna, on the lateral aspect of the distal radial epiphysis. The lateral pin should be directed from distolaterally to proximomedially and the tip of the pin should be seated in the medial cortex of the distal radial metaphysis/diaphysis. The pin ends can be cut short and countersunk or bent over and cut short. Distal radial physeal fractures often result in closure of the distal radial physis. Continued growth of the distal ulnar physis, in patients with an isolated fracture of the distal radial physis may result in an antebrachial angular limb deformity and elbow incongruency. For these reasons the authors advocate that a distal ulnar partial ostectomy (removal of

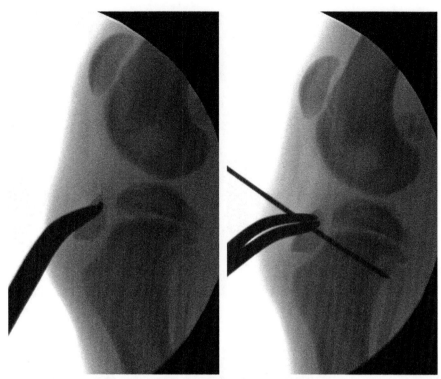

Fig. 7. Lateral-projection intraoperative fluoroscopic images demonstrating reduction of a Salter-Harris type I proximal tibial physeal fracture using a pointed reduction forceps and initial stabilization of the tibial epiphysis with a K-wire inserted through the tibial apophyseal segment into the proximal tibial metaphysis.

approximately 1 cm of the distal ulnar diaphysis just proximal to the distal ulnar physis) be performed in patients who appear to have significant growth potential left in the distal ulnar physis at the time of distal radial physeal fracture stabilization.

IMMEDIATE POSTOPERATIVE CARE

Fracture reduction and pin placement are carefully assessed on postoperative radiographs. For all cases, parenteral analgesia is administered for up to 12 hours to address immediate postoperative pain. Because of the limited soft tissue trauma induced by surgery, analgesic requirements are expected to be substantially lower than if the procedure was performed with a traditional open approach. There are very few risk factors for infection (clean procedures, young patients, minimal surgical exposure), hence postoperative prophylactic antibiotics are not indicated with routine percutaneous pinning. Local cryotherapy and passive range-of-motion exercises can be instituted in the immediate postoperative period for stabilized fractures at the level of the shoulder, hip, and stifle. Range-of-motion exercises of the stifle for distal femoral physeal fractures are especially important to minimize the risk of quadriceps contracture. Distal tibial and radial physeal fracture repairs must be protected from failure with external coaptation.

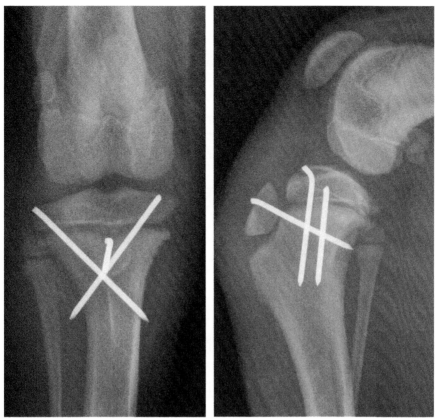

Fig. 8. Orthogonal-view postoperative radiographs of a proximal tibial Salter-Harris type I fracture stabilized with 3 pins inserted using percutaneous pinning technique. The pins have been cut short and countersunk to the level of the subchondral bone.

REHABILITATION AND RECOVERY

Early return to weight bearing and good limb function is anticipated following percutaneous pinning. Because the minimum size and number of pins that will provide adequate stability are typically used, cage rest should be strictly enforced until complete union of the fracture is documented. If strict crate rest is not enforced, these repairs are at high risk for implant failure and pin migration. With preservation of surrounding soft tissue structures and the tremendous capacity for healing inherent in young animals, clinical union is expected within 3 to 4 weeks. The authors advocate obtaining recheck radiographs of the repair every 2 weeks to identify potential complications and assess fracture healing early. For distal tibial and radial physeal fractures, external coaptation should be maintained until clinical union. Bandages should be checked and changed on a weekly basis to minimize the risk of bandage-associated morbidity, such as pressure sores.

Precise application of pins may be more difficult with percutaneous pinning than with a traditional open approach, potentially resulting in a higher chance that implant removal may be required for cases of percutaneous pinning. Even very mild protrusion of pins beyond the articular cartilage surface can cause persistent lameness

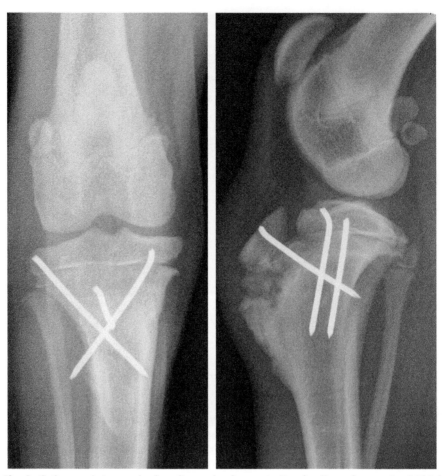

Fig. 9. Orthogonal-view recheck radiographs demonstrating healing of a proximal tibial Salter-Harris type I fracture treated with percutaneous pinning 4 weeks after fixation.

and pin loosening, and initiate osteoarthritis. Overly long pins extending into surrounding extra-articular soft tissues can predispose to local irritation and seroma formation. Owners should be informed that pin migration or irritation could still occur even after clinical union of the physeal fracture, which would require future pin removal.

CLINICAL RESULTS

Percutaneous pinning for tibial and femoral fractures was first described in 1989, although it was performed in a "blind" manner without intraoperative fluoroscopy.[17] Osseous union was achieved in 55 of 56 fractures treated in this manner. Age, body weight, fracture type, and time from injury to repair were found to influence overall outcome in these cases. A small retrospective case series on percutaneous pinning under fluoroscopic guidance was described in abstract format.[7] In this report, 3 dogs were treated for distal femoral fracture (Salter-Harris type II) and 2 dogs were treated for proximal humeral fracture (Salter-Harris type II). The mean age

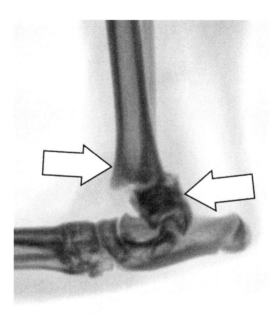

Fig. 10. Lateral-projection intraoperative fluoroscopic image of a Salter-Harris type I distal tibial fracture. Arrows indicate the direction of force applied on the fracture segments for closed reduction.

at presentation was 6 months. Breeds included English springer, Yorkshire terrier, and mixed breeds. The mean duration from trauma was 2 days. All fractures were closed and mildly to moderately displaced. Mean duration of surgery was 67 minutes. Mean time to radiographic union was 3.5 weeks. No major complications occurred. Mild rotational malalignment occurred in one of the humeral

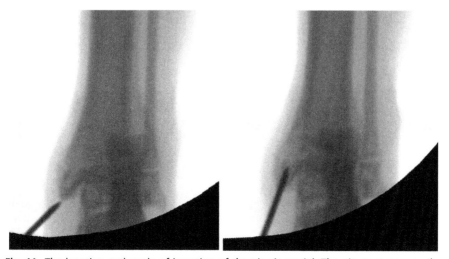

Fig. 11. The location and angle of insertion of the pins is crucial. The pin must engage the medial malleolus without entering the tarsocrural joint.

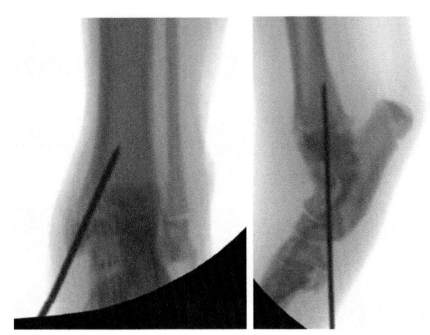

Fig. 12. Orthogonal fluoroscopic views are necessary to accurately assess pin positioning.

fractures. Good function (subjectively evaluated by the clinician and by the owner) was achieved in all cases. A multi-institutional retrospective study evaluated outcomes after closed reduction and fluoroscopically guided percutaneous pinning stabilization of 42 physeal fractures in 41 patients (37 dogs and 4 cats).[1] Mean

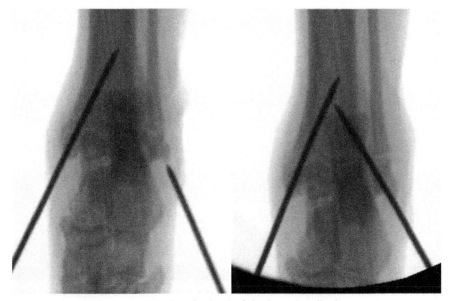

Fig. 13. The second pin is inserted at the level of the lateral malleolus.

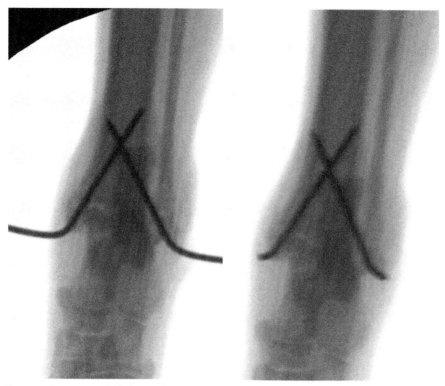

Fig. 14. Pins are carefully bent, then trimmed to beneath the surface of the skin.

patient age in this study was 6.9 months. Physes affected included proximal tibia (20), distal femur (8), distal tibia (7), proximal humerus (3), distal radius (3), and femoral capital physis (1). All fractures were Salter-Harris types I or II. Seventy-six percent of fractures were treated with cross-pinning and 24% were treated with parallel pins. Pin numbers used per fracture ranged from 2 to 6 with a median of 2 pins. Median pin diameter was 1.1 mm. Operative times ranged from 4 to 119 minutes with a mean of 42 minutes. Overall complication rate was 15% with 12% major and 3% minor complications. Major complications included infection, implant migration, or implant-associated soft tissue irritation requiring pin removal. Forty-one percent of patients in this study underwent elective pin removal after fracture union. Radiographic union was achieved in all patients for which radiographic follow-up was available. Of patients for which radiographic follow-up on both the fractured and contralateral bone was available, 78% experienced shortening of the fractured relative to the contralateral bone (mean of 5.7% shorter). Follow-up data on patient functional outcome were available for 37 patients, with 92% of patients returning to full function and 8% returning to acceptable function with a mean follow-up duration of 16 months.[1] A single institution retrospective case series evaluated the outcome of percutaneous pinning performed to treat tibial physeal fractures in 17 patients (14 dogs and 3 cats).[2] Physes fractured including tibial apophyseal (11), distal tibial physis (6), and proximal tibial physis (1). Intraoperative fluoroscopy or digital radiography was used to guide fracture reduction and pin insertion in all cases. Mean time to return to full function was

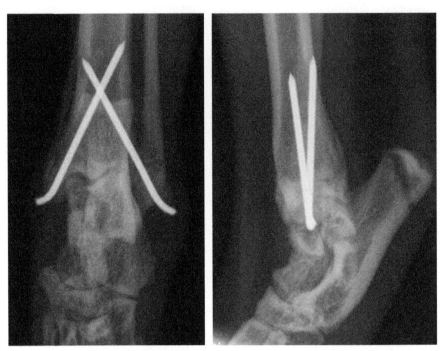

Fig. 15. Orthogonal-view recheck radiographs showing complete healing of a distal tibial Salter-Harris type I fracture treated with percutaneous pinning 3 weeks after fixation.

1.9 ± 1.6 weeks. Overall complication rate was 18% and consisted of soft tissue irritation from a pin, development of medial patellar luxation, and tibial apophyseal partial reavulsion after stabilization. Long-term follow-up was available at a mean of 40.6 months. Long-term outcome was graded as excellent in 82% and good in 18% of patients.[2]

SUMMARY

Percutaneous pinning is a feasible and safe method for stabilizing selected Salter-Harris type I and II physeal fractures in dogs and cats. Surgical intervention must be performed soon after the time of trauma, otherwise closed reduction cannot be achieved. The procedure is technically demanding; surgeon experience, intraoperative fluoroscopy, appropriate surgical instrumentation, and strict case selection are all required for consistent successful outcomes. Although clinical comparisons between open and closed pinning have not been described, percutaneous pinning may offer the advantages of decreased postoperative morbidity, earlier return to normal function, and decreased risk of infection. Prospective clinical studies should be performed to better define the role of this minimally invasive method of fracture repair in dogs and cats.

REFERENCES

1. Boekhout-Ta CL, Kim SE, Cross AR, et al. Closed reduction and fluoroscopic-assisted percutaneous pinning of 42 physeal fractures in 37 dogs and 4 cats. Vet Surg 2017;46(1):103–10.

2. Pfeil von DJF, Glassman M, Ropski M. Percutaneous tibial physeal fracture repair in small animals: technique and 17 cases. Vet Comp Orthop Traumatol 2017; 30(4):279–87.
3. Brioschi V, Langley-Hobbs SJ, Kerwin S, et al. Combined physeal fractures of the distal radius and ulna: complications associated with K-wire fixation and long-term prognosis in six cats. J Feline Med Surg 2017;19(8):907–14.
4. Parker RB, Bloomberg MS. Modified intramedullary pin technique for repair of distal femoral physeal fractures in the dog and cat. J Am Vet Med Assoc 1984; 184(10):1259–65.
5. Presnell KR. Pins versus plates: the orthopedic dilemma. Vet Clin North Am 1978; 8(2):213–7.
6. Campbell JR. The technique of fixation of fractures of the distal femur using Rush pins. J Small Anim Pract 1976;17(5):323–9.
7. Pozzi A, Thieman KM. Percutaneous pinning of growth plate fractures in dogs. Vet Comp Orthop Traumatol 2011;32(4):A13–4.
8. Fischer HR, Norton J, Kobluk CN, et al. Surgical reduction and stabilization for repair of femoral capital physeal fractures in cats: 13 cases (1998–2002). J Am Vet Med Assoc 2004;224(9):1478–82.
9. Saglam M, Kaya Ü. Treatment of proximal tibial fractures by cross pin fixation in dogs. Turk J Vet Anim Sci 2004;28(5):799–805.
10. Laer von L. General observations on treatment, . Pediatric fractures and dislocations. Stuttgart (Germany): Thieme; 2004. p. 69–77.
11. Cheng JC, Lam TP, Shen WY. Closed reduction and percutaneous pinning for type III displaced supracondylar fractures of the humerus in children. J Orthop Trauma 1995;9(6):511–5.
12. Kaewpornsawan K. Comparison between closed reduction with percutaneous pinning and open reduction with pinning in children with closed totally displaced supracondylar humeral fractures: a randomized controlled trial. J Pediatr Orthop B 2001;10(2):131–7.
13. de Buys Roessingh AS, Reinberg O. Open or closed pinning for distal humerus fractures in children? Swiss Surg 2003;9(2):76–81.
14. Skaggs DL. Extra-articular injuries of the knee. In: Beaty JH, Kasser JR, editors. Rockwood and Wilkins' fractures in children. 5th edition. Philadelphia: Lippincott Williams and Wilkins; 2001.
15. Guiot LP, Dejardin LM. Fractures of the femur. In: Johnston SA, Tobias KM, editors. Veterinary surgery small animal. St Louis (MO): Elsevier; 2018. p. 1019–71.
16. Piermattei DL, Flo GL, Decamp CE. Fractures in growing animals. In: Handbook of small animal orthopedics and fracture repair. St Louis (MO): Saunders Elsevier; 2006. p. 737–46.
17. Newman ME, Milton JL. Closed reduction and blind pinning of 29 femoral and tibial fractures in 27 dogs and cats. J Am Anim Hosp Assoc 1989;25(1):61–8.

Minimally Invasive Osteosynthesis Techniques for Humerus Fractures

Karl C. Maritato, DVM[a,b,*], Gian Luca Rovesti, DVM[c]

KEYWORDS

- Minimally invasive osteosynthesis • Humerus • Fracture • Condyle • Dog • Cat

KEY POINTS

- A thorough knowledge of humeral anatomy is critical to performing minimally invasive techniques.
- Fluoroscopy, when available, is invaluable in optimizing fracture repair with minimally invasive techniques.
- Minimally invasive approaches decrease morbidity and allow an earlier return to function.
- Minimally invasive fracture repair is performed using implant systems similar to open approaches.
- Minimally invasive osteosynthesis techniques for the humerus.

Humeral fractures account for 8% to 10% and 5% to 13% of fractures in dogs and cats, respectively.[1–4] Fracture locations along the bone are commonly divided into proximal, diaphyseal/metaphyseal, supracondylar, and condylar. In dogs, most fractures are in the distal portions of the humerus (supracondylar/condylar), whereas in the cat, fractures are more commonly mid-diaphysis.[5]

Humerus fractures are often associated with high-impact trauma so it is critical that the entire patient be evaluated and not simply focus on the fracture. Thoracic trauma, including pneumothorax and hemothorax, are present in many patients.[6,7] Brain and neck injuries, as well as brachial plexus and more distal nerve injuries, can occur and may critically impact patient morbidity and long-term outcomes and should therefore be thoroughly evaluated for.

There are several advantages to the use of minimally invasive fracture repair (MIFR) techniques in treatment of humeral fractures. These include less patient

---

Disclosure Statement: No conflicts of interest to disclose.
a Department of Surgery, MedVet Medical and Cancer Centers for Pets, 3964 Red Bank Road, Cincinnati, OH 45227, USA; b Department of Surgery, MedVet Medical and Cancer Centers for Pets, Dayton, OH, USA; c Department of Orthopedics, Clinica Veterinaria M. E. Miller, Via della Costituzione 10, Cavriago, Reggio Emilia 42025, Italy
* Corresponding author. 3964 Red Bank Road, Cincinnati, OH 45227.
E-mail address: kmaritato@medvet.com

Vet Clin Small Anim 50 (2020) 123–134
https://doi.org/10.1016/j.cvsm.2019.08.005
vetsmall.theclinics.com

morbidity from surgical dissection and manipulation, less disruption of the fracture environment, and improved fracture healing. Humeral fractures are frequently comminuted, and these fracture environments have sustained severe trauma leading to damage to the perifracture environment, most importantly, blood supply. The significant amount of muscle mass surrounding the humerus necessitates extensive dissection during traditional open approaches to expose the fracture site and apply implants. This further traumatizes the already injured muscle and blood supply, which can lead to delays in bone healing and increased risk of implant failure and infection.[8]

The aim of this article was to describe the techniques associated with MIFR using various implants for different types of humeral fractures.

ANATOMY

The humerus is an S-shaped bone that is eccentrically loaded with the tension surface of the bone being the craniolateral aspect. The "S" is more pronounced in the dog than in the cat. There are several landmarks important to the surgeon performing MIFR, because a thorough knowledge of the topography of the brachium is critical when repairing a fracture without full visualization of the bone, as is available with an open approach. Important bony landmarks of the humerus include the greater tubercle on the craniolateral proximal aspect, the intertubercular groove containing the tendon of origin of the biceps brachii along with the transverse humeral ligament, the tricipital line from proximal to distal until reaching the deltoid tuberosity, and the palpable epicondyles (**Fig. 1**).

The cortical bone caudally along the tricipital line is thicker, which is helpful in terms of screw-holding strength.[9] The epicondyles are the attachment sites of ligaments and tendons. Dogs have a supratrochlear foramen, which is closed by a thin membrane. Cats differ from dogs in that they have a supracondylar foramen proximal to the medial epicondyle and no supratrochlear foramen. The median nerve and brachial artery pass through the supracondylar foramen. The medullary canal tapers distally in the bone, which can make placement of large intramedullary pins difficult in certain patients with very distal fracture locations.[10]

Understanding the relationship between the proximal and distal aspects, as well as the internal torsion and S shape of the humerus, will allow the surgeon to place the implants correctly. The proximal aspect lies more cranial topographically to the distal aspect. These proximal and distal anatomic relationships facilitate dissection, as the bony landmarks are palpable, and any important structures can be predictably avoided. The radial nerve courses distally on the lateral aspect and the median and ulnar nerves and the brachial artery reside on the medial aspect just proximal to the epicondyle.

SURGICAL APPROACH

Traditional open techniques with dynamic compression plates (DCP) are typically approached from the medial side of the humerus because of the relative flatness of the bone on that surface. This allows for easier and better contouring of the plate on the medial surface, which is important in fracture stability repaired with a DCP. The size of the shaft and the epicondyle are the same and it is possible to use the same-length screws. By contrast, this is not always possible on the lateral epicondyle because it is much narrower than the diaphysis. Because precise contouring is not required with locking implants, the lateral aspect of the bone is commonly used in minimally invasive plate osteosynthesis (MIPO). This allows for more flexible patient positioning and easier approaches to the bone.

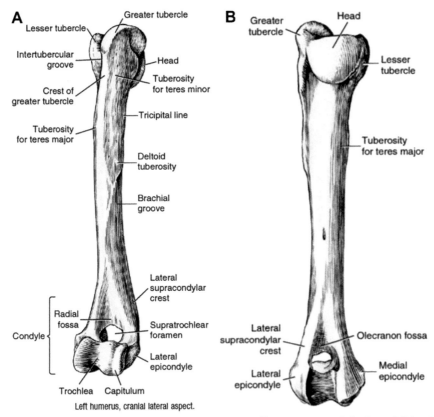

A

Lesser tubercle

Greater tubercle

Intertubercular groove

Crest of greater tubercle

Tuberosity for teres major

Head

Tuberosity for teres minor

Tricipital line

Deltoid tuberosity

Brachial groove

Lateral supracondylar crest

Radial fossa

Condyle

Supratrochlear foramen

Lateral epicondyle

Trochlea   Capitulum

Left humerus, cranial lateral aspect.

B

Greater tubercle

Head

Lesser tubercle

Tuberosity for teres major

Lateral supracondylar crest

Lateral epicondyle

Olecranon fossa

Medial epicondyle

Fig. 1. (*A, B*) The canine humerus. (*From* H. Evans. Miller's Anatomy of the Dog, Edition 3. Saunders; 1993; with permission.)

Most fractures amenable to MIFR techniques are located in the mid to distal diaphysis. When using MIPO, the strategies dictate the use of long plates that span the length of the bone, so portal incisions are located proximally and distally (**Fig. 2**A, B). The proximal incision is 2 to 3 cm long and is located on the craniolateral aspect of the proximal humerus in the region of the metaphysis after palpating the crest of the greater tubercle. The craniolateral surface is exposed after elevating and reflecting the cleidobrachialis, brachialis, lateral head of the triceps, and acromial head of the deltoid muscles. The axillobrachial vein (caudal) and the cephalic vein (deep) should be avoided.

The distal incision is made caudolaterally over the lateral aspect of the epicondylar ridge. The surgeon should be cautious, as the superficial branches of the radial nerve are present before branching at the level of the elbow. Both the lateral head of the triceps and the origin of the extensor carpi radialis muscle are elevated to expose the ridge. Many distal diaphyseal/metaphyseal/supracondylar fractures can easily be visualized by simply extending this distal portal proximally as minimally as necessary to achieve visualization (see **Fig. 2**).

To visualize a mid-diaphyseal fracture (if the aid of fluoroscopy is not available), a third small incision can be made over the fracture site. Dissection either through or between muscle bellies to expose the fracture ends will facilitate the passage of an intramedullary (IM) pin or interlocking nail, all while being diligent to minimize trauma to the fracture site by disturbing it as little as is possible.

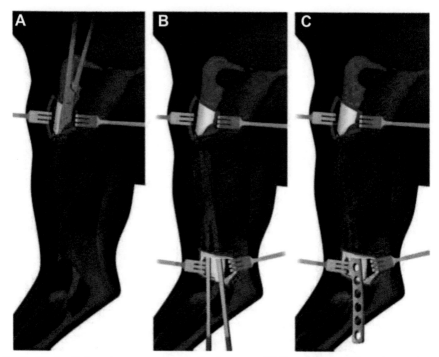

Fig. 2. Minimally invasive approaches to the humerus. (*A*) Proximal incision to the proximo-lateral humerus. (*B*) Distal incision to the distolateral humerus with creation of tunnel with metzenbaum scissors. (*C*) Placement of the plate from distal to proximal from the distal inci-sion. (*From* A. Pozzi; D. D. Lewis. Surgical approaches for minimally invasive plate osteosyn-thesis in dogs. VCOT 2009; with permission.)

REDUCTION TECHNIQUES

When a fracture is comminuted, additional strength and stability are gained by the placement of an IM pin. It also aids in the restoring the bone length and alignment, as anatomic reconstruction is typically not possible, nor necessary, provided the bone length is maintained and the adjacent joints are in good orientation. The pins can be placed either normograde (pin placement that begins at a bone end and exits the fracture site) or retrograde (pin placement that begins at the fracture site and exits a bone end) fashion.

Normograde placement of pins can begin either proximally or distally. When placing normograde proximally, the pin is inserted from the greater tubercle, being careful to avoid the biceps brachii tendon in the intertubercular groove. As the pin is driven distally, the distal fracture fragment is moved into alignment by the use of bone-holding forceps via the distal incision portal. The pin is visualized exiting the proximal and entering the distal fracture site either with fluoroscopy or through the third skin portal as previously described. The pin is then driven distally toward the medial epi-condyle and trochlea, ensuring not to breach the supratrochlear foramen. When placing a pin normograde from the distal insertion point, the pin is placed entering the lateral epicondylar ridge, driven to the fracture site, and once again, the fracture is aligned by the use of bone forceps and visualizing the fracture ends. It is important to pay close attention to the pin proximally and proceed slowly so that it does not exit and damage the biceps brachii tendon in the intertubercular groove because the exact location of an exit site can be difficult to predict. Complete exit of the pin through the proximal cortex is unnecessary. Removal of the sharp trocar tip is helpful to avoid breaching the bone. This can be done by either cutting the tip off as it exits the proximal fracture fragment before distal insertion or after creating the insertion hole by removing the pin, cutting the tip off, and then reinserting the pin and driving it through the medullary canal. In cats, it has been shown that normograde placement from distal to proximal is the most ideal.[11]

Retrograde placement of pins requires a third portal to be created for mid-diaphyseal fractures that are not reachable by either of the initial proximal or distal incisions. The pin is placed in the proximal or distal segment fracture end, driven into the bone and out the proximal or distal aspect. The exposed pin tip is then grasped with a drill or hand chuck, backed up further into it, is recessed to the fracture and then driven into the corresponding fracture segment. Again, be cautious when driving the pin so as to not damage structures as it exits the bone. As previously described, the trocar tip of the pin can be removed before entry into the final fragment to help prevent cortex penetration. Retrograde pinning has been criticized by 2 studies that showed damage to periarticular soft tissues, articular cartilage, and ulnar nerve entrapment.[11,12] Specific attention to the radial nerve should be paid as well, if not already isolated and protected.

For transverse or short oblique fractures, the surgeon may aim for direct bone apposition and compression for primary bone healing via rigid fixation. This too can be achieved by utilization of the 3 incision portals as described previously. Using the "fracture site portal," reduction of the fracture is attained and maintained by bone-holding forceps or with a small temporary trans-fracture pin after the fracture is reduced using the proximal and distal incisions for instrument placement. The goal is to disturb the fracture site as little as possible. An IM pin also can be placed to aid in reduction as well as increase the overall strength of the repair if needed. In this situation, either a locking plate or DCP can be used.

PLATE PLACEMENT

Once the portals have been made and the fracture reduced as desired, the plate is placed. One of the many advantages of locking implants in MIFR applications is the fact that less precise contouring is not needed compared with DCPs. Some contouring of the plate to the general shape of the bone is still recommend by the author because it allows more accurate placement of screws with a shorter working length, thereby increasing the stability of the construct.[13] It also can aid in fracture reduction by using a cortical screw as the first screw instead of a locking screw. The epiperiosteal bone tunnel is then made with the aid of Metzenbaum scissors and elevators and the plate is passed into the tunnel from either proximally or distally. The plate is then laid on the bone in the desired position and the screws placed. Using the principles of locking fixation, no more than 50% of the holes should be filled with screws for comminuted fractures. The author typically uses 2 to 3 screws per segment at the most proximal and distal ends of the plate. For transverse/short oblique fractures, no more than a 40% hole fill ratio is recommended. The length of the plate should be a minimum of 2 to 3 times the length of the fracture segment in comminuted fractures and 8 to 10 times the length of a simple fracture segment.[14]

In the distal aspect of the humerus, it is important ensure that implants do not breach the foramen or the joint. In this area, monocortical screws may be needed, particularly in supracondylar fractures, which is yet another advantage of locking implants.[13] In this situation, the longest possible monocortical screw is used, as studies have shown a linear relationship between screw length and axial pullout strength in the distal humerus.[15] When possible, a transcondylar bicortical screw has been shown to increase construct strength.[16]

See **Fig. 3** for series example of mid-diaphyseal fracture repair.

CONDYLAR FRACTURES

Condylar fractures represent a common but special subset of humeral fractures and represent 41% of all humeral fractures in a survey of 107 fractures.[5] Because these

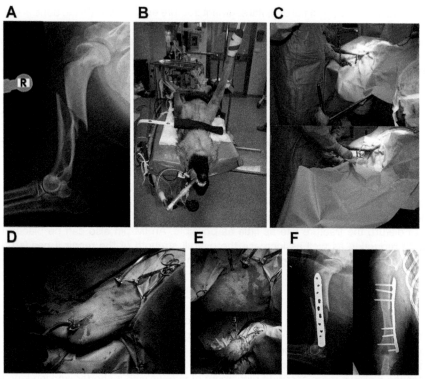

Fig. 3. Series of mid-diaphyseal fracture repair. (*A*) A 7-year-old German shepherd with a mid-diaphyseal humeral fracture and concomitant fracture of contralateral shoulder. (*B*) Positioning for scrubbing. The retention belts are padded to avoid soft tissue lesions. The belt passing over the neck is passed on the support to avoid excessive compression on the neck. The position for scrubbing allows the limb to be prepared surgically and then abducted for medial approach. (*C*) Once prepared, the limb is abducted and a traction stirrup is connected. The stirrup is connected to a traction bar. (*D*) A proximal humeral stirrup is used to counteract the distraction force. This is needed for the humerus, because the shoulder is loosely connected to the thorax by means of muscles and tendon attachments. Very often it will displace distally without achieving a satisfactory bone alignment if not counteracted by the proximal stirrup. (*E*) Once the fracture is correctly aligned, the periosteal elevation along the bone allows for introducing the plate underneath the soft tissues. While the fracture is held in place by the distraction forces, the plate is connected to the bone fragments by a minimally invasive, fluoroscopy-assisted technique. (*F*) Postoperative radiographs. Although the fracture reduction is not anatomical, the axis of the humerus is maintained and the mutual position of the adjacent joints is correct.

fractures are articular, anatomic reconstruction is critical. The lateral aspect (capitulum) is fractured more commonly, accounting for 34% to 67% of fractures of the humeral condyle and for 37% of all distal humeral fractures.[5,17–20] Fractures of the medial aspect of the humeral condyle (trochlea) occur in 6.9% to 11%, and bicondylar fractures (also known as "T" or "Y" fractures) represent 25.9% to 35.0% of fractures affecting the humeral condyle.[5,17,18] Most fractures occur in puppies because closure of growth plates occurs between 5 and 8 months of age and relatively minor trauma during this time can cause fractures.[20,21] Specific diseases may predispose to condylar fracture, as is the case for incomplete ossification of the humeral condyle in spaniels.[22]

Reduction techniques can be performed using either open or closed approaches. The main difference compared with other humeral fractures is the absolute necessity for good reduction of the joint surface under direct visual or fluoroscopy-assisted guidance. The latter is more amenable to preserving the vascular supply to bone and soft tissues.[23,24]

One study reported that 43% of patients treated with open surgery developed degenerative joint disease (DJD) and varying degrees of postoperative lameness.[25] Much of this may be due to the initial trauma to the joint; however, the extensive dissection associated with open approaches may add to the long-term DJD development and therefore MIFR techniques should be investigated and considered.

The reduction technique described here uses skeletal traction performed by a traction stirrup[26] and a minimally invasive approach to fracture stabilization. The rationale is that when the epicondylar fracture is perfectly reduced, in noncomminuted fractures, the articular fracture of the condyle should be correctly reduced as well. Fluoroscopy is required for success.

The dog is positioned in lateral recumbency with the limb to be operated on in the uppermost position for fractures of the capitulum and in lowermost position for fractures of the trochlea. The dog's body is stabilized by means of padded traction bands (Ad Maiora, Cavriago, Italy) as previously described.[26,27] Two fluoroscopic images are taken before any reduction attempt, so as to define the exact magnitude of dislocation. The lateral projection of the condyle is straightforward, with the C-arm in vertical position. For the sagittal projection, the rotation of the C-arm in the horizontal plane can be very time-consuming. A specifically designed technique was developed to perform the sagittal with the C-arm in vertical position as for the lateral projection to dramatically reduce the time needed for visualization. Extreme pronation of the humerus is induced together with the antebrachium and the images taken as for the lateral.

A 1.0-mm to 1.5-mm Kirschner wire (K-wire) is placed orthogonally through the proximal ulna, just distally to the elbow on the axis of the humerus and connected to a traction stirrup. The stirrup is made by 2 mobile arms with a joint and a threaded bar with a nut (**Fig. 4**). Acting on the nut, the arms can be separated from each other in a progressive way. The extremities of the arms hold bolts with a perforated screw that can lock a K-wire up to 1.5 mm in diameter. Once the K-wire is locked at both extremities, acting on the nut opens the arms, thus tensioning the wire. The tensioned wire will not bend, thus preventing cutting through surrounding soft tissues.

A 3-cm to 4-cm surgical approach to the lateral or medial epicondyle is performed, and the fractured epicondyle exposed. Traction is manually applied to the stirrup to displace the ulna caudally, thus avoiding any interference with the reduction of the condylar fragments. Furthermore, the muscle and tendon attachments between the ulna and the fractured humeral condyle bring the fractured portions back to their original location using the principles of ligamentotaxis.[28] Specific attention is paid to achieve anatomic reduction of the epicondylar fracture without opening the elbow joint

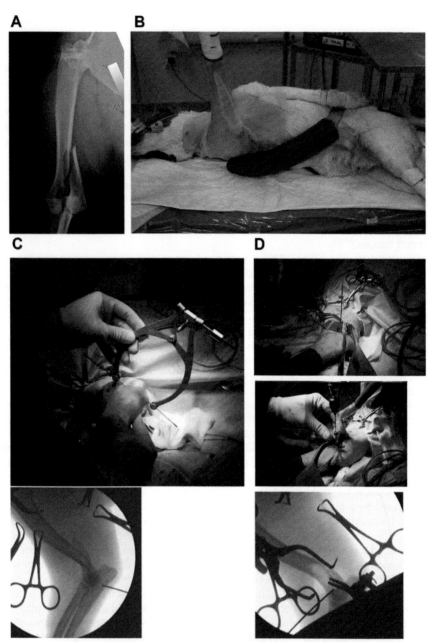

Fig. 4. Series of humeral condylar fracture repair. (*A*) Fracture involving the joint surface and metaphyseal area of the distal humerus. (*B*) Positioning for scrubbing. Same philosophy as **Fig. 3**B. (*C*) Location and positioning of the traction stirrup on the proximal ulna. (*D*) Preliminary stabilization of the fracture through a small distal approach for visualization of the epicondylar fracture line. The fracture is stabilized by a K-wire NOT in the center of the humeral condyle and a pointed reduction forceps. (*E*) A cortical compression screw is first positioned on the long part of the epicondyle under visual control. (*F*) The insertion and locking of the screw is performed by the same minimally invasive, fluoroscopy-assisted procedure as described in **Fig. 3**E. (*G*) Sequence of locking screw placement in the plate. (*H*) Postoperative radiographs showing reduction. Note the small hole in the proximal ulna where the stirrup was connected for intraoperative traction.

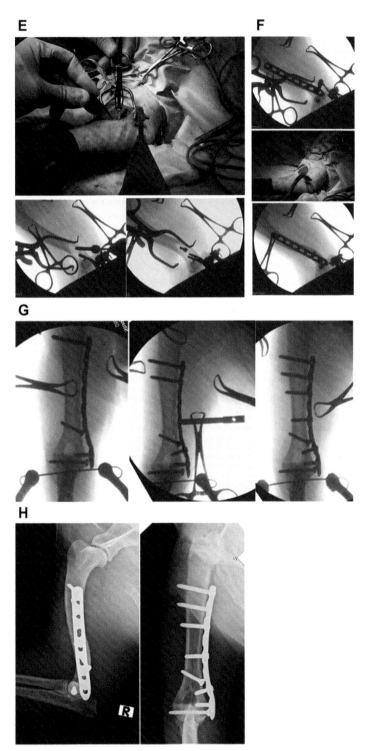

Fig. 4. (*continued*).

to visually check for proper reduction. Then, a pointed reduction forceps is applied on the medial and lateral aspects of the humeral condyle to stabilize the fracture, and 2 orthogonal fluoroscopic pictures are taken to confirm proper anatomic reduction.

If the fluoroscopic pictures show an unsatisfactory reduction, the clamp is released, the fracture reduction of the epicondyle revised, and the clamp applied again. A 1.0-mm to 1.5-mm K-wire, depending on the dog's size, is used to stabilize the epicondylar fracture first once reduction is appropriate. The condylar fracture is then stabilized while maintaining the reduction forceps in place.

The technique has shown to be consistently repeatable with good fracture reduction. It can be considered a potential alternative to standard open reduction and fixation techniques. It has a steep learning curve, linked to the appropriate use of the instruments and the patient's positioning for intraoperative confirmation of fracture reduction. See **Fig. 4** for series example of condylar fracture repair.

POSTOPERATIVE CARE

The intensity of postoperative management is dependent on the patient status at the time of fracture repair, and a deep discussion on the management of polytrauma is beyond the scope of this article. However, proper postoperative management of the fractured limb is imperative.

Adequate postoperative pain management is of paramount importance to the health and well-being of the patient. Opioids and nonsteroidal anti-inflammatories are the mainstay of treatment. Brachial plexus nerve blocks can be used for fractures of the distal third of the humerus. The author also highly recommends the use of liposomal bupivacaine (Nocita; Aratana Therapeutics, Leawood, KS) in the surgery site for extended postoperative pain relief.

It is critical that the owners understand the importance of confinement and exercise restriction to lessen the risk of implant failure. Confinement to a cage or small area with only leash-controlled walks and avoidance of strenuous activity (eg, running, jumping, playing) is recommended. Restrictions should be maintained until at least 6 weeks postoperatively in patients 6 months and older (1 week of confinement per month of age until 6 months of age), when the first radiograph to assess fracture healing is typically made. Most fractures have adequate healing at this time and a slow return to normal exercises can be gradually achieved over the following 4 to 6 weeks. However, some patients of advanced age or with severely comminuted fractures may not be sufficiently healed to begin more advanced exercises at 6 weeks, with osseous bridging present, but not robust. As long as there is load sharing between the bone and the plate, there is less stress on the plate and slightly increased activities can enhance bone formation, as based on Wolf's law.

Physical rehabilitation under veterinary supervision should be instituted as soon as is possible. Underwater treadmill therapy, controlled land exercises, and energy therapy, such as therapy lasers, shockwave, and radiofrequency can aid in the recovery.

COMPLICATIONS

General surgical complications and complications unique to MIFR can all be encountered in these patients. In all patients with fractures, potential complications include infection, implant failure, nonunion, delayed union, and malunion. Also, specific to the humerus, iatrogenic neurovascular injury is of particular concern.

In MIFR patients, the risk of malalignment is increased because of the limited view of the bone. That is why a solid working knowledge of the topography of the limb and its landmarks is important, ensuring the limb is properly aligned during fixation. Fluoroscopy can aid in viewing alignment intraoperatively, if available. If malalignment is noted immediately postoperatively, it should be corrected immediately.

REFERENCES

1. Hill FW. A survey of bone fractures in the cat. J Small Anim Pract 1977;18:457.
2. Johnson J, Austin C, Breur GJ. Incidence of canine appendicular musculoskeletal disorders in 16 veterinary teaching hospitals from 1980 through 1989. Vet Comp Orthop Traumatol 1994;7:56.
3. Ness M, Abercromby R, May C, et al. A survey of orthopaedic conditions in small animal veterinary practice in Britain. Vet Comp Orthop Traumatol 1996;9:43.
4. Phillips IR. A survey of bone fractures in the dog and cat. J Small Anim Pract 1979;20:661.
5. Bardet J, Hohn R, Rudy R, et al. Fracture of the humerus in the dog and cat: a retrospective study of 130 cases. Vet Surg 1983;12:73.
6. Selcer B, Buttrick M, Barstad R, et al. The incidence of thoracic trauma in dogs with skeletal injury. J Small Anim Pract 1987;28:1.
7. Simpson AM. Fractures of the humerus. Clin Tech Small Anim Pract 2004;19:120.
8. Moens N. The biology of locking plate applications. In: Barnhart MD, Maritato KC, editors. Locking plates in veterinary orthopedics. Hoboken (NJ): Wiley; 2018. p. 13–24.
9. Moses PA, Lewis DD, Lanz OI, et al. Intramedullary interlocking nail stabilisation of 21 humeral fractures in 19 dogs and one cat. Aust Vet J 2002;80:336.
10. Langley-Hobbs SJ, Straw M. The feline humerus: an anatomical study with relevance to external skeletal fixator and intramedullary pin placement. Vet Comp Orthop Traumatol 2005;18:1.
11. Cohen L, Israeli I, Levi S, et al. Normograde and retrograde pinning of the distal fragment in feline humeral fractures. Vet Surg 2012;41:604–10.
12. Milgram J, Hod N, Benzioni H. Normograde and retrograde pinning of the distal fragment in humeral fractures of the dog. Vet Surg 2012;41:671–6.
13. Biedrzycki AH. Dynamic compression vs. locking plating – is one better? A review of biomechanical principles and in vitro testing. In: Barnhart MD, Maritato KC, editors. Locking plates in veterinary orthopedics. Hoboken (NJ): Wiley; 2018. p. 25–40.
14. Schmierer P, Pozzi A. Minimally invasive plate osteosynthesis. In: Barnhart MD, Maritato KC, editors. Locking plates in veterinary orthopedics. Hoboken (NJ): Wiley; 2018. p. 41–50.
15. Vaughan DP, Syrcle JA, Ball JE, et al. Pullout strength of monocortical and bicortical screws in metaphyseal and diaphyseal regions of the canine humerus. Vet Comp Orthop Traumatol 2016;29(6):466–74.
16. Hurt RJ, Syrcle JA, Elder SA, et al. A biomechanical comparison of unilateral and bilateral string of pearl locking plates in a canine distal humeral metaphayseal gap model. Vet Comp Orthop Traumatol 2014;27:186–91.
17. Denny HR. Condylar fractures of the humerus in the dog: a review of 133 cases. J Small Anim Pract 1983;24:185–97.
18. Rorvik A. Risk factors for humeral condylar fractures in the dog: a retrospective study. J Small Anim Pract 1993;34:277.
19. Vannini R, Olmstead ML, Smeak DD. Humeral condylar fractures caused by minor trauma in 20 adult dogs. J Small Anim Pract 1988;24:335–62.
20. Vannini R, Smeak D, Olmstead M. Evaluation of surgical repair of 135 distal humeral fractures in dogs and cats. J Am Anim Hosp Assoc 1988;24:537.

21. Sumner-Smith G. Observations on epiphyseal fusion in the canine appendicular skeleton. J Small Anim Pract 1966;7(4):303–6.
22. Marcellin-Little DJ, DeYoung DJ, Ferris KK, et al. Incomplete ossification of the humeral condyle in spaniels. Vet Surg 1994;23:475–87.
23. Herron MR. Lateral condylar fracture of the humerus: a method of closed repair. Canine Pract 1975;30–4.
24. Cook JL, Tomlinson JL, Reed AL, et al. Fluroscopically guided closed reduction and internal fixation of fractures of the lateral portion of the humeral condyle: prospective study of the technique and results in ten dogs. Vet Surg 1999;28: 315–21.
25. Gordon WJ, Besancon MF, Conzemius MG, et al. Frequency of post-traumatic osteoarthritis in dogs after repair og a humeral condylar fracture. Vet Comp Orthop Traumatol 2003;16:1–5.
26. Rovesti GL, Margini A, Cappellari F, et al. Intraoperative skeletal traction in the dog: a cadaveric study. Vet Comp Orthop Traumatol 2006;19(1):9–13.
27. Peirone B, Rovesti GL, Boero Baroncelli A, et al. Minimally invasive plate osteosynthesis. fracture reduction techniques in small animals. Vet Clin North Am Small Anim Pract 2012;42(5):873–95.
28. Tartaglia N, Vicenti G. The treatment of distal third humeral diaphyseal fractures: is there still a place for the external fixation? Musculoskelet Surg 2016;100(Suppl 1):45–51.

Minimally Invasive Plate Osteosynthesis
Radius and Ulna

Caleb C. Hudson, DVM, MS[a],*, Daniel D. Lewis, DVM[b],
Antonio Pozzi, DMV, MS[c]

KEYWORDS

- Plate osteosynthesis • MIPO • Fracture • Radius • Ulna

KEY POINTS

- Minimally invasive plate osteosynthesis for radius and ulna fractures is performed by reducing the radius in a closed, indirect fashion and by applying a dorsal bone plate through 2 small plate insertion incisions remote from the fracture site.
- The surgical approach for minimally invasive plate osteosynthesis of the radius preserves the soft tissue structures and vascular supply supporting the fracture site, which results in rapid bone healing.
- A simple circular fixator frame is an excellent tool for assisting the closed reduction and alignment of radius and ulna fractures before minimally invasive plate stabilization.
- Minimally invasive plate osteosynthesis is most suited for acute, comminuted radius and ulna fractures, but can be applied to chronic fractures or simple fractures in selected cases.
- Open reduction and internal fixation may be a better surgical option than minimally invasive plate osteosynthesis for most simple oblique, open, or chronic malaligned radius and ulna fractures.

INTRODUCTION

Surgical management of radius and ulna fractures in dogs and cats most commonly consists of the application of a bone plate and screws to stabilize the radius.[1,2] Bone plates have traditionally been applied to the cranial, or less commonly, the medial

Disclosure Statement: The authors have nothing to disclose.
The article is an update of "Hudson CC, Lewis DD, Pozzi A. Minimally invasive plate osteosynthesis in small animals: radius and ulna fractures.Vet Clin North Am Small Anim Pract 2012; 42(5):983-96."
[a] Gulf Coast Veterinary Specialists, 8042 Katy Fwy, Houston, TX 77024, USA; [b] Small Animal Surgery, Canine Sports Medicine and Comparative Orthopedics, Department of Small Animal Clinical Sciences, College of Veterinary Medicine, University of Florida, 2015 Southwest 16th Avenue, PO Box 100126, Gainesville, FL 32610-0126, USA; [c] Clinic for Small Animal Surgery, Vetsuisse Faculty, University of Zurich, Zurich CH-8057, Switzerland
* Corresponding author.
E-mail address: Caleb.hudson@me.com

surface of the radius using an open surgical approach and direct fracture reduction.[3–5] More recently, minimally invasive bone plating techniques have been developed that minimize iatrogenic soft tissue trauma and vascular disruption at the fracture site.[6–11] The technique of stabilization of a fractured bone with a bone plate and screws, which are applied without performing an extensive open surgical approach to directly expose, reduce, and stabilize the fracture, is referred to as minimally invasive plate osteosynthesis (MIPO). When MIPO is performed, the major fracture segments are aligned using closed, indirect reduction techniques. Small plate insertion incisions are made over the anticipated (intended) locations of the proximal and distal ends of the bone plate. An epiperiosteal tunnel is developed, extending from 1 plate insertion incision to the other and spanning the fracture site, adjacent to the periosteal surface of the fractured bone and subjacent to the overlying soft tissues. The bone plate is inserted through the epiperiosteal tunnel and fixed proximally and distally with bone screws placed through the plate insertion incisions. Small screw incisional incisions can be created over unexposed, more centrally located plate holes to facilitate insertion of additional screws if necessary. MIPO techniques can result in superior preservation of periosteal vascular supply around the fracture site,[6,12–14] less disruption of supporting soft tissue structures, and potentially a faster return to function and more rapid bone healing than would be achieved with an open surgical approach to facilitate bone plating.[15]

ANATOMY OF THE RADIUS AND ULNA

The closed reduction techniques and small plate insertion incisions used when performing MIPO do not allow direct observation of the muscles, tendons, fascia layers, and neurovascular structures in the limb segment being stabilized. A thorough knowledge of the anatomy of the antebrachium is essential when performing MIPO to stabilize radial fractures efficiently and with minimal morbidity.

The radius and ulna articulate by means of a proximal radioulnar joint, a distal radioulnar joint, and along their length are bound together by a strong interosseous ligament. The combination of the joints and supporting ligaments permits minimal translational motion between the radius and the ulna, while some rotational motion, known as pronation and supination of the distal limb, is allowed.[16] The caudal interosseous branch of the common interosseous artery, which originates from the median artery, runs in the interosseous space between the radius and ulna and branches to provide a nutrient artery to both the radius and the ulna. The nutrient arteries perforate the cortex and enter the medullary canal of the radius and ulna at the junction between the proximal and middle thirds of both bones.[17]

Deep to the skin, the antebrachium is surrounded by a delicate superficial antebrachial fascia layer. Deep to and protected by the superficial antebrachial fascia, the cephalic vein along with 2 branches of the cranial superficial antebrachial artery and 2 branches of the superficial radial nerve course together on the dorsomedial aspect of the antebrachium. During the surgical approach to the distal aspect of the radius, the superficial fascia is incised lateral to the cephalic neurovascular bundle, after which the neurovascular bundle is gently retracted medially. Under the superficial antebrachial fascia is a deep antebrachial fascia layer, which surrounds and protects the antebrachial muscles. The deep antebrachial fascia will also be incised during the surgical approach to the radius to expose the underlying antebrachial muscles.

The shape of the radius in dogs and cats is ideal for performing MIPO. The flat cranial surface allows the plate to slide easily under the tendons, requiring only minimal contouring. The radius has mild torsion distally, which is more pronounced in cats that may lead to rotational malalignment when a long plate is applied craniomedially. By applying the plate craniolaterally, the effect of the shape of the distal radius is minimized, decreasing the risk of intraoperative malalignment.

INDICATIONS AND DECISION MAKING
Simple Versus Comminuted

Proper case selection is important to achieve successful outcomes with MIPO. MIPO is not the optimal surgical technique for all radius and ulna fractures. When MIPO is performed to stabilize a radius fracture, the bone plate is typically applied in a bridging fashion, and secondary bone healing with proliferative callus formation is expected.[18] The ideal radius and ulna fracture configuration for MIPO would be a closed, minimally displaced, mildly comminuted diaphyseal fracture with minimal associated soft tissue trauma. Fractures that adhere perfectly into these narrowly defined criteria are unfortunately rare. In the authors' experience, almost all comminuted radius fractures can be successfully managed using the MIPO technique. Simple transverse fractures may benefit from direct, anatomic reduction and application of a bone plate in compression fashion; however, simple fractures that can be anatomically reduced using indirect reduction techniques can also be managed quite successfully using MIPO (**Fig. 1**).

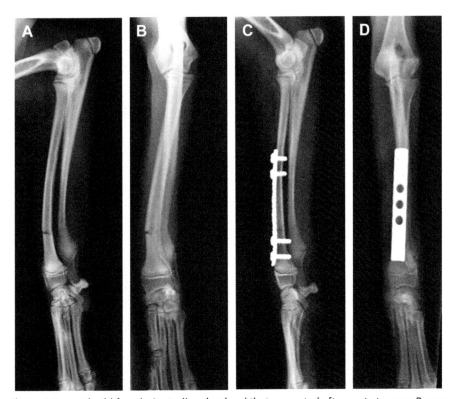

Fig. 1. A 5-month-old female Australian shepherd that presented after acute trauma. Preoperative (*A*) lateral and (*B*) craniocaudal radiographic projections demonstrate a simple transverse fracture of the distal radial diaphysis. The fracture was reduced in an indirect, closed fashion, and a 7-hole plate was applied with MIPO technique. Postoperative (*C*) lateral and (*D*) craniocaudal radiographic projections demonstrate that near anatomic reduction of the fracture segments has been achieved.

Diaphyseal Versus Metaphyseal Fractures

MIPO is well suited for diaphyseal fractures of the radius. Distal metaphyseal fractures, more commonly encountered in toy breed dogs, can also be managed successfully with MIPO, but indirect fracture reduction and screw placement may be more challenging because of the short length of the distal radius segment. In some fractures that involve the distal metaphysis or epiphysis of the radius, the length of the distal segment may not be sufficient to allow appropriate screw purchase to be suitable for bone plate application. A good rule of thumb is that at least 2 bicortical screws should be placed in each of the major fracture segments. Metaphyseal or epiphyseal radius fractures, which are not suitable for bone plate application, may be more appropriately stabilized in a minimally invasive fashion with the use of a circular or linear-circular hybrid external skeletal fixator.[19]

Acute Versus Chronic

In the authors' experience, MIPO can be effectively applied to most acute fractures, but may not be the best option for fractures in which treatment has been delayed long enough for fibrosis to develop. Chronic overriding fractures may require direct open reduction because the organizing callus may not allow distraction of the fracture segments unless some type of fixator is used to elongate the limb segment.[20–22] Minimally displaced chronic fractures with acceptable bone alignment may be amenable to MIPO. In these minimally displaced, chronic fractures, the minimally invasive approach of MIPO may be more efficacious than exposing the fracture site and disrupting the ongoing healing process.

Open Versus Closed Fractures

Closed fractures are the optimal candidates for MIPO, because the soft tissue envelope around the fracture site is intact before surgery and MIPO technique allows stabilization of the fracture with minimal disruption of the soft tissue envelope. Open fractures have already sustained disruption of the soft tissues around the fracture site, and the open wound may result in extensive contamination of the fracture site. The authors have successfully used MIPO to stabilize open fractures, but recommend that open fractures stabilized with MIPO technique have minimal soft tissue envelope disruption (Gustilo-Anderson type I) with minimal evidence of contamination. More severe open fractures (Gustilo-Anderson type II or III) and open fractures with gross wound contamination typically benefit from an open surgical approach to allow thorough lavage and debridement of the wound. When using the MIPO technique to stabilize open fractures, the authors recommend the potential need for plate explant after fracture healing be discussed in advance with the owner. External skeletal fixation may be a preferable option to plating in open fractures with severe soft tissue disruption or significant contamination.[23]

Locking Versus Nonlocking Plates

Implant selection is important to maximize successful outcomes. MIPO can be performed with standard or locking bone plates. The advantage of using nonlocking bone plates for MIPO of radius and ulna fractures is that the plate can be used to reduce and align the fracture in the sagittal plane. The relatively flat cranial surface of the radius allows precise reduction of the proximal and distal fracture segments as long as the plate has been appropriately contoured before application to the radius. Precise plate contouring can be performed preoperatively using radiographs of the contralateral normal limb or a bone model. Locking bone plates provide the advantage of not requiring precise contouring because the screws lock into the bone plate and the fracture fragments are not displaced as the screws are tightened, even when the plate is not in contact with the bone. Because of the angular stability achieved by the screws locking into the plate, locking constructs function as internal fixators.[24] The major disadvantages of using locking implants are the inability to vary the angle of screw insertion through the bone plate (unless using a variable angle locking plate system) and the increased cost of locking implants compared with standard plates and screws. Many locking plates also allow the insertion of nonlocking (cortical) screws into the plate holes. If a locking plate is precontoured and initially applied to the radius using a cortical screw in the proximal and distal fracture segment, then the locking plate can be used to align the radius in the sagittal plane similarly to a nonlocking plate. Once sagittal plane alignment is obtained, the remaining screws inserted can be locking screws. The cortical screws that were initially inserted may be left in place or removed and replaced by locking screws. The authors routinely use both nonlocking (round or oval hole) and locking plates for MIPO of the radius. Specially designed "L," "Y," or "T" plates have proven to be very useful for MIPO stabilization of distal diaphyseal or metaphyseal fractures of the radius, which would normally be difficult to stabilize using straight plates.

PREOPERATIVE PLANNING

Careful preoperative planning is critical to facilitate any MIPO procedure. Well-positioned craniocaudal and mediolateral projection radiographs of the fractured and the contralateral antebrachium should be obtained. The radiographs should be scaled to actual size. Computed tomographic (CT) scan of the forelimbs followed by virtual 3-dimensional (3D) reconstruction or 3D printing of the fractured and contralateral radii can also be used to facilitate preoperative surgical planning and plate contouring. Measurements of the diameter and length of the fractured radius, obtained from the preoperative images, are used in combination with the weight, age, breed, and activity level of the animal to select the appropriate implant type and size. Proper plate selection is important because using undersized implants increases the risk of implant failure, whereas applying overly stiff implants can result in stress protection and delayed healing. Screw diameter should not exceed 40% of the diameter of the fractured radial diaphysis as measured on the craniocaudal projection radiograph.[25] When performing MIPO, the bone plate is applied in bridging fashion in most cases. Long plates, which span the length of the radius, are preferred because longer plates provide mechanical advantages, including an increased plate-bridging ratio, an increased plate span ratio, and the potential for an increased plate working length.[26–30] Long plates also allow the plate insertion incisions to be made remote to the fracture site. Preoperative planning should include the position and order of insertion of all of the screws that will be placed. In most cases, the authors prefer to insert the first screw distally to center the plate in the distal segment. The most proximal screw is then placed in the proximal fracture segment to align the radius and stabilize the fracture. Additional screws are inserted and used to reduce the radius to the plate. When using a precontoured locking plate, the authors recommend that a cortical screw be placed in both the distal and the proximal bone segments to draw the bone to the plate, further aligning the radius in the sagittal plane. After stabilizing the fracture with the 2 nonlocking screws, locking screws are sequentially placed.

Preoperative bone plate contouring is another strategy to streamline the MIPO technique intraoperatively. Preoperative plate contouring can be performed using contralateral limb antebrachium radiographs, if the contralateral radius is intact. The digital radiographic projections should be magnification corrected to real size on the screen. Using the mediolateral radiographic projection of the intact radius, the bone plate can be contoured to match the normal procurvatum of the radius in the sagittal plane. The rotational alignment of the cranial surface of the canine radius (also referred to as "torsion profile") changes from proximal to distal.[31] To optimally match the shape of the cranial aspect of the radius, a small amount of torsional plate contouring can be performed to optimize the shape of the bone plate to conform to the cranial surface of the radius and to direct the screws through the center of the diaphysis in the fracture segments. A CT study found that applying 6° of external torsion to the plate from the proximal to the distal end of the radius would approximate the cranial cortical torsional profile of the canine radius.[31] Preoperative plate contouring can also be performed using a bone model or anatomic specimen from a similarly sized dog if available. If a CT scan of the forelimbs is available, then a 3D printer can be used to fabricate models of the fractured and/or contralateral radius. The printed bone model of the intact radius can be used to allow accurate preoperative plate contouring.

Availability of intraoperative fluoroscopy is invaluable when performing MIPO. Fluoroscopy allows fracture reduction, accuracy of plate contouring, and location of screws relative to the fracture site and joint surfaces to be assessed. If MIPO is performed without intraoperative fluoroscopy, there is a higher risk of obtaining suboptimal fracture reduction, less than ideal plate application, as well as a risk of inserting screws too close to the fracture site or into a joint. The authors routinely use intraoperative fluoroscopy when performing MIPO on radial fractures and think that the use of intraoperative fluoroscopy results in shorter surgery times and superior fracture reduction and implant placement than would have been achieved without the use of fluoroscopy during the procedure. Intraoperative fluoroscopy should be used judiciously during MIPO procedures to avoid exposure of the animal and operating room personnel to unnecessary amounts of radiation.

PREPARATION AND POSITIONING

In preparation for surgery, the fractured forelimb should be clipped from dorsal midline to digits, and a dirty scrub should be performed in routine fashion. In the operating room, the animal should be positioned in dorsal recumbency with a foam pad under the shoulder of the fractured limb. The fractured limb should be sterilely scrubbed using a hanging limb technique. The limb should be draped so that both the brachium and the antebrachium are in the surgical field to allow intraoperative manipulation of the limb and facilitate positioning of the limb in the fluoroscopy unit. The entire manus on the fractured limb should be scrubbed in sterile fashion or the manus can be wrapped with a barrier drape. If a barrier drape is used to cover the manus, the drape should not extend proximal to the carpometacarpal joint to allow manipulation of the carpus intraoperatively and to allow the distal plate insertion incision to be created without interference. Both the elbow and the carpus need to be included in the surgical field so both joints can be flexed and extended simultaneously to assess limb alignment during and after fracture reduction.

INDIRECT REDUCTION TECHNIQUES

Indirect reduction refers to the reduction of a fracture by application of distraction forces to fracture segments applied distant from the fracture site. Indirect reduction techniques allow for fracture segment alignment without direct exposure of the fracture.[32,33] Indirect reduction techniques are used when performing MIPO because the fracture site is never exposed. The goals of indirect reduction are to restore the fractured radius to normal length and to properly align the elbow and carpal joints. In general, the authors do not attempt to anatomically reduce radius fractures before performing MIPO, nor do they attempt to manipulate any small, comminuted fracture fragments. Reduction efforts are focused on aligning the major fracture segments, and smaller intermediate fragments are left to be incorporated in the fracture callus and remodeled over time. The exceptions to this rule are the cases in which MIPO is used in simple transverse radius fractures. Simple transverse fractures can, in some animals, be reduced anatomically or nearly anatomically using indirect reduction techniques.

Several techniques have been described to assist in the closed, indirect reduction of radius and ulna fractures. These techniques include hanging limb technique, use of a circular fixator to distract the fracture, the Minimally Invasive Reduction Instrumentation System (Depuy Synthes Trauma, West Chester, PA, USA), or placement of an ulnar intramedullary pin. See Bruno Peirone and colleagues' article, "Minimally Invasive Plate Osteosynthesis Fracture Reduction Techniques in Small Animals," in this issue for an in-depth description of reduction techniques.

The hanging limb technique involves suspending the fractured forelimb from the paw. The animal's body weight provides the distraction force to stretch contracted muscles and return the fractured limb segment to normal length.[33,34] Despite being an effective indirect technique, the authors find the vertical orientation of the antebrachium when using the hanging limb technique to be a somewhat cumbersome orientation in which to approach the radius minimally invasively and apply a bone plate and screws.

The authors commonly use a simple 2-ring circular fixator to distract the antebrachium out to length and facilitate radial alignment. Rings should be selected that allow at least 1 cm of clearance, and preferably more, between the inner circumference of the rings and the circumference of the limb. Rings that are oversized relative to the diameter of the animal's limb make the surgical approach and plate application easier to perform. A single Kirschner wire is inserted from medial to lateral through the distal radial epiphysis, perpendicular to the longitudinal axis of the distal radius, roughly parallel to the radiocarpal articulation. A second Kirschner wire is inserted in the proximal radial diaphysis, perpendicular to the longitudinal axis of the proximal radial segment, roughly parallel with the articular surface of the radial head (**Fig. 2**). Each Kirschner wire is attached to its respective ring using a pair of fixation bolts and with the radius centered in the rings (**Fig. 3**). The rings are articulated with 2 or

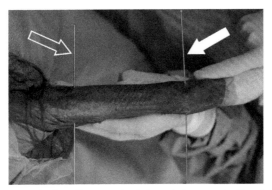

Fig. 2. Antebrachium with the elbow to the left and the paw to the right demonstrating proper positioning of 2 Kirschner wires inserted parallel to the radiocarpal joint (*solid white arrow*) and the proximal radial articular surface (*open white arrow*).

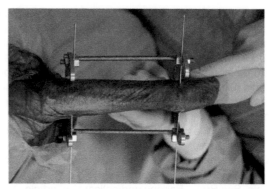

Fig. 3. A 2-ring circular fixator frame (Imex Veterinary Inc, Longview, TX, USA) using incomplete 5/8 rings and 2 connecting rods has been applied to the antebrachium. The Kirschner wires are fixed to the rings using cannulated/slotted fixation bolts. The circular frame facilitates closed, indirect fracture distraction and reduction as well as limb alignment.

3 segments of threaded rod. The rods are secured in corresponding holes in each of the rings and are positioned craniolaterally (craniomedially if using a craniolateral surgical approach), caudolaterally, and caudomedially. This configuration provides a stable construct, and the rods will not impede intraoperative imaging. Omitting placement of a rod in the craniomedial quadrant (craniolateral for a craniolateral surgical approach) provides an open space for unobstructed plate placement. The nuts on the segments of threaded rod on the interior of the construct are serially rotated in a clockwise direction to distract the rings and the fractured limb segment to the desired length (**Fig. 4**). Once the desired length is achieved, the nuts on the threaded rod on the exterior of the construct are tightened to maintain the position of the rings and secured limb segment. With the limb distracted, the fracture is indirectly reduced using closed digital manipulation of the 2 major radial fracture segments. Limb alignment should be assessed in the frontal and sagittal planes. If necessary, the fracture segments can be translated along the Kirschner wires using digital pressure to improve frontal plane alignment.[19] Sagittal plane angulation, often a result of inadequate restoration of antebrachial length, can be improved by additional distraction of the fixator.

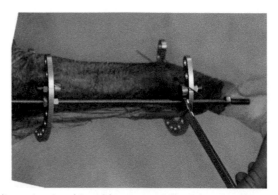

Fig. 4. Fracture distraction is achieved by sequentially tightening the connecting rod nuts on the inside of the circular rings. Once sufficient distraction has been achieved, the nuts on the outside of the circular rings are tightened down to secure the fixator frame.

Application of a properly contoured plate to the cranial surface of the radius will also improve sagittal plane alignment. The elbow and carpus should be flexed and extended to assess rotational alignment. Rotational alignment can be adjusted by altering the position of the Kirschner wire about the circumference of the distal ring. The nuts on the fixation bolts securing the Kirschner wire on the distal ring are removed. The Kirschner wire securing the distal radial segment is rotated about the surface of the ring until appropriate rotational alignment is achieved. The fixation bolts are then reinserted to maintain the position of the distal limb segment. The fixator is left in place to maintain reduction and alignment as the surgical approach is developed and the bone plate is applied. Alternatively, the plate insertion incisions can be created, and the epiperiosteal tunnel can be developed before fixator application because working within the confines of the construct can sometimes be cumbersome.

The Minimally Invasive Reduction Instrumentation System (Depuy Synthes Trauma, West Chester, PA, USA) is another external fixator construct that has been used to perform indirect reduction before MIPO of radius fractures in dogs (**Fig. 5**).[35] This unilateral, linear fixator system includes cannulated reduction handles, which are slid over and secured to implanted half-pins. The half-pins are placed laterally, 1 pin in each major fracture segment. The handles, which afford greater leverage when manipulating the secured major fracture segments, are used to traction the antebrachium out to length. After the fracture is distracted and aligned, a carbon fiber connecting

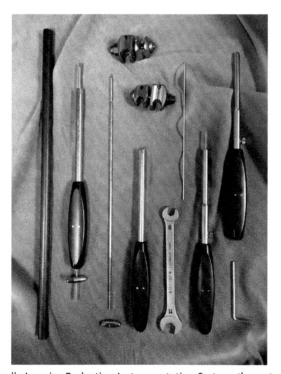

Fig. 5. The Minimally Invasive Reduction Instrumentation System: the system includes 2 sets of cannulated reduction handles, which slide over end-threaded half-pins. The smaller handles are secured to 2.8-mm end-threaded half-pins using a set screw, while the larger handles are secured to 5-mm end-threaded half-pins with an elliptical adjusting nut. The double connecting clamps, which secure the carbon fiber rod to the shaft of the reduction handles, are spring loaded, which facilitates rapid system assembly and positioning adjustments.

rod is secured to each of the reduction handles with quick coupling connecting clamps. When the clamps are tightened, the articulated reduction handles maintain fracture reduction and alignment. The clamps are designed to allow rapid loosening and tightening, simplifying adjustments. A properly positioned system should allow unobstructed MIPO implant placement. A recent canine cadaveric study compared the use of the Minimally Invasive Reduction Instrumentation System and a 2-ring circular construct to facilitate alignment and reduction during MIPO applications in a comminuted radius and ulna fracture model.[22] The Minimally Invasive Reduction Instrumentation System–facilitated procedures had faster reduction times with simplified plate placement, while yielding comparable fracture reduction and alignment to fractures, which were reduced and stabilized with a 2-ring circular construct.[22,35] Clinical experience with the Minimally Invasive Reduction Instrumentation System has mirrored observations made in the cadaveric study, that the unilateral position of the construct offers an unobstructed field for epiperiosteal tunnel development and plate placement. Insertion of a half-pin in the proximal radius can be problematic because of the sharply convex topography of the proximolateral radial metaphysis, but the pin can be effectively placed in the olecranon if needed and still provide effective leverage for performing indirect reduction.[22,35] The Minimally Invasive Reduction Instrumentation System is probably better suited for acute fractures, and indirect reduction can typically be more effectively performed with a 2-ring circular construct once fibrous tissue has begun to organize at the fracture site.[22]

In dogs with a relatively straight ulnar diaphysis, an ulnar intramedullary pin can be used to assist in radius fracture reduction and temporary stabilization during plate application. The ulnar intramedullary pin can be inserted in retrograde or normograde fashion.[36] To insert in normograde fashion, the use of intraoperative fluoroscopy is typically necessary to guide pin insertion. A small stab incision is created over the proximal aspect of the olecranon with the elbow in a flexed position. A bone-holding forceps can be introduced through a small incision to secure and manipulate the proximal ulna and facilitate pin placement. An intramedullary pin smaller than the narrowest diameter of the ulnar medullary canal in the region the pin will occupy is selected. The pin is introduced through the stab incision and inserted near the caudal aspect of the proximal end of the olecranon. The pin is inserted using a drill set to oscillate. Once the pin enters the medullary canal, the pin can be withdrawn and the pin's tip can be blunted. The pin is then reinserted into the ulna and driven to the level of the fracture site in the ulna. The ulna segments are aligned using the intramedullary pin to manipulate the proximal ulnar segment. The pin is then driven across the fracture site and into the distal ulnar segment. The pin is seated into the distal ulnar diaphysis or metaphysis. The ulnar pin can also be inserted using a retrograde technique by performing a caudolateral approach to the ulna at the site of the ulnar fracture.[36] Reduction of the ulnar fracture and insertion of the ulnar intramedullary pin typically aligns or partially aligns the fractured radius. The ulnar pin helps maintain radial alignment while the bone plate is applied to the radius. After the radius is stabilized, the ulnar intramedullary pin can be removed, but is generally left in place, functioning as a plate-rod construct.[36] If the ulnar pin is not removed, the proximal end of the pin should be cut short and countersunk in the olecranon or bent over close to the cortex to minimize irritation to the triceps muscles.[36]

SURGICAL APPROACH

A craniomedial surgical approach, as has been previously described, is most commonly used when performing MIPO of the radius.[37] The limb is extended caudally alongside the thorax for the surgical approach. The surgical approach should begin by making the distal plate insertion incision. Digital palpation is combined with flexion of the carpus and, if necessary, insertion of a 25-gauge hypodermic needle to locate the antebrachiocarpal joint. A 2- to 4-cm-long skin incision is made, starting at the antebrachiocarpal joint and extending proximally. The incision should be centered over the cranial aspect of the radius. The skin edges are retracted laterally and medially using Senn retractors or a small Gelpi retractor. The incision is continued through the superficial and then the deep antebrachial fascia between the tendon of the extensor carpi radialis and the tendon of the common digital extensor muscles (**Fig. 6**). The cephalic neurovascular bundle should be gently retracted medially if necessary. The tendon of insertion of the abductor pollicus longus can be transected where the tendon obliquely crosses the distal radius to simplify positioning the bone plate. The anticipated location of the proximal portion of the plate over the radius can be marked on the skin on the craniomedial aspect of the antebrachium. A 2- to 4-cm skin incision is created at the previously marked location. The skin edges are retracted, similarly to the distal incision, and the incision is continued through the deep antebrachial fascia between the extensor carpi radialis and the pronator teres muscles. The extensor carpi radialis muscle belly is retracted laterally to expose the shaft of the radius (**Fig. 7**). An epiperiosteal soft tissue tunnel is developed, typically from distal to proximal, along the cranial surface of the radius using Metzenbaum scissors or a freer periosteal elevator (**Fig. 8**). It may be necessary to finish the tunnel by inserting the instrument from proximal to distal, particularly if the fracture is not yet completely reduced. Alternatively, a craniolateral proximal plate insertional incision may be used for MIPO of the radius.[36] The authors find the proximal craniolateral approach useful for proximal radial fractures, because the proximal radius is located lateral in the antebrachium. To perform the craniolateral approach, the distal radius is approached as described above for the craniomedial approach. The anticipated location of the proximal portion of the plate over the radius is marked on the skin on the craniolateral aspect of the antebrachium. A 2- to 4-cm skin incision is created at the previously marked location. The skin edges

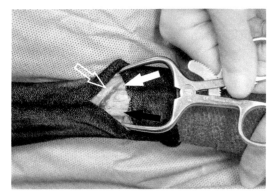

Fig. 6. The distal plate insertion incision is 2 to 4 cm in length extending proximally from the antebrachiocarpal joint. The incision extends through skin, superficial antebrachial fascia, and deep antebrachial fascia. Gelpi retractors can be used to provide better exposure. The surgical approach is between the extensor carpi radialis tendon (*solid white arrow*) and the common digital extensor tendon (*black arrow*). The abductor pollicus longus tendon (*open white arrow*) runs obliquely across the distal radius and extensor carpi radialis tendon from proximolateral to distomedial and may be released to facilitate exposure of the distal radius and plate insertion. The manus is to the right in this image.

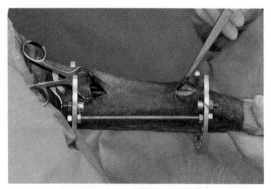

Fig. 7. A Gelpi retractor exposes the proximal shaft of the radius through the proximal plate insertion incision, whereas the distal end of the radius is exposed with a baby Hohman retractor through the distal plate insertion incision (craniomedial surgical approach). The circular fixator maintains the antebrachial alignment and fracture reduction during the surgical approach.

are retracted, similarly to the distal incision, and the incision is continued through the deep antebrachial fascia between the extensor carpi radialis and the common digital extensor muscles. The extensor carpi radialis muscle belly is retracted medially to expose the proximal radius. The epiperiosteal tunnel is developed as previously described.

SURGICAL PROCEDURE

Limb alignment and fracture reduction should be assessed immediately before plate insertion. Limb alignment can be assessed visually, and the elbow and carpus should be simultaneously flexed and extended to ensure that rotational alignment is correct. Fracture reduction is assessed with intraoperative fluoroscopy, if available, or by digital palpation of the fracture site. Adjustments to alignment and reduction are made if necessary using the previously described techniques. The precontoured bone plate is inserted through one of the insertion incisions and slid along the cranial surface of the

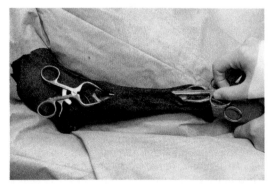

Fig. 8. A pair of Metzenbaum scissors is used to create an epiperiosteal soft tissue tunnel starting at the distal plate insertion incision and extending to the proximal plate insertion incision (craniolateral surgical approach). The tip of the Metzenbaum scissors is visible in the proximal incision.

radius through the previously developed epiperiosteal tunnel until the end of the plate is appropriately positioned in the second insertion incision (**Figs. 9** and **10**). The authors have found that it is easiest to insert the plate through the distal insertion incision and slide the plate toward the proximal insertion incision, especially if the proximal plate insertional incision is positioned near the elbow. Alternatively, the plate can be inserted from the proximal incision toward the distal incision, which may be necessary if the distal radial segment is caudally displaced and the distal end of the proximal fracture segment impedes advancement of the plate from the distal plate insertional incision.[37] If a locking implant is used, the drill guide can be secured in the terminal plate hole and used as a handle to insert and position the bone plate. The position of the bone plate on the radius can be assessed with fluoroscopy. Once the position of the plate is deemed appropriate, a screw is inserted through the most distal hole in the bone plate into the distal radius segment (**Fig. 11**). Care should be taken to ensure that the screw is centered in the radius. The screw should be secure, but not fully tightened so that the position of the plate on the proximal radial segment can still be adjusted. Limb alignment and fracture reduction are again assessed. The plate's position is adjusted so that the proximal portion of the plate is centered over the radius. A screw is then inserted into the proximal radius segment through the most proximal hole in the bone plate (**Fig. 12**). The proximal screw is tightened securely, and then the first screw that was placed in the distal end of the plate is also tightened securely. Limb alignment and fracture reduction are again assessed. One or 2 additional screws are then sequentially inserted into both the most proximal and the most distal holes in the bone plate. The authors typically insert 3 screws in the proximal segment and either 2 or 3 screws (length of the segment permitting) in the distal segment of the radius. All screws should obtain bicortical bone purchase if possible. Typically, the 2 insertion incisions are sufficient for placing all the necessary screws because a Senn retractor can be used to shift the end of the incisions either proximally or distally as necessary to expose additional holes in the bone plate. If a screw needs to be placed in a plate hole that cannot be accessed through the insertion incisions, then a stab incision can be created over the desired plate hole using fluoroscopic guidance. Once the fracture has been adequately stabilized with the plate, both insertion incisions and any additional stab incisions are closed in routine fashion using a 3-layer closure (deep fascia, subcutaneous tissue, and skin). Tendonorrhaphy of the previously transected abductor pollicus longus tendon is not necessary. The closure should be performed meticulously to prevent postoperative incisional dehiscence, which could result in exposure of the bone plate and surgical site infection.

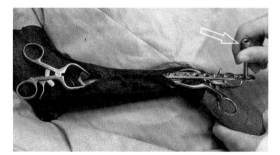

Fig. 9. Plate insertion starts at the distal insertion incision. The plate will then be slid proximally through the epiperiosteal soft tissue tunnel. The handle of the locking drill guide (*arrow*) can be used to direct and slide the plate.

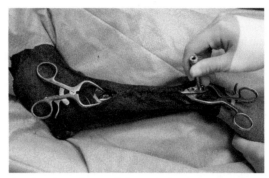

Fig. 10. A locking plate has been inserted through the epiperiosteal soft tissue tunnel into final position. The proximal end of the plate is visible in the proximal insertion incision.

IMMEDIATE POSTOPERATIVE CARE

Postoperative radiographs should be obtained with the animal still anesthetized so that revision surgery can be performed immediately if necessary. The alignment of the elbow and carpal joints as well as apposition at the fracture site and the presence of iatrogenic limb angulation should be assessed on orthogonal view radiographs of the antebrachium. Bone plate positioning on the radius should be assessed, and verification that screws have not been placed in either the carpal or the elbow joints should be obtained. If any significant problems are noted, the animal should be returned to the operating room so the problem can be corrected.

Once satisfactory radiographs have been obtained and assessed, the animal can be recovered from anesthesia. A soft padded bandage may be placed for the first night after surgery; alternately, the limb can be left unbandaged so that cold compresses

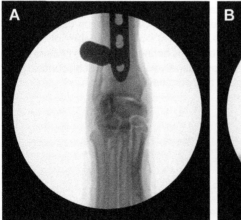
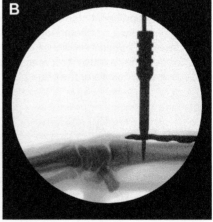

Fig. 11. Intraoperative fluoroscopy images of the distal radius with a bone plate positioned over the distal radial metaphysis before screw application. A locking drill guide is inserted in the terminal plate hole. The craniocaudal projection (A) demonstrates that the plate is centered over the distal radial metaphysis in the frontal plane. The mediolateral projection (B) shows a drill bit inserted through the locking drill guide to drill the first hole in the distal radial segment.

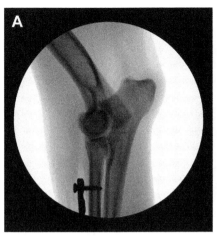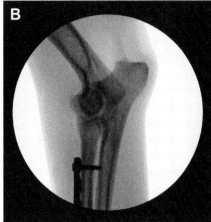

Fig. 12. Intraoperative fluoroscopy images of the proximal radius with a precontoured bone plate positioned over the cranial cortex of the proximal radial diaphysis as a cortical screw is inserted through the proximal plate hole. (*A*) The precontoured bone plate is initially positioned cranial to the proximal radial diaphysis. (*B*) As the cortical screw is tightened, the proximal radial cortex is pulled into contact with the proximal end of the plate.

can be applied over the surgical sites. The authors typically administer an injectable opioid and a nonsteroidal anti-inflammatory agent as analgesia for the first 12 to 18 hours following surgery.

MANAGEMENT DURING THE POSTOPERATIVE CONVALESCENT PERIOD

Dogs and cats are typically hospitalized overnight following MIPO stabilization of a radius and ulna fracture and then discharged the following day. Animals are typically sent home with a 7- to 10-day supply of oral tramadol or oral gabapentin, and dogs are also dispensed a 7- to 10-day course of an oral nonsteroidal anti-inflammatory agent. Some animals are discharged with a 2-week course of oral cephalexin depending on surgeon preference.

The authors do not routinely apply a bandage and splint to the antebrachium after MIPO stabilization of radial fractures, unless the implants appear to have been severely undersized relative to the size of the animal. The authors have seen problems, particularly in toy breeds, with stress shielding and delayed union when splints are used as adjunctive stabilization for radius fractures stabilized with bone plates. The authors typically apply a light, adhesive, sterile dressing to cover the incisions rather than a full antebrachium bandage.

Animals should be confined to a crate following surgery until clinical and radiographic documentation of bone healing has been obtained. Owners should be instructed to restrict the pet's activity to short walks on a leash, mainly for the purposes of urinating and defecating. The authors advocate the use of a support sling placed under the thorax to assist larger dogs when leash walking for the first 2 to 3 weeks following surgery.

ASSESSMENT OF REPAIR AND OUTCOME

Recheck orthopedic examinations and radiographs should be performed at 3 weeks postsurgery and at subsequent 3-week intervals until radiographic evidence of

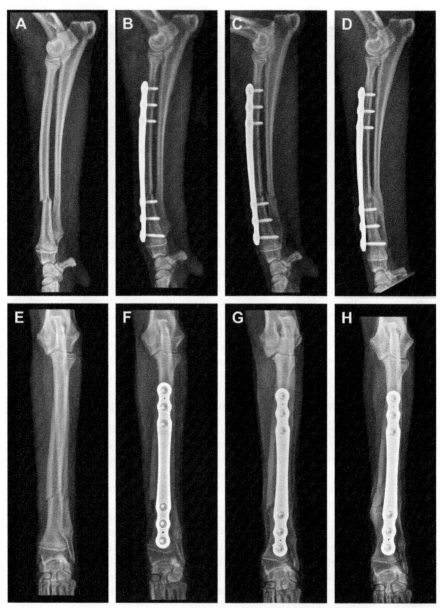

Fig. 13. A 6-month-old female spayed Australian shepherd presented for non-weight-bearing left forelimb lameness. Preoperative (*A*) mediolateral and (*E*) craniocaudal projections reveal a short oblique fracture of the distal diaphysis of the radius and ulna. The fracture was reduced in an indirect, closed fashion and a 6-hole locking bone plate was placed using MIPO technique. Immediate postoperative radiographs reveal (*B*) good alignment in the sagittal plane on the mediolateral projection and (*F*) the presence of a small translational malalignment in the frontal plane on the craniocaudal projection. Four-week postoperative recheck radiographs demonstrate mild bone end resorption at the fracture site with concurrent early osseous callus formation on (*C*) the mediolateral and (*G*) the craniocaudal projections. Eight-week postoperative recheck radiographs demonstrate bridging osseous callus formation at both the radial and ulnar the fracture sites on both (*D*) the mediolateral and (*H*) the craniocaudal projections.

osseous union is obtained. Repeat radiographs are recommended every 3 weeks because in the authors' experience some radius fractures treated with MIPO are healed in as short a time as 3 weeks and many fractures are healed by 6 weeks.[20] Radiographs should consist of craniocaudal and mediolateral projections of the antebrachium. Additional oblique views of the antebrachium may be desirable in small or toy breeds if the plate obscures assessment of radius fracture healing in the craniocaudal projection radiograph. Many radius fractures treated using MIPO have not been anatomically reduced, and the majority are plated in buttress fashion, meaning that most of these fractures heal with bridging, secondary callus formation. Once bone bridging is noted on mediolateral and craniocaudal projections of the radius and the animal is clinically bearing weight on the stabilized limb without lameness, the fracture is pronounced healed, and the animal is allowed to return to normal activity over a period of 2 weeks (**Fig. 13**).

SUMMARY

MIPO has become an accepted approach to fracture reduction and stabilization, which prioritizes fracture biology and is applicable to many radius and ulna fractures. Appropriate knowledge of antebrachial anatomy and careful preoperative planning are prerequisites for obtaining successful outcomes. The initial technical difficulty associated with the inability to directly observe the fracture segments during surgery tends to decrease as experience and familiarity with the procedure are attained. Based on the authors' experience, good outcomes, including rapid time to union and pain-free function, can be expected when MIPO is applied to radius and ulna fractures.

REFERENCES

1. Harasen G. Common long bone fracture in small animal practice–part 2. Can Vet J 2003;44(6):503–4.
2. Fox DB. Radius and ulna. In: Johnston SA, Tobias KM, editors. Veterinary surgery small animal. St Louis (MO): Elsevier; 2018. p. 896–920.
3. Harrison JW. Fractures of the radius and ulna. In: Brinker WO, Hohn RB, Prieur WD, editors. Manual of internal fixation in small animals. New York: Springer-Verlag; 1984. p. 144–51.
4. Sardinas JC, Montavon PM. Use of a medial bone plate for repair of radius and ulna fractures in dogs and cats: a report of 22 cases. Vet Surg 1997;26(2): 108–13.
5. Piermattei D, Flo G, Decamp C. Handbook of small animal orthopedics and fracture repair. 4th edition. St Louis (MO): Saunders Elsevier; 2006. p. 359–81.
6. Garofolo S, Pozzi A. Effect of plating technique on periosteal vasculature of the radius in dogs: a cadaveric study. Vet Surg 2013;42(3):255–61.
7. Miclau T, Martin RE. The evolution of modern plate osteosynthesis. Injury 1997; 28(Suppl 1):A3–6.
8. Tong GO, Bavonratanavech S. AO manual of fracture management. Davos, Switzerland: Thieme/Ao; 2007.
9. Krettek C, Müller M, Miclau T. Evolution of minimally invasive plate osteosynthesis (MIPO) in the femur. Injury 2001;32(Suppl 3):SC14–23.
10. Schmökel H, Stein S, Radke H. Treatment of tibial fractures with plates using minimally invasive percutaneous osteosynthesis in dogs and cats. J Small Anim Pract 2007;48(3):157–60.
11. Schmökel HG, Hurter K, Schawalder P. Percutaneous plating of tibial fractures in two dogs. Vet Comp Orthop Traumatol 2003;16(3):191–5.

12. Farouk O, Krettek C, Miclau T, et al. Effects of percutaneous and conventional plating techniques on the blood supply to the femur. Arch Orthop Trauma Surg 1998;117(8):438–41.
13. Farouk O, Krettek C, Miclau T, et al. Minimally invasive plate osteosynthesis: does percutaneous plating disrupt femoral blood supply less than the traditional technique? J Orthop Trauma 1999;13(6):401–6.
14. Borrelli JJ, Prickett W, Song E, et al. Extraosseous blood supply of the tibia and the effects of different plating techniques: a human cadaveric study. J Orthop Trauma 2002;16(10):691–5.
15. Baumgaertel F, Buhl M, Rahn BA. Fracture healing in biological plate osteosynthesis. Injury 1998;29(Suppl 3):C3–6.
16. Evans HE. Arthrology. In: Evans HE, editor. Miller's anatomy of the dog. 3rd edition. Philadelphia: WB Saunders Company; 1993. p. 219–57.
17. Evans HE. The heart and arteries. In: Evans HE, editor. Miller's anatomy of the dog. 3rd edition. Philadelphia: WB Saunders Company; 1993. p. 586–681.
18. Pozzi A, Risselada M, Winter MD. Assessment of fracture healing after minimally invasive plate osteosynthesis or open reduction and internal fixation of coexisting radius and ulna fractures in dogs via ultrasonography and radiography. J Am Vet Med Assoc 2012;241(6):744–53.
19. Anderson G, Lewis D. Circular external skeletal fixation stabilization of antebrachial and crural fractures in 25 dogs. J Am Anim Hosp Assoc 2003;39(5):479–98.
20. Pozzi A, Hudson CC, Gauthier CM, et al. Retrospective comparison of minimally invasive plate osteosynthesis and open reduction and internal fixation of radius-ulna fractures in dogs. Vet Surg 2013;42(1):19–27.
21. Boero Baroncelli A, Peirone B, Winter MD, et al. Retrospective comparison between minimally invasive plate osteosynthesis and open plating for tibial fractures in dogs. Vet Comp Orthop Traumatol 2012;25(5):410–7.
22. Gilbert ED, Lewis DD, Townsend S, et al. Comparison of two external fixator systems for fracture reduction during minimally invasive plate osteosynthesis in simulated antebrachial fractures. Vet Surg 2017;46(7):971–80.
23. Millard RP, Towle Millard HA. Open fractures. In: Johnston SA, Tobias KM, editors. Veterinary surgery small animal. St. Louis (MO): Elsevier; 2018. p. 649–54.
24. Schütz M, Südkamp NP. Revolution in plate osteosynthesis: new internal fixator systems. J Orthop Sci 2003;8(2):252–8.
25. Johnson A, Houlton J, Vannini R. AO principles of fracture management in the dog and cat. New York: Thieme; 2005. p. 1–546.
26. Gautier E, Sommer C. Guidelines for the clinical application of the LCP. Injury 2003;34(Suppl 2):B63–76.
27. Wagner M, Frigg R. Background and methodological principles. In: Buckley R, Gautier E, Schütz M, et al, editors. AO manual of fracture management: internal fixators. Stuttgart (Germany): Thieme; 2006. p. 1–57.
28. Weiss DB, Kaar SG, Frankenburg EP, et al. Locked versus unlocked plating with respect to plate length in an ulna fracture model. Bull NYU Hosp Jt Dis 2008; 66(1):5–8.
29. Sanders R, Haidukewych GJ, Milne T, et al. Minimal versus maximal plate fixation techniques of the ulna: the biomechanical effect of number of screws and plate length. J Orthop Trauma 2002;16(3):166–71.
30. Morris AP, Anderson AA, Barnes DM, et al. Plate failure by bending following tibial fracture stabilisation in 10 cats. J Small Anim Pract 2016;57(9):472–8.

31. Abrams B, Hudson C, Beale B. Assessment of canine cranial radial cortex torsion profile using computed tomography. Vet Comp Orthop Traumatol 2018;31(S 02): A1–25.
32. Palmer RH. Biological osteosynthesis. Vet Clin North Am Small Anim Pract 1999; 29(5):1171–85.
33. Johnson AL. Current concepts in fracture reduction. Vet Comp Orthop Traumatol 2003;16(2):59–66.
34. Aron DN, Johnson AL, Palmer RH. Biologic strategies and a balanced concept for repair of highly comminuted long bone fractures. Comp Cont Edu Small Anim 1995;17:35–47.
35. Townsend S, Lewis DD. Use of the minimally invasive reduction instrumentation system for facilitating alignment and reduction when performing minimally invasive plate osteosynthesis in three dogs. Case Rep Vet Med 2018;2018(3): 2976795–8.
36. Witsberger TH, Hulse DA, Kerwin SC, et al. Minimally invasive application of a radial plate following placement of an ulnar rod in treating antebrachial fractures. Technique and case series. Vet Comp Orthop Traumatol 2010;23(6):459–67.
37. Pozzi A, Lewis D. Surgical approaches for minimally invasive plate osteosynthesis in dogs. Vet Comp Orthop Traumatol 2009;22(4):316–20.

Minimally Invasive Osteosynthesis Techniques of the Femur

Michael P. Kowaleski, DVM

KEYWORDS

• Femur • Fracture • Minimally invasive osteosynthesis

KEY POINTS

- A thorough working knowledge of the anatomic landmarks of the femur facilitates anatomic alignment during minimally invasive osteosynthesis (MIO).
- A variety of fixation techniques, including plate, plate-rod, and interlocking nail, are well suited for stabilization of femoral shaft fractures with MIO techniques.
- Axis and torsional alignment can be assessed with various intraoperative techniques to ensure that anatomic alignment is obtained.

CLINICAL ANATOMY OF THE FEMUR

The proximal end of the femur is composed of the nearly hemispherical femoral head, which caps the dorsocaudal and medial aspects of the femoral neck. The neck is about as long as the diameter of the femoral head, and is slightly compressed from cranial to caudal.[1] Femoral neck anteversion describes the cranial (anterior) projection of the femoral head and neck relative to the anatomic axis of the femur. The anteversion angle in normal dogs has been reported to be 12° to 40°, with a mean value of 27°[2] (**Fig. 1**). Femoral inclination angle is the angle formed between the anatomic axis of the femur and the long axis of the femoral head and neck (**Fig. 2**A). The range of motion of the hip joint in healthy Labrador retrievers, as determined by goniometry, was 50° ± 2° of flexion to 162° ± 3° of extension. The hip joint angle was measured at the intersection of the longitudinal axis of the femur and a line that joined the tuber sacrale and ischiadicum.[3] The normal range of motion of the hip in rotation is approximately 45° of internal rotation and 90° of external rotation. These values are important in assessing correct

Disclosure: Dr. M.P. Kowaleski has acted indirectly through the AO Foundation as a consultant on product development for DePuy Synthes Vet as a member and Chairman of the Veterinary Expert Group (VEEG) of the AO Technical Commission (AOTK).
The article is an update of "Kowaleski MP. Minimally invasive osteosynthesis techniques of the femur. Vet Clin North Am Small Anim Pract 2012;42(5):997-1022."
Department of Clinical Sciences, Cummings School of Veterinary Medicine, Tufts University, 200 Westboro Road, North Grafton, MA 01536, USA
E-mail address: mike.kowaleski@tufts.edu

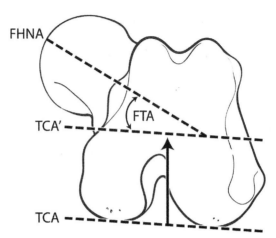

Fig. 1. The anteversion angle is the angle formed by the cranially projecting femoral head and neck and the femoral shaft. In an axial view of the femur, femoral anteversion and femoral torsion are quantified together as the femoral torsion angle (FTA) at the intersection of the femoral head and neck axis (FHNA) and the transcondylar axis (TCA). Note that the TCA is translated vertically (TCA') to highlight the intersection of the axes within the image.

femoral torsional alignment intraoperatively. For instance, if following femoral diaphyseal fracture reduction the range of motion in internal rotation is less than 45°, and the range of motion in external rotation is more than 90°, then it is likely that external femoral torsion (decreased angle of anteversion) has been induced, and assessment of alignment using local landmarks or image intensification is warranted.

The greater trochanter is positioned directly lateral to the femoral head and neck; it is connected to the femoral head medially by a ridge of bone referred to as the

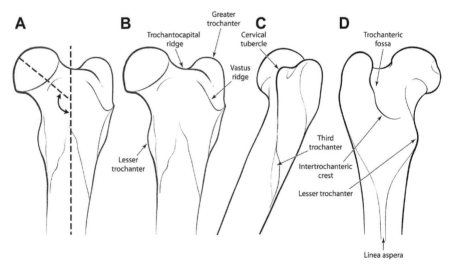

Fig. 2. The femoral inclination angle is the angle formed by the anatomic axis of the femur and the long axis of the femoral head and neck (*curved arrow, A*). The anatomic landmarks of the femur are shown in the (*B*) cranial, (*C*) lateral, and (*D*) caudal views.

trochantocapital ridge (**Fig. 2**). The trochanteric fossa is caudal to the trochantocapital ridge. A dorsally arched ridge of the bone, known as the transverse line, runs across the cranial surface of the trochantocapital ridge, reinforcing the femoral neck and connecting the femoral head to the laterally placed greater trochanter (see **Fig. 2**). The lesser trochanter is a distinct pyramidal eminence that projects from the caudomedial surface of the femoral metaphysis, near the junction with the proximal diaphysis. It is connected to the greater trochanter by a low but wide arciform crest, known as the intertrochanteric crest (see **Fig. 2**). The most craniolateral eminence of the greater trochanter is known as the cervical tubercle. A crest of bone, known as the vastus ridge, arches distocaudally from the cervical tubercle, terminating at the third trochanter.[1]

The femoral shaft is nearly circular in cross section and is straight proximally, and curved from cranial to caudal distally, yielding the normal procurvatum of the femur. The medial, cranial, and lateral surfaces cannot be identified from each other, but the caudal surface is flatter than the others. The caudal surface is marked by a finely roughened surface, the linea (facies) aspera, which is narrow in the middle, and wider at both ends. This slightly roughened face is bounded by the medial and lateral lips, which diverge proximally, running into the lesser and greater trochanters respectively (see **Fig. 2**).[1] This anatomic feature is useful in confirming the correct torsional alignment of the femoral shaft following reduction of shaft fractures.

The quadrangular distal end of the femur protrudes caudally, and contains 3 major articular areas, 1 each on the medial and lateral femoral condyles and the third within the femoral trochlea on the cranial surface. The medial and lateral femoral condyles are thick, rollerlike surfaces that are convex in both the sagittal and transverse planes, and are separated by the intercondyloid fossa. The femoral trochlea is the smooth, wide, articular groove on the cranial surface of the distal femur, which is continuous with the condyles distally.[1]

FEMORAL CAPITAL PHYSEAL AND FEMORAL NECK FRACTURE
Patient Positioning and Surgical Approach

The patient is positioned on a radiolucent operating table in dorsal or dorsolateral recumbence, with the affected leg uppermost. A modified approach to the greater trochanter and subtrochanteric region of the femur is performed to access the region of the third trochanter of the femur[4–8] (**Fig. 3**). A 1-cm to 2-cm incision is made beginning 3 to 4 cm distal to the greater trochanter. The skin and subcutaneous tissue are retracted and the superficial leaf of the fascia lata is incised along the cranial border of the biceps femoris muscle. The biceps muscle is retracted caudally and the fascia lata is retracted cranially with sharp Volkmann rake or Senn retractor; care should be taken during caudal retraction of the biceps muscle to avoid damage to the sciatic nerve. The deep fascia lata is incised cranial to its insertion on third trochanter and caudal to the vastus lateralis, leaving enough fascia for closure. The origin of the vastus lateralis is partially incised and elevated from the vastus ridge. The vastus lateralis is retracted cranially with a Hohmann retractor to expose the third trochanter and lateral aspect of the femur.

Reduction

Pointed reduction forceps are placed on the greater trochanter through the surgical approach or skin. The fracture is reduced with a combination of distal and lateral traction, internal rotation, and abduction of the femur. The preoperative and intraoperative position of the bone segments can be used to predict what manipulations will be necessary. Once reduced, medial pressure on the greater trochanter is used to

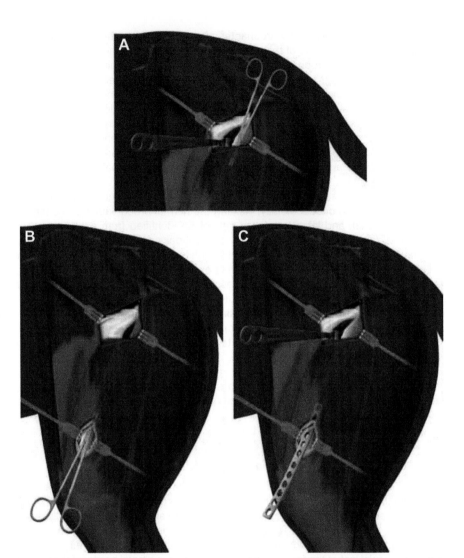

Fig. 3. (*A–C*) Modified approach to the greater trochanter and subtrochanteric region of the femur and modified approach to the (*B, C*) distal femur through a lateral incision. (*From* Pozzi A, Lewis DD. Surgical Approaches for Minimally Invasive Plate Osteosynthesis in Dogs. Vet Comp Orthop Traumatol 2009; 22: 316-320; with permission.)

maintain reduction. Anatomic reduction is confirmed with image intensification or radiographic images in both the craniocaudal and lateral views.

Implants and Fixation

A Kirschner wire is positioned at the distal end of the third trochanter and directed through the lateral femoral cortex parallel to the calcar of the femur, through the femoral neck, and into the femoral head, ensuring that both the inclination and ante-version of the femoral neck are accounted for during Kirschner wire insertion. Image intensification is used to assess the alignment of the Kirschner wire during insertion as well as the depth of insertion. Two more Kirschner wires are placed parallel to the first and seated in the femoral head.

Alternatively, a bone screw placed in lag fashion and antirotational Kirschner wire can be used to stabilize the fracture. Once the fracture is reduced, a Kirschner wire is placed as described earlier to maintain reduction. A second Kirschner wire is placed parallel to the first in the proximal aspect of the femoral neck. A cannulated bone screw is placed over the first Kirschner wire to achieve compression of the fracture.

The Kirschner wires are bent over and cut at the lateral femoral cortex, hip joint range of motion is assessed to ensure there is no crepitus from inadvertent joint penetration with implants, and reduction is confirmed with image intensification or orthogonal radiographic images. The biceps fascia, subcutaneous tissues, and skin are closed routinely (**Fig. 4**). Further details on percutaneous pinning are presented in Caleb C. Hudson and colleagues' article, "Percutaneous Pinning for Fracture Repair in Dogs & Cats," in this issue.

FEMORAL DIAPHYSEAL, PROXIMAL, AND DISTAL METAPHYSEAL FRACTURES
Patient Positioning and Surgical Approach

The patient is positioned on a radiolucent operating table in dorsal or dorsolateral recumbence, with the affected leg uppermost. A foam pad or vacuum bag should be placed under the hip on the affected side to elevate the surgical site from the surface of the table. A modified approach to the greater trochanter and subtrochanteric region of the femur[4,8] is combined with a modified approach to the distal femur and stifle joint through a lateral incision (see **Fig. 3**).[5,8]

To create the proximal portal, a 2-cm to 4-cm incision is made starting 1 to 2 cm distal to the greater trochanter. The skin and subcutaneous tissue is retracted and the superficial leaf of the fascia lata is incised along the cranial border of the biceps femoris muscle. The biceps muscle is retracted caudally and the fascia lata is retracted cranially with sharp Volkmann rake or Senn retractors; care should be taken during caudal retraction of the biceps muscle to avoid damage to the sciatic nerve. The deep fascia lata is incised cranial to its insertion on the third trochanter and caudal to the vastus lateralis, leaving enough fascia for closure. The origin of the vastus lateralis is partially incised and elevated from the vastus ridge. The vastus lateralis is retracted cranially with a Hohmann retractor to expose the third trochanter and lateral aspect of the femur.

To create the distal portal, a 2-cm to 4-cm incision is made extending from just proximal and 1 cm lateral to the base of the patella. The biceps fascia is incised along the same line, just cranial to the cranial border of the biceps femoris muscle. The biceps muscle is retracted caudally and the fascia lata is retracted cranially with sharp Volkmann rake or Senn retractors. The aponeurotic septum of the fascia lata is incised and the vastus lateralis muscle is retracted cranially with Hohmann retractors to expose the femur.

Alternatively, an approach to the shaft of the femur[6] can be used with an open but do not touch technique (**Fig. 5**). A skin incision is made along the craniolateral border of the shaft of the femur extending from the greater trochanter to 1 cm lateral to the base of the patella. The skin and subcutaneous tissue are retracted and the superficial leaf of the fascia lata is incised along the cranial border of the biceps femoris muscle. The biceps muscle is retracted caudally and the fascia lata is retracted cranially with sharp Volkmann rake or Senn retractor; care should be taken during caudal retraction of the biceps muscle to avoid damage to the sciatic nerve. The skin and/or fascial incisions can be made as discrete portals as described earlier (see **Fig. 5**). The aponeurotic septum of the fascia lata is incised and the vastus lateralis muscle

Preop

Intraop

Postop

6 wk

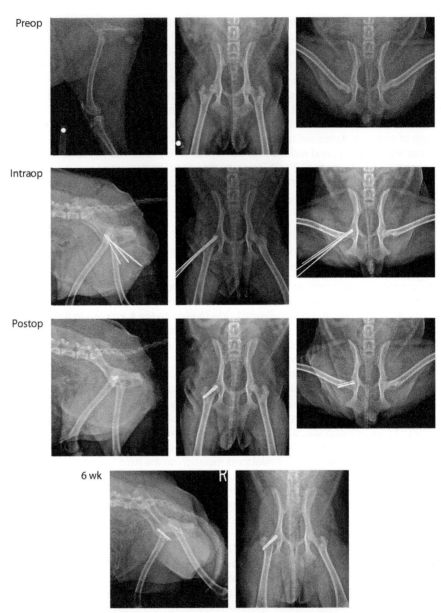

Fig. 4. Femoral capital physeal fracture in a young dog. Note that the proximal femoral epiphysis is minimally displaced in the ventrodorsal view, and much more noticeably displaced in the mediolateral and frog-leg views. Intraoperative (Intraop) images show Kirschner wire placement. Postoperative (Postop) views were obtained after confirming appropriate Kirschner wire placement and cutting the Kirschner wires. Radiographic union is evident in the 6-week follow-up radiographs. Preop, preoperative. (*Courtesy of* B. S. Beale, DVM, Houston, TX.)

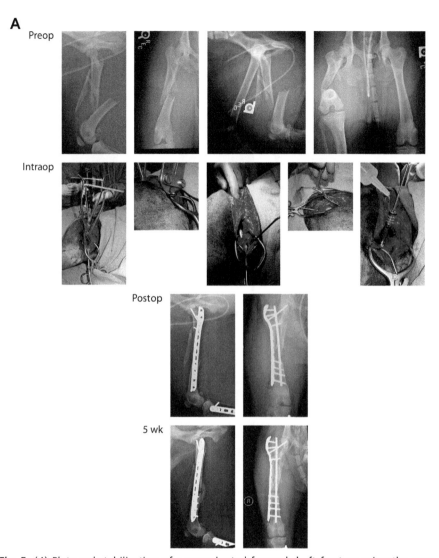

Fig. 5. (*A*) Plate-rod stabilization of a comminuted femoral shaft fracture using the open but do not touch approach. The intraoperative views show anatomic alignment of the femoral shaft using Kern bone holding forceps, and normograde, proximal to distal intramedullary pin placement. The tip of the pin is exposed at the fracture site and cut off to mitigate inadvertent penetration into the stifle joint. An epiperiosteal tunnel is created, the plate is slid along the bone within the tunnel, and locking screws are inserted into the plate; the locking drill guide is used to align the drill bit within the plate hole. Clinical union has been obtained at 5 weeks postoperatively. (*B*) Minimally displaced, mid-diaphyseal tibial fracture in the same patient as in (*A*) stabilized in a minimally invasive plate osteosynthesis (MIPO) fashion with a locking compression plate. Clinical union has been obtained at 5 weeks postoperatively.

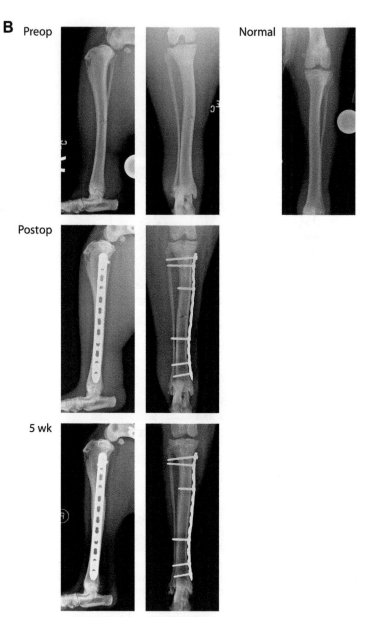

Fig. 5. (*continued*)

is retracted cranially with Hohmann retractors to expose the femoral shaft, ensuring that the soft tissue attachments of fracture fragments and the fracture hematoma are not disturbed.

METHODS OF REDUCTION

In multifragmentary metaphyseal and diaphyseal fractures, it is only essential to achieve functional reduction, which consists of restoration of length, mechanical and/or anatomic axis, and torsional alignment of the major bone segments that are attached to the joint surfaces. Precise anatomic reduction of each bone fragment is not necessary, and doing so may jeopardize the blood supply to these fragments and/or the main bone segments. Stabilization of the 2 major bone segments with relative stability, without disturbing the multifragmentary zone and its vascularity, promotes indirect bone healing within 4 to 8 weeks.[9]

In contrast, simple metaphyseal or diaphyseal fractures, such as transverse, oblique, or spiral fractures, should be treated with absolute stability achieved by anatomic reduction and compression fixation. Absolute stability with anatomic reduction and compression reduces the risk of implant failure from stress concentration.

In minimally invasive osteosynthesis (MIO), the goals are to achieve fracture reduction and fixation without exposure of the fracture site or, at a minimum, without disturbance of the vascularity and fracture hematoma within the zone of comminution (see **Fig. 5**). Thus, whenever possible, indirect reduction techniques should be used. However, the quality of reduction should never be sacrificed simply for the sake of minimally invasive techniques. If adequate reduction cannot be achieved by indirect techniques, then it is necessary to resort to direct reduction to achieve the desired accuracy of reduction. Even if direct reduction techniques are used, small incisions with minimal soft tissue dissection will still achieve the goals of MIO.

Ideally, the choice of reduction technique should be made during preoperative planning. If adequate reduction cannot be achieved with a closed technique and indirect reduction, conversion to direct reduction can be performed. Even with direct methods, there are a variety of techniques, instruments, and implants that can be used to minimize intraoperative trauma to the soft tissues surrounding the fracture. The key to MIO is to leave a small footprint, or the least possible damage at the fracture zone.[9]

Indirect Reduction

The primary indications for indirect reduction are multifragmentary metaphyseal and diaphyseal fractures, although some long oblique and spiral fractures, and some minimally displaced simple articular fractures, are also amenable to these techniques. An image intensifier is essential to assess the quality of reduction, whereas arthroscopy can be used in selected articular fractures.

Using indirect reduction techniques, the fracture site is not exposed, thus it remains covered by the surrounding soft tissues and fracture hematoma, resulting in maximal preservation of the biology intrinsic to the fracture site and bone fragments. Indirect reduction is accomplished using instruments or implants introduced distant to the fracture zone. Reduction is achieved by applying traction along the long axis of the limb as well as rotation, angulation, and translation as necessary. Bone fragments in the zone of comminution are indirectly reduced by ligamentotaxis; the application of longitudinal force in order to bring fracture fragments into reduction. In order for ligamentotaxis to be successful, soft tissue attachments must be present on the bone fragments to pull and guide the fragments into reduction. Because there is no direct visualization or fixation of these fragments, their reduction is usually not anatomic, and healing occurs by callus formation.

Direct Reduction

The primary indications for direct reduction are simple transverse and oblique fractures, most long oblique and spiral fractures, and most articular fractures. Absolute stability is achieved with anatomic reduction and interfragmentary compression, resulting in direct bony healing. Using direct reduction, the fracture site is exposed and the fracture fragments are directly manipulated. Because all maneuvers are directly visualized, image intensification is not necessary, although it can still be useful. With direct reduction techniques, fracture reduction is typically more precise and easier than when indirect reduction techniques are used. However, the surgical approach and application of reduction instrumentation may damage soft tissues and/or their attachments to bone, affecting the vascularity of the bone fragments. Thus, when using direct reduction techniques, the surgical exposure should be adequate for direct reduction to be used, with minimal stripping of the periosteum or soft tissue attachments. The remainder of the fixation can be done percutaneously to achieve the goals of MIO.

TECHNIQUES OF INDIRECT REDUCTION FOR DIAPHYSEAL FRACTURES OF THE FEMUR

Indirect reduction of diaphyseal fractures is a demanding technique, because the fracture fragments are neither directly visualized nor manipulated. A clear understanding of normal anatomy is necessary for surgeons to accurately restore limb length, axis, and rotation. Various methods must be used to assess the accuracy of reduction. Preoperative, intraoperative, and/or postoperative comparison with the intact opposite limb is useful to establish the normal anatomic shape of the limb and relationship of the joints, particularly considering the variety of patient sizes and shapes that are common in small animal practice. Radiographs of the intact opposite limb can be used to determine the correct length of bone plate and size of intramedullary pin, and can be used as a guide to precontour the bone plate; alternatively, a similarly sized plastic or cadaveric bone can be used to precontour the bone plate.

Traction

Application of traction is essential to achieve indirect reduction, because it restores limb length and can be used to correct torsional and angular malalignment. Traction is the basis for ligamentotaxis, and, in order for ligamentotaxis to be successful, the soft tissue attachments to the fracture fragments must be intact and preserved. In addition, the fracture must be relatively acute, otherwise soft tissue contracture may prevent effective indirect reduction.

Traction can be applied with a variety of methods. A traction table or external traction device can be used (see Bruno Peirone and colleagues' article, "Minimally Invasive Plate Osteosynthesis Fracture Reduction Techniques in Small Animals," in this issue). This method is particularly useful when surgical assistance is limited. Disadvantages include difficulty in fine adjustments of the reduction; difficulty in assessing adjacent joint orientation, because the joint cannot be flexed and extended while traction is applied; and difficulty comparing with the opposite limb.

In many cases manual traction is adequate to achieve reduction. A fracture distractor or temporary external skeletal fixator can be used to apply and maintain traction and reduction. Once reduction is achieved, the bolts on the distractor or fixator are tightened, locking the fracture fragments in position, and the definitive fixation is applied.

Supports and Pads

Muscular forces usually determine the displacement of fracture segments. Although traction is useful to correct limb length, it may exacerbate torsional or axial malalignment. A supporting pad may be used to correct angular or torsional alignment. For instance, because the distal aspect of the pelvic limb is thinner than the proximal aspect, external femoral torsion is common if the limb is laid flat on the surgical table.

Elevation of the tarsus off the table with a pad or support corrects the torsional deformity.

External Fixators and Fracture Distractors

External fixators and fracture distractors can be used to achieve and maintain fracture reduction, and therefore they are indispensable tools for MIO of multifragmentary fractures of the diaphysis. These devices can be used to apply longitudinal traction to the bone segments, manipulate the segments into reduction, correct axial and torsional malalignment, and maintain reduction. The primary difference between the two is that the fracture distractor can be used to both distract and compress fractures using the integral threaded rod and nuts. Manual traction must be applied to an external skeletal fixator, unless a threaded rod is used as a connecting bar.

Once the limb is prepped and draped, threaded fixation pins are inserted into the bone ends opposite the fracture site through stab incisions. Placing both pins in the same anatomic plane, perpendicular to the axis of the bone, facilitates reduction, because alignment of the pins parallel to each other essentially aligns the bone segments. Manipulation of the fracture is performed, and reduction is assessed with image intensification and/or local landmarks. Once satisfactory reduction is obtained, the clamps on the external fixator or distractor are tightened to maintain reduction.

Push-Pull Technique

The push-pull technique is used to adjust length and reduction once a bone segment has been secured to an implant; typically a bone plate. A tension device, bone spreader, or bone clamp is applied to the nonsecured end of the bone plate. The bone plate and attached bone segment is pushed away from the opposite segment to achieve reduction. Pulling on the bone plate can be used to achieve compression. An independent screw can be placed as an anchor point for the tensioner, bone spreader, or bone clamp.

Reduction by Implants

Anatomically shaped implants can be used to achieve reduction. Although there is a paucity of precontoured, anatomically shaped implants available to veterinary surgeons, precontouring available implants yields an anatomic shape and can easily be achieved using a radiograph of the unaffected opposite limb or a bone model or cadaver bone. The appropriate plate length and position on the bone can be determined, and the plate can be accurately contoured and sterilized, saving time and facilitating intraoperative reduction. The bone plate is secured in the correct position to 1 bone segment. Often standard cortex screws are placed first to pull the bone segment to the bone plate. Once the plate is positioned accurately on the first bone segment, an additional standard or locking head screw is placed to stabilize the bone segment to the bone plate. Next, the bone-plate construct is reduced to the other bone segment. A standard cortex screw can be used to pull the bone plate to the bone; this is known as a reduction screw (**Fig. 6** shows reduction screws in distal segment). Alternatively, a push-pull reduction device can be used for this purpose. Minor degrees of angulation and translation can be corrected at this time, because only a single point of fixation has been applied; however, torsional malalignment cannot be corrected, thus it is imperative to achieve correct torsional alignment before applying fixation to the second bone segment. If adequate alignment cannot be achieved, the screw or push-pull fixation device can be removed, and reduction can be improved. Once proper reduction is achieved, the fixation can be completed by the placement of additional standard or locking head screws in each bone

Preop

Postop

7 wk

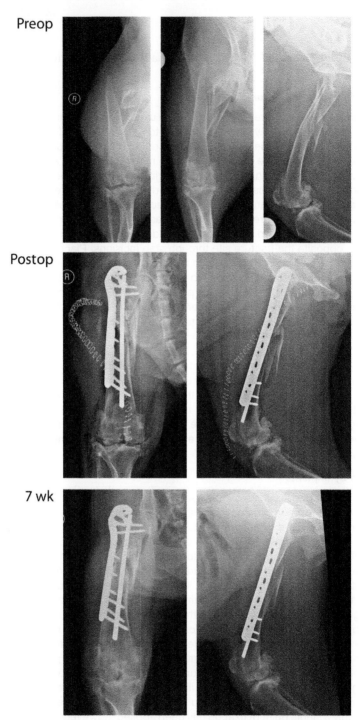

Fig. 6. A comminuted proximal diaphyseal femoral fracture stabilized with a plate-rod construct. Note that the plate is contoured to the proximal extent of the greater trochanter in order to obtain multiple, converging screw fixation of the proximal segment. Standard cortex screws were used distally to draw the bone plate to the bone; screws used in this fashion are referred to as reduction screws. After reduction, additional locking screws were added. Stable implants and clinical union is evident at 7 weeks postoperatively.

segment. When locking head screws are used, it is imperative to ensure that accurate reduction has been obtained before placing the locking screws. Otherwise, a poorly reduced fracture will be maintained in suboptimal position once the locking head screws are placed.

Cerclage Wires

Cerclage wiring is a useful technique for the reduction of large butterfly (wedge) fragments, and displaced long oblique or spiral fractures, particularly when the degree of displacement is large enough to delay bone healing. In addition, cerclage wires can be used to neutralize fissure fractures (**Fig. 7**). Cerclage wires should be carefully placed using a wire passer, ensuring that there is minimal denuding of soft tissues from the bone segments. Cerclage may be used as temporary reduction aids, or can remain as part of the definitive fixation; most commonly they remain as definitive fixation.

IMPLANTS AND FIXATION
Bone Plates with Compression or Neutralization Function

Standard and locking bone plates can be placed with a neutralization function and many of these implants can be placed with a compression function; the compression function is typically indicated for the stabilization of transverse or short oblique fractures. The bone plate is precontoured using a bone model, cadaveric bone, and/or radiograph of the unaffected opposite limb; the bone plate is then sterilized before surgery. Because of the normal procurvatum of the femur (**Fig. 8**A), a long, straight bone plate cannot be applied along the entire length of the lateral aspect of the bone (**Fig. 8**B). Doing so would create a recurvatum deformity in the bone (**Fig. 8**C). In order to place a bone plate along the length of the femur, the plate must be twisted to match the local anatomy and applied in a helical fashion: so-called helical plating (**Fig. 8**D). For instance, in the case of a distal diaphyseal fracture, the plate can be applied relatively caudal on the lateral femoral condyle to avoid interference with the patella and parapatellar fibrocartilage, and contoured such that it extends to the craniolateral aspect of the proximal femur (see **Fig. 8**D).

Following development of proximal and distal portals, a pathway for the introduction of the bone plate is prepared in a submuscular, epiperiosteal plane using a periosteal elevator, a blunt pair of scissors, a tunneler, or the bone plate itself. A locking bone plate can be attached to a plate holder, which is used as a handle to hold the plate for percutaneous insertion. Usually the screw at the proximal end of the plate is placed first. The fracture is reduced, if it has not been reduced already, the accuracy of plate contouring is confirmed, and the screw at the distal end of the plate is placed. The quality of reduction is assessed using image intensification and/or local landmarks, and minor adjustments in angular and translational alignment are made as needed. The remainder of the bone screws are placed in the plate holes, accessible through the proximal or distal portals, or through separate stab incisions, based on the preoperative plan.

The sequence of screw insertion can be altered as needed. If both standard and locking head screws are to be placed, it is recommended that the standard screws are placed first. These screws should be placed in plate holes in which the plate is well contoured and lying directly on the bone, or they can be used as reduction screws to pull the bone to a well-contoured bone plate, as long as adequate plate-bone contact occurs with screw tightening. If a standard screw must be place after a locking screw has been placed, it is recommended that all the locking screws in that bone

Preop

Postop

5 wk

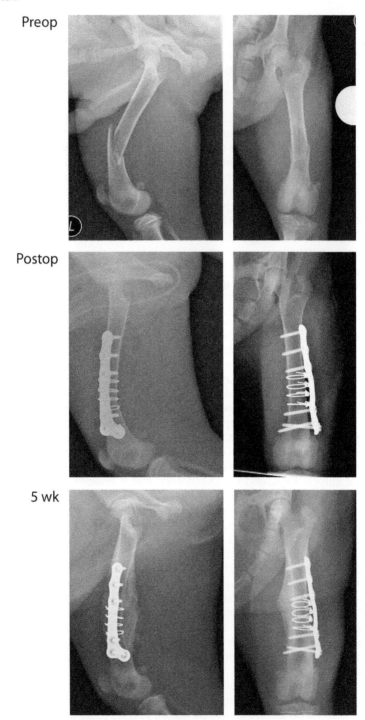

Fig. 7. Distal diaphyseal fracture in an immature dog. Following an open but do not touch approach, reduction was obtained and maintained with loop cerclage wires. A Fixin locking plate in a neutralization function was used to stabilize the fracture. Abundant bridging periosteal callus, stable implants, and considerable longitudinal bone growth are radiographically evident at 5 weeks postoperatively.

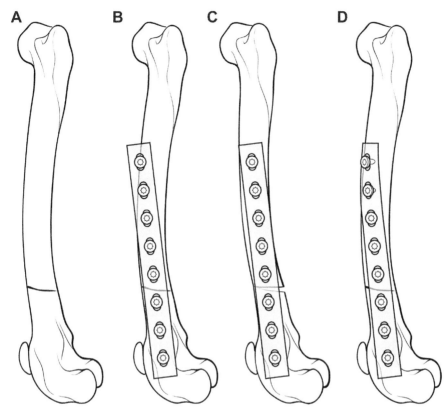

Fig. 8. (*A*) Procurvatum is normally present in the canine femur. (*B*) Because of the normal procurvatum of the femur, a straight bone plate cannot be applied along the entire length of the lateral aspect of the femur because this would cause the plate to be malaligned proximally, which may result in the inability to direct the bone screws into the bone at the proximal extent of the bone plate. (*C*) Alignment of the femur along the straight bone plate can result in a recurvatum deformity. Application of the distal end of the plate on the caudal aspect of the femoral condyle prevents interference with the parapatellar fibrocartilage. (*D*) The proximal extent of the plate can be twisted to lie on the craniolateral aspect of the femur; this technique is known as helical plating. Using the helical plating technique, a straight bone plate can be applied along the entire length of the lateral aspect of the femur while maintaining anatomic alignment.

segment are loosened until they are fully unlocked from the plate before placing the standard screw; the locking head screws are then retightened. The portals are closed routinely.

Screws Placed in Lag Fashion

Independent lag screws, or lag screws placed through the bone plate, can be used to produce and/or maintain reduction and generate interfragmentary compression. Although the placement of a lag screw requires exposure of the fracture site, such screws can be placed with minimally invasive techniques. Lag screws are used to create absolute stability in articular or reconstructable fractures of the metaphysis or diaphysis.

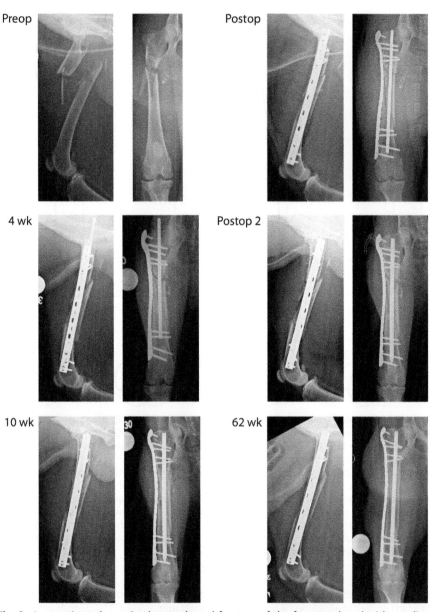

Fig. 9. A comminuted, proximal metaphyseal fracture of the femur reduced with an alignment pin that was cut short and countersunk below the greater trochanter; the alignment pin remains as part of the plate-rod fixation. At 4 weeks, the pin has migrated, indicating motion at the fracture site. Inadequate bone healing is present for the pin to be safely removed at this time. The pin was removed and a larger pin was placed to improve stability at the fracture site. In addition, the larger pin has greater contact with the bone screws, mitigating the risk of pin migration. The new pin has been cut short and countersunk below the greater trochanter. Clinical union is evident at 10 weeks, and fracture site remodeling and stable implants are evident at 62 weeks.

Bone Plates with Bridging Function

Bridging plates are used to span nonreconstructable fractures. Initially, indirect reduction is achieved with manual traction, an alignment pin, and/or the aid of a distractor or external skeletal fixator. The pin, distractor, or external skeletal fixator can be used to maintain reduction once it has been achieved. Alternatively, the plate itself can be used as an additional or the sole indirect reduction tool. To use the plate as a reduction tool, it must be well contoured to the intact proximal and distal bone segments. Contouring the plate anatomically to the nonreconstructable portion of the fracture also aids in the fitment of the device to the local anatomy, particularly within the soft tissue envelope. Placement of standard cortex screws should be done only in areas in which the bone plate is well contoured and lying directly on the bone; these screws should be place before the placement of locking bone screws. If locking screws are used, the plate contour does not need to be as precise; however, the closer the bone plate is applied to the bone, the greater the construct strength. Standard bone screws can be used as reduction screws to pull the bone to a well-contoured bone plate, as long as adequate plate-bone contact occurs with screw tightening. If a standard screw must be placed after a locking screw has been placed, it is recommended that all the locking screws in that bone segment are loosened until they are fully unlocked from the plate before placing the standard screw; the locking head screws are then retightened.

Appropriate proximal and distal portals are developed, a submuscular, epiperiosteal tunnel is created, and the plate is inserted as described earlier. The bone plate is generally secured to the proximal bone segment first, because it is usually easier to adjust the reduction of the distal limb if adjustments are necessary. The adequacy of reduction is assessed, and temporary fixation of the distal segment with a monocortical or bicortical bone screw or bone clamp placed over the plate is applied. The accuracy of reduction is confirmed using image intensification and/or local landmarks such as axis alignment and range of motion of the adjacent joints, reduction is adjusted as necessary by removing and replacing the bone screw or bone clamp, and the remaining bone screws are placed through the portals or additional stab incisions. If conventional bone screws are placed, they should be placed in the buttress position using the neutral end of the appropriate load/neutral drill guide, or a universal drill guide. Placement of the bone screws in the buttress position eliminates the potential for screw migration toward the fracture site during limb loading, by placing the screw head adjacent to the edge of the bone plate hole near to the fracture site. If an alignment pin is used it is generally withdrawn slightly, cut, and seated back to its original depth with a mallet and pin punch or similar device after 2 to 3 bone screws are placed in each major bone segment (**Fig. 9**). As a greater number of bone screws are placed, the interference of the screws with the pin may make withdrawing the pin for cutting difficult or impossible. Withdrawing the pin enables it to be cut to the desired length without interference from anatomic structures adjacent to the pin entry site. The portals and stab incisions are closed routinely.

INTERLOCKING NAIL

The interlocking nail is ideally suited to minimally invasive, percutaneous osteosynthesis, because it can be placed through small stab incisions. In addition, the large diameter fills a considerable amount of the medullary cavity; thus, the placement of the nail from the medullary cavity of one major segment into the other achieves good reduction. A nail can be placed normograde from proximal to distal, or normograde from distal to proximal. The latter requires an approach to the stifle joint, and placement

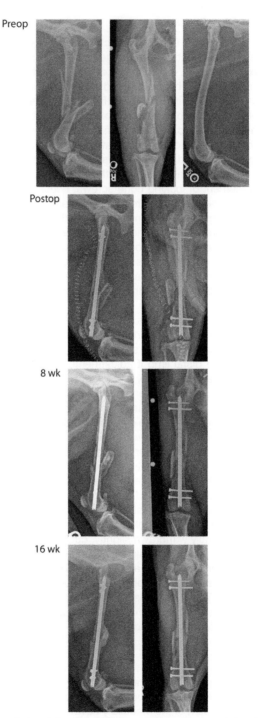

Fig. 10. A comminuted, distal diaphyseal fracture of the femur stabilized with an interlocking nail. A radiograph of the intact, opposite femur was obtained to facilitate preoperative planning. Note the normal procurvatum of the intact femur, and the slight recurvatum of

of the nail through the articular surface in the non–weight-bearing distal portion of the trochlear groove. The nail is countersunk below the cartilage surface, and secured with locking bolts. This technique is particularly well suited to fractures of the distal femoral diaphysis or distal metaphysis in which anatomic axis alignment precludes adequate depth of nail placement in the distal segment (**Fig. 10**). Slight over-reduction of the distal segment (intentional creation of slight recurvatum) is performed such that the medullary canal of the distal segment is axially aligned with that of the proximal segment to facilitate nail placement (see **Fig. 10**; **Fig. 11**).

The diameter, length, hole pattern, depth of insertion, and bolt position of the inter-locking nail are determined by preoperative planning (see **Fig. 11**). A radiograph of the opposite intact femur is invaluable for planning purposes (see **Fig. 11**). The angle-stable interlocking nail (AS-ILN) (**Fig. 12**) features rigid interaction between the nail and locking devices, resulting in significantly less angular deformation in bending and torsion, resulting in more rapid healing and less lameness compared with stan-dard interlocking nails, as described in Loïc M. Déjardin and colleagues' article, "Interlocking Nails and Minimally Invasive Osteosynthesis," in this issue. A small approach to the greater trochanter and trochanteric fossa is performed, which is a modification of the approach to the craniodorsal and caudodorsal aspects of the hip joint by osteotomy of the greater trochanter.[7] A 1-cm to 2-cm incision is made from proximal to distal, centered over the greater trochanter. The subcutaneous tissue is retracted with the skin, and the superficial leaf of the biceps fascia is incised along the cranial border of the biceps femoris muscle. An incision in the deep leaf of the biceps fascia is made caudal to or through the superficial gluteal muscle with a muscle-splitting technique. The nail is introduced medial to the medial border of the greater trochanter, is aligned along the anatomic axis of the femur, and is inserted into the medullary canal of the proximal segment. The nail is directed into the distal segment using fluoroscopic guidance, closed palpation, or an open but do not touch approach to the fracture site as described earlier. The accuracy of reduction is confirmed using image intensification and/or local landmarks such as axis alignment and range of motion of the adjacent joints; reduction is adjusted as necessary. When using an interlocking nail, the axis alignment in the coronal and sagittal planes is usually good owing to the intramedullary location and canal fill of the device; torsional alignment must be carefully assessed to prevent torsional deformity. Once adequate reduction is confirmed, the locking bolts are placed from proximal to distal through stab incisions (see Loïc M. Déjardin and colleagues' article, "Interlocking Nails and Minimally Invasive Osteosynthesis," in this issue), and the incisions are closed routinely.

EXTERNAL SKELETAL FIXATION

External skeletal fixation is well suited to provide distraction and temporary stabiliza-tion during implant (typically bone plate) placement. Because of the overlying muscle mass of the femur and the associated morbidity with long-term application of fixation pins, external skeletal fixation is not typically the first choice of definitive fixation for most femoral fractures. In select cases, particularly metaphyseal or diaphyseal

---

the affected femur following repair with a straight interlocking nail. Because of the distal location of the fracture, the interlocking nail was inserted normograde from distal to prox-imal through a non–weight-bearing portion of the femoral articular surface, just proximal to the intercondylar notch. Slight over-reduction (recurvatum deformity) is introduced, then the nail is passed into the proximal bone segment. Clinical union has been obtained at 16 weeks postoperatively.

Preop

Postop

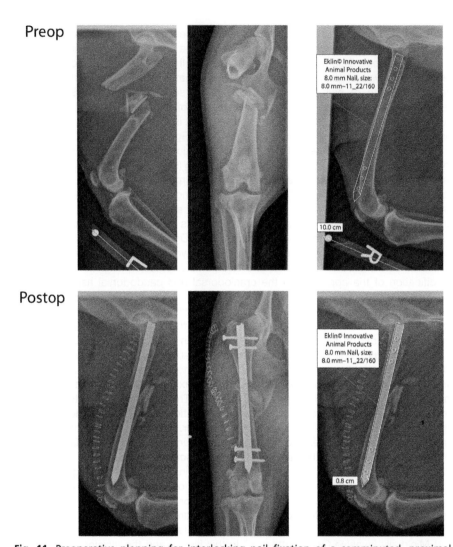

Fig. 11. Preoperative planning for interlocking nail fixation of a comminuted, proximal diaphyseal femoral fracture. A radiograph of the intact, opposite femur was obtained to facilitate preoperative planning. Note that the straight interlocking nail template does not fit into the medullary canal of the intact, curved femur because of the normal procurvatum of the femur. Slight over-reduction (recurvatum deformity) of the femur is necessary to insert the interlocking nail, and this is evident in the postoperative lateral view. A digital template applied to the postoperative lateral view reveals an exact match of the digital template and the interlocking nail.

fractures in feline or small canine patients, an alignment pin can be used in a tie-in configuration with a laterally applied type I external skeletal fixator for definitive stabilization.

ELASTIC PLATE OSTEOSYNTHESIS

Several factors must be considered when stabilizing femoral shaft fractures in growing animals. The growth plates must be preserved for normal growth to occur;

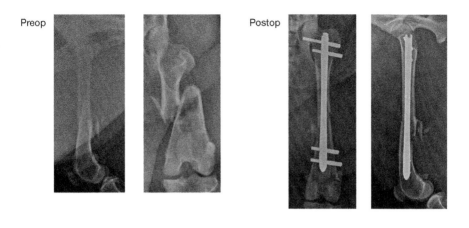

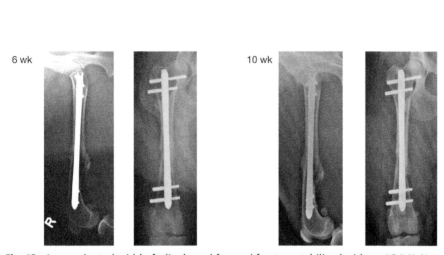

Fig. 12. A comminuted midshaft diaphyseal femoral fracture stabilized with an AS-ILN. Note the callus formation evident at the 6-week follow-up radiographic examination, and bridging callus formation evident at the 10-week postoperative radiographic examination, denoting clinical union.

ideally, the periosteum should not be damaged during the surgical approach or application of fixation, and the cortices are thin, therefore the purchase of bone screws is poor. In a review of 8 cases of femoral diaphyseal fracture in young, growing dogs treated by intramedullary pin fixation, 7 of 8 puppies had radiographic evidence of alteration of the coxofemoral joint, including subluxation of the hip joint and/or malformations of the femoral head and neck following the procedure.[10] These abnormalities were likely caused by disruption of proximal femoral physis during pin insertion, thus intramedullary pin fixation of such fractures should be performed with caution, or avoided. Application of bone plates in the standard manner may result in fixation failure caused by screw pullout, owing to the high stress imposed on bone screws by rigid implants, and the poor screw holding power of the thin cortices in young dogs. In order to overcome the limitations of standard plate fixation, Cabassu[11] described the application of an elastic implant, the veterinary cuttable plate, with 2 screws in the proximal and distal segments, as far from the fracture site as possible, known as elastic plate osteosynthesis. Using this technique, 21 puppies aged 6 to 20 weeks were successfully treated,[11] with bone healing. In another report, 17 cases of femoral and tibial fractures in puppies were successfully managed.[12] The elasticity of the implant coupled with the young age of the patient leads to the rapid formation of a large periosteal callus in these cases. The most common complication seems to be plate bending,[12] thus this technique is best applied to young puppies in which cortical bone thinness creates concern for adequacy of bone screw holding power. In addition, patient factors such as body weight, age, activity level, and presence of other injuries in other limbs must be considered when considering this technique.[12] In older, larger puppies with adequate cortical thickness and thus bone screw holding power, conventional rigid fixation bone plate may be more safely used than elastic fixation (see **Fig. 7**).

ASSESSMENT OF AXIS AND TORSION WITH LOCAL LANDMARKS

Intraoperative image intensification is the ideal method to assess limb alignment and adequacy of reduction. However, this modality is not available to every veterinary surgeon. Therefore, surgeons must be well versed in several intraoperative methods to assess alignment of the limb using local landmarks and anatomic features.

HIP ROTATION TEST

The hip rotation test is a clinical method that compares the hip range of motion with the unaffected normal side, or normal range-of-motion values. The technique is easy to perform, and does not require fluoroscopy. However, the estimation of range of motion may be incorrect, and depends on the position of the pelvis on the surgical table. Ideally, the range of motion of the unaffected normal hip is assessed preoperatively in both internal and external rotation. To perform this test, the hip is flexed to a normal standing angle of $120°$[13,14] and the stifle is extended to a normal standing angle of $135°$[13]; the hip range of motion in both internal and external rotation is assessed. The normal range of motion of the hip of the dog is approximately $45°$ of internal rotation and $90°$ of external rotation. Increased internal rotation and diminished external rotation indicate an internal femoral torsion malalignment, whereas increased external rotation and diminished internal femoral rotation indicate an external femoral torsion malalignment.

LESSER TROCHANTER SHAPE SIGN

The lesser trochanter shape sign is an intraoperative radiological or palpation assessment in which the shape of the lesser trochanter is compared with that of the contralateral femur. Obtain a true craniocaudal view of the contralateral femur using a horizontal beam, angled beam, or elevated torso view[15]; alternatively, an image can be taken and stored in the image intensifier. Before fixing the distal main fracture segment to the proximal main segment, the patella is oriented cranially, and the proximal segment is rotated until the shape of the lesser trochanter on the ipsilateral side matches the shape of the contralateral lesser trochanter.

In cases of external torsion of the distal segment, the lesser trochanter is smaller and partially hidden behind the proximal femoral shaft. In cases of internal torsion of the distal segment, the lesser trochanter appears enlarged. If intraoperative fluoroscopy or radiography is not available, this assessment can be made clinically by palpation or radiologically on the immediate postoperative radiographs.

GREATER TROCHANTER POSITION SIGN

The position of the greater trochanter can be used in a fashion similar to that of the shape of the lesser trochanter to assess rotational alignment of the 2 main bone segments. With the distal femur positioned such that the patella faces cranially, the greater trochanter is typically in a true lateral position, which can be confirmed by preoperative palpation of the unaffected contralateral limb, and/or by assessment of the mediolateral radiograph of the unaffected contralateral limb.

In cases of external torsion of the distal segment, the greater trochanter is positioned cranial to the proximal femoral shaft. In cases of internal torsion of the distal segment, the greater trochanter is positioned caudal to the proximal femoral shaft. If intraoperative fluoroscopy or radiography is not available, this assessment can be made clinically by palpation or radiologically on the immediate postoperative radiographs.

CORTICAL STEP SIGN

The correct rotation of simple transverse or oblique fractures may be assessed by the thickness of the cortices of the proximal and distal segments. This assessment is accurate when considerable torsional deformity is present in human patients,[16] but is not likely as accurate in dogs and cats because the femoral cortices are thin.

DIAMETER DIFFERENCE SIGN

Assessment of the similarity in periosteal (clinical) or endosteal (radiological) diameter of the proximal and distal main bone segments is useful to diagnose rotational alignment and malalignment in reducible simple transverse or oblique fractures. This test is only relevant in areas in which the cross section of the bone is oval rather than round; this is known as the diameter difference sign. This sign is positive in the presence of rotational malalignment, and the diameters of the 2 bone segments differ at the fracture site.

FEMORAL HEAD AND NECK VERSION SIGN

In a normal femur, approximately one-half of the femoral head projects cranial to the greater trochanter, which can be confirmed preoperatively by assessment of the mediolateral view of the unaffected contralateral femur. With the distal femur positioned such that the patella faces cranially, palpation of the femoral head and neck through the proximal portal can be used to clinically evaluate the version of the femoral head and neck. In addition, intraoperative fluoroscopy, if available, can be used to assess version.

In cases of external torsion of the distal segment, less than half of the femoral head projects cranial to the greater trochanter. In cases of internal torsion of the distal segment, more than half of the femoral head projects cranial to the greater trochanter. The findings of palpation and/or intraoperative fluoroscopy are confirmed radiologically on the immediate postoperative radiographs.

RADIOGRAPHS OF INTACT OPPOSITE LIMB

A mediolateral view and a true craniocaudal view of the contralateral femur using a horizontal beam, angled beam, or elevated torso view[15] are invaluable for preoperative planning and intraoperative reference (**Fig. 13**). The mediolateral view is more useful for assessing limb length than the craniocaudal view, because it is more likely that

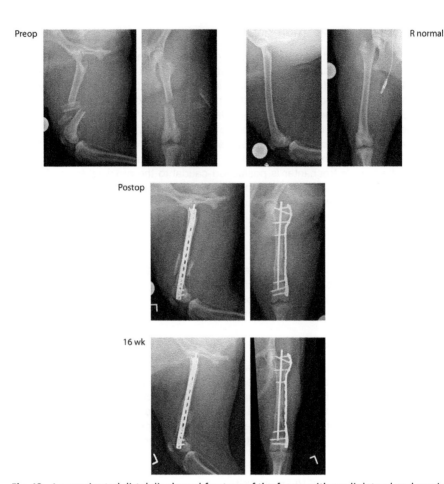

Fig. 13. A comminuted distal diaphyseal fracture of the femur with mediolateral and cranio-caudal views of the intact opposite femur for preoperative planning. The metallic sphere in the image is a 30-mm diameter magnification marker, situated at the same distance from the digital detector as the femur; this marker is used to quantify magnification and calibrate the digital image. The fracture has been stabilized with a plate-rod construct in an MIPO fashion. Clinical union is evident at the 16-week follow-up radiographic examination.

the femur is parallel to the radiographic cassette or detector in this view, mitigating the likelihood of foreshortening caused by malposition. In addition, the mediolateral view is useful to assess the greater trochanter position and femoral head and neck version. The craniocaudal view is useful to assess the lesser trochanter shape, and can be used as a guide for precontouring a bone plate.

PREVENTION OF FEMORAL TORSION

- Keep in mind that this complication is a common pitfall, and aim to prevent it.[16]
- Be familiar with the various methods to detect this complication intraoperatively so it may be addressed before application of final fixation.
- If possible, use a radiolucent operating table and intraoperative fluoroscopy to assess alignment rather than a traction table. Although a traction table can be

used to maintain length of the limb, the torsional alignment cannot be assessed clinically while traction is applied. If a traction table is used, radiological methods of torsional assessment, such as the lesser trochanter sign, must be relied on to assess alignment.
- If a radiolucent table is used, torsional alignment should be assessed with the hip rotation test following preliminary fixation of the proximal and distal segments, and adjusted as needed.
- Drape both lower limbs into the surgical field if possible to compare the hip rotation and measure length. Alternatively, obtain a lateral radiographic projection of the unaffected opposite femur to measure length, and measure and record the hip range of motion of the opposite limb before surgery for intraoperative reference.

Intraoperative correction or early revision of any torsional deformity is essential. It is much easier, less time consuming, and preferable to correct a malreduced fracture than a malunion. In addition, the patient can return to normal function earlier.

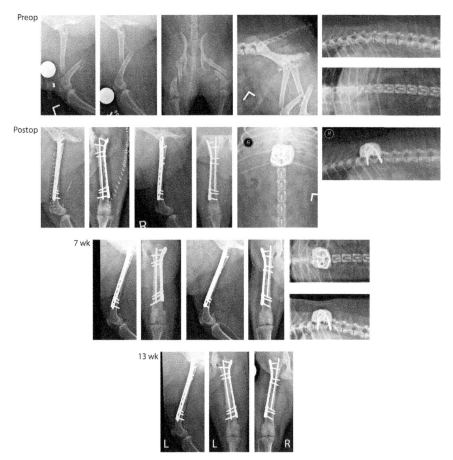

Fig. 14. Case study. A young mixed-breed dog sustained vehicular trauma resulting in bilateral comminuted femoral fractures and a T12-T13 vertebral fracture luxation. The femoral fractures were stabilized with plate-rod constructs using MIPO techniques, and the vertebral fracture was stabilized with direct reduction, pins, and polymethylmethacrylate. Progressive bony union is evident at 7 weeks and clinical union is apparent at 13 weeks.

CORONAL PLANE: VARUS-VALGUS MALALIGNMENT

Coronal plane malalignment occurs more commonly in metaphyseal fractures than diaphyseal fractures because the metaphyseal cortex is not as straight as that in the diaphysis. Therefore, the bone plate must be accurately precontoured and positioned on the bone in the same location as during the precontouring process. An intraoperative technique to assess coronal plane alignment of the pelvic limb is the cable technique.[16] In this technique, image intensification and a sterile marking pen are used to identify and mark the center of the femoral head and the distal intermediate ridge of the tibia. A cautery cable is spanned between the center of the femoral head and the distal intermediate ridge of the tibia, and a radiographic image of the stifle is obtained. The position of the cautery cable relative to the center of the stifle joint indicates the axial deviation in the coronal plane. Although this is a reliable method, it is radiation dependent.

SAGITTAL PLANE: PROCURVATUM-RECURVATUM MALALIGNMENT

In proximal femoral fractures with the lesser trochanter attached to the proximal segment, the proximal segment has a tendency to be positioned in flexion, abduction, and external rotation because of the strong pull of the gluteals and external rotators. Counteracting these forces is necessary for accurate anatomic reduction of this segment. This reduction can be achieved with bone holding forceps and manual reduction, an external skeletal fixator or fracture distractor, or a so-called joystick (a pin placed in the proximal segment, manipulated to counteract the muscle pull).

Sagittal plane alignment of femoral diaphyseal fractures can be assessed clinically by visual inspection or radiologically with intraoperative lateromedial radiographs or fluoroscopy. Because of normal procurvatum of the femur, fixation of a simple fracture with a bone plate that is centered on the lateral cortex tends to create a recurvatum deformity (see **Fig. 8**C). To avoid this, the ends of the bone plate should be positioned roughly centered on the lateral cortex, and the plate could be positioned closer to the caudal cortex near the fracture; however, this may not result in adequate alignment of the bone plate and femur if a long bone plate is chosen or the normal procurvatum of the femur is profound. Another strategy to accommodate the normal procurvatum of the femur is to contour the bone plate in the coronal plane to create a cranial to caudal curvature. Alternatively, the plate must be twisted to match the local anatomy and applied in a helical fashion: so-called helical plating. Twisting the plate such that it begins on the craniolateral cortex proximally and ends on the lateral cortex distally (see **Fig. 8**D) achieves an anatomic contour; this is known as helical plating.

LIMB LENGTH DISCREPANCY

The femur is more commonly affected by limb length discrepancy than the tibia or radius/ulna because of the difficulty in evaluation of overall length caused by the overlying muscle mass. The most common form of limb length discrepancy is shortening, whereas lengthening rarely occurs. Clinical or radiological comparison with the unaffected contralateral limb is an accurate and reproducible method to determine limb length. The overall length of the femur from the greater trochanter to the femoral condyle is measured on the mediolateral view of the contralateral femur, and compared with a clinical measurement of the ipsilateral femur made with a sterilized ruler. The meter-stick technique involves the measurement of the femoral length from the top of the femoral head to the distal margin of the lateral femoral condyle using a radiographic ruler or meter stick and fluoroscopic guidance.

SUMMARY

Indirect reduction techniques (**Fig. 14** case study, right femur) and carefully planned and executed direct reduction techniques (see **Fig. 14** case study, left femur) result in maximal preservation of the biology of the fracture site and bone fragments. These techniques, coupled with the use of small soft tissue windows for the insertion of instruments and implants, result in minimal additional trauma to the soft tissues and fracture fragments. Without direct visualization, MIO techniques are more demanding than open reduction and internal fixation; however, the biological advantages are vast. As such, MIO techniques represent a fascinating addition to the armamentarium in fracture fixation.

REFERENCES

1. Evans HE. The skeleton, arthrology, the muscular system. In: Evans HE, editor. Millers anatomy of the dog. 3rd edition. Philadelphia: WB Saunders; 1993. p. 122–384.
2. Nunamaker DM, Beiry DN, Newton CD. Femoral neck anteversion in the dog: its radiographic measurement. Am J Vet Rad Soc 1973;14:45–8.
3. Jaegger G, Marcellin-Little DJ, Levine D. Reliability of goniometry in Labrador retrievers. Am J Vet Res 2002;63:979–86.
4. Johnson KA. Approach to the greater trochanter and subtrochanteric region of the femur. In: Johnson KA, editor. Piermattei's atlas of surgical approaches to the bones and joints of the dog and cat. 5th edition. Philadelphia: Saunders; 2014. p. 369.
5. Johnson KA. Approach to the distal femur and stifle joint through a lateral incision. In: Johnson KA, editor. Piermattei's atlas of surgical approaches to the bones and joints of the dog and cat. 5th edition. Philadelphia: Saunders; 2014. p. 388.
6. Johnson KA. Approach to the shaft of the femur. In: Johnson KA, editor. Piermattei's atlas of surgical approaches to the bones and joints of the dog and cat. 5th edition. Philadelphia: Saunders; 2014. p. 372.
7. Johnson KA. Approach to the craniodorsal and caudodorsal aspects of the hip joint by osteotomy of the greater trochanter. In: Johnson KA, editor. Piermattei's atlas of surgical approaches to the bones and joints of the dog and cat. 5th edition. Philadelphia: Saunders; 2014. p. 343.
8. Pozzi A, Lewis DD. Surgical approaches for minimally invasive plate osteosynthesis in dogs. Vet Comp Orthop Traumatol 2009;22:316–20.
9. Leung FKL, Chow SP. Reduction techniques. In: Tong GO, Bavonratanavech S, editors. Minimally invasive plate osteosynthesis (MIPO). New York: Georg Thieme Verlag; 2007. p. 67–77.
10. Black AP, Withrow SJ. Changes in the proximal femur and coxofemoral joint following intramedullary pinning of diaphyseal fractures in young dogs. Vet Surg 1979;8:19–24.
11. Cabassu JP. Elastic plate osteosynthesis of femoral shaft fractures in young dogs. Vet Comp Orthop Traumatol 2001;14:40–5.
12. Sarrau S, Meige F, Autefage A. Treatment of femoral and tibial fractures in puppies by elastic plate osteosynthesis. Vet Comp Orthop Traumatol 2007; 20:51–8.
13. Hottinger HA, DeCamp CE, Olivier B, et al. Noninvasive kinematic analysis of the walk in healthy large breed dogs. Am J Vet Res 1996;57:381–8.

14. Hudson CC, Pozzi A, Lewis DD. Minimally invasive plate osteosynthesis: applications and techniques in dogs and cats. Vet Comp Orthop Traumatol 2009;22: 175–82.
15. Kowaleski MP, Boudrieau RJ, Pozzi A. Stifle joint. In: Johnston SA, Tobias KM, editors. Veterinary surgery: small animal. 2nd edition. St Louis (MO): Elsevier; 2018. p. 1071–168.
16. Apivatthakakul T. Complications and solutions. In: Tong GO, Bavonratanavech S, editors. Minimally invasive plate osteosynthesis (MIPO). New Yorkw: Georg Thieme Verlag; 2007. p. 67–77.

Minimally Invasive Fracture Repair of the Tibia and Fibula

Brian Beale, DVM[a,b,]*, Ryan McCally, DVM[c]

KEYWORDS

- Tibia • Fracture • Minimally invasive plate osteosynthesis • Dog • Cat

KEY POINTS

- Tibial fractures are often amenable to repair using minimally invasive fracture repair (MIFR) technique.
- The rationale for MIFR is preservation of blood supply to encourage more rapid healing, lower patient morbidity, and a more rapid return to function.
- Locking bone plates are often used with MIFR because of a lack of a need for anatomic contouring of the plate, preservation of periosteal blood supply below the plate, greater screw security, and an enhanced ability to prevent collapse of the fracture gap.
- MIFR repair of tibial fractures uses indirect reduction to return the limb to normal length and establish proper limb alignment.

INTRODUCTION

Fracture of the tibia and fibula is common in dogs and cats.[1–4] Tibial fractures occur most commonly as a result of substantial trauma. Common causes include vehicular trauma, rough play, sports-related injury, and gunshot.[3,4] Fractures may be closed or open, but tibial fractures have a higher incidence of open fractures compared with other bones because of the sparse soft tissue covering medially. Fracture treatment is determined after careful consideration of mechanical, biologic, and patient compliance factors.[5] Nonsurgical treatment of tibial fractures may be possible with minimally displaced fractures, particularly in immature patients.[3,4] Nonsurgical stabilization includes casting or splinting. Surgical stabilization of tibial and fibular fractures is more commonly required.[3,4] The goal of repair is stabilization of the tibia only. The fibular fracture is rarely repaired. Minimally invasive techniques have become popular for repair of most types of tibial fractures in recent years.[6–9] The rationale for using minimally invasive fracture repair (MIFR) is preservation of blood supply to encourage

Disclosure Statement: None.
[a] Gulf Coast Veterinary Specialists, Houston, TX, USA; [b] Department of Surgery, The Beale Clinic, 38 Cheshire Bend Drive, Sugar Land, TX, 77479, USA; [c] Veterinary Specialty, Center of Tucson, 4909 N. La Canada Drive, Tucson, Arizona 85704, USA
* Corresponding author. 38 Cheshire Bend Drive, Sugar Land, TX, 77479, USA.
E-mail address: brianbeale@me.com

more rapid healing, lower patient morbidity, and a more rapid return to function.[6–13] Surgical trauma is minimized during the stabilization procedure in an effort to preserve blood supply to the fracture fragments.[13–21] Less invasive surgical approaches include a closed approach, the "open but don't touch" approach, and the minimally invasive surgical (MIS) approach.[6–13,21] MIFR has been associated with decreased surgical times and this can lead to a lower risk of infection.[13] Use of a bone plate with the MIS approach is referred to as minimally invasive plate osteosynthesis (MIPO).[13,15,21]

Surgical stabilization using MIS technique can be achieved using a variety of implant systems, including external fixator, interlocking nail, plate-rod construct, clamp-rod internal fixator, and bone plate and screws.[3,4,11,14,15] Two types of bone-plating systems are commonly used for MIPO. Traditional bone plates, such as the veterinary cuttable plate, dynamic compression plate, and limited contact dynamic compression plate, can be placed using cortical screws in compression, neutralization, and buttress modes, as previously described.[4,12] Locking plates, also known as internal fixators, can be applied using locking or cortical screws.[4] Locking screws provide fixed-angle stabilization.[4] Locking bone plates have certain advantages, including the lack of a need for anatomic contouring of the plate, preservation of periosteal blood supply below the plate, greater screw security, and an enhanced ability to prevent collapse of the fracture gap.[20,22,23] Bone plates are traditionally applied to the medial surface of the tibia using direct or indirect reduction of the fracture.[3,4,21] Occasionally, a second plate is applied to the cranial surface of the tibia to supplement the fixation. Application of locking plates also has been reported in a supracutaneous position similar to placement of an external fixator to maintain fracture biology.[9]

Certain tibial fractures are amenable to repair using closed technique and application of an external fixator. External fixators commonly used to stabilize tibial fractures include linear, circular, and hybrid fixators. Closed reduction and fracture stabilization results in the least amount of iatrogenic surgical trauma to the tibia and regional soft tissues. When using closed or MIFR techniques, it is imperative to restore proper length and alignment to the limb.

ANATOMY OF THE TIBIA AND FIBULA

The proximal aspect of the tibia is triangular with its apex facing cranially (**Figs. 1** and **2**). The proximal articular surface lies on the medial and lateral condyles. A sagittal, nonarticular region and 2 eminences called the intercondyloid eminence separate the condyles (see **Fig. 1**; **Fig. 3**).[24] This nonarticular region is not covered with hyaline cartilage. The eminences are called the medial and lateral intercondylar eminences.[24] The meniscal ligaments attach just cranial and caudal to the intercondyloid eminence.[24] The medial condyle is oval in shape and the lateral condyle is circular.[24] The extensor groove (or muscular groove) of the tibia is a small notch in the cranial aspect of the lateral condyle, through which the tendon of the extensor digitorum longus courses.[24] The popliteal notch is found on the caudal aspect of the proximal tibia between the condyles.[24] The head of the fibula attaches to a flat area at the caudolateral aspect of the proximal tibia. The tibial tuberosity is a large, quadrangular process found at the proximal and cranial aspect of the tibia. The patellar tendon and portions of the biceps femoris (lateral) and sartorius (medial) muscles insert on the tibial tuberosity.[24] The extension of the tibial tuberosity distally along the cranial edge of the tibia is called the cranial border (formerly known as the tibial crest).[24] Portions of the gracilis, semitendinosus, sartorius (medial), and biceps femoris (lateral) muscles insert on the tibial crest.[24]

The tibia shaft is triangular in the proximal half and cylindrical in the distal half. The medial surface of the tibia is relatively flat along it entire length and is an ideal location

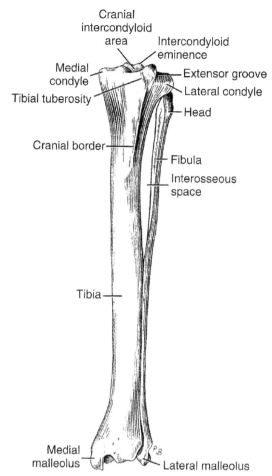

Cranial
intercondyloid
area   Intercondyloid
eminence

Medial
condyle

Extensor groove

Lateral condyle

Tibial tuberosity

Head

Cranial border

Fibula

Interosseous
space

Tibia

Medial
malleolus

P.B.

Lateral malleolus

Fig. 1. Cranial aspect of tibia and fibula. (*From* Schutz M, Sudkamp NP. Revolution in plate osteosynthesis: new internal fixator systems. J Orthop Sci 8:252-8, 2003; with permission.)

for placement of a bone plate. The medial surface of the bone is easily accessed due to the sparse soft tissue covering in this region. The popliteus muscle lies along the caudal surface of the tibia and attaches to the caudomedial edge at the intersection of the proximal and middle thirds.[24] The flexor hallucis longus, tibialis posterior, and flexor digitorum longus muscles lie lateral to the popliteus on the caudal aspect of the tibia and course the length of the bone.[24] The tibialis cranialis muscle arises from the craniolateral aspect of the tibia and courses along the lateral surface of the tibia along its entire length.[24] The distal third of the tibial shaft has a slight degree of torsion. A slight twist in the distal end of the bone plate may be needed if the plate extends the entire length of the tibia.

The distal end of the tibia is quadrilateral and larger than the adjacent shaft.[24] The distal articular surface is formed by 2, nearly sagittal arciform groves called the tibial cochlea tibiae.[24] The grooves are separated by an intermediate ridge. The medial aspect of the tibia extends more distal than the lateral end and is called the medial malleolus. The medial collateral ligament complex of the tarsus originates from the medial

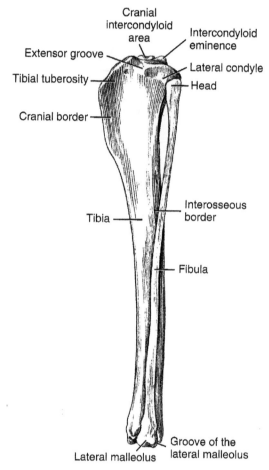

Fig. 2. Lateral aspect of tibia and fibula. (*From* Schutz M, Sudkamp NP. Revolution in plate osteosynthesis: new internal fixator systems. J Orthop Sci 8:252-8, 2003; with permission.)

malleolus. A large sulcus for the tendon of the flexor hallucis longus muscle lies on the caudal aspect of the distal tibia. No muscles attach to the distal half of the tibia.[24]

The fibula is long and thin and attaches to the proximal and distal aspects of the tibia laterally. The head of the fibula is flattened and broader than the shaft. The head of the fibula serves as the insertion of the lateral collateral ligament of the stifle and a portion of the origin of the flexor digitorum longus, tibialis caudalis, peroneus brevis, and peroneus longus muscles.[24] The shaft of the fibula is slender and irregular and is the site of attachment of a portion of the origin of the flexor hallucis longus muscle.[24] The distal end of the fibula is known as the lateral malleolus, which is the origin for the lateral collateral ligament complex of the tarsus.

The saphenous artery and vein course along the medial aspect of the tibia and have a cranial and caudal branch. The cranial branch courses over the medial surface of the tibia in a distocranial direction near the mid to distal third of the diaphysis. The caudal saphenous artery is the direct continuation of the saphenous artery and it lies between the tibia and the medial head of the gastrocnemius muscle.[24] The popliteal artery is a continuation of the femoral artery.[24] It courses caudal to the stifle and divides into the

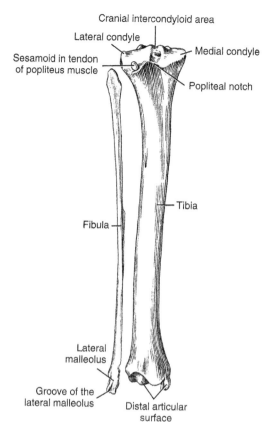

Fig. 3. Caudal aspect of tibia and fibula. (*From* Schutz M, Sudkamp NP. Revolution in plate osteosynthesis: new internal fixator systems. J Orthop Sci 8:252-8, 2003; with permission.)

cranial tibial and caudal tibial arteries.[24] The cranial tibial artery runs between the tibia and fibula distally.[22] Many muscular branches arise from the cranial tibial artery supplying the extensor hallucis longus and tibialis cranialis muscles.[24] The caudal tibial artery runs adjacent to the flexor hallucis longus and supplies a branch that forms the nutrient artery of the tibia.[24]

The sciatic nerve branches into the tibial and common peroneal nerves.[24] The tibial nerve runs caudal to the tibia between the semimembranosus and the biceps femoris muscles.[24] The common peroneal nerve lies below the terminal part of the deep portion of the biceps femoris muscle and it courses over the lateral head of the gastrocnemius muscle.[24] It continues to run distally between the flexor hallucis longus and extensor digitorum lateralis muscles caudally and the peroneus longus cranially.[24] The common peroneal nerve divides into a superficial and deep branch slightly distal to the stifle.[24] The superficial peroneal nerve courses toward the cranial aspect of the crus.[24] The tibial nerve courses toward the plantar aspect of the crus.[24]

INDICATIONS

Most tibial fractures requiring surgical fixation are amenable to MIFR (**Fig. 4**). An exception would be articular fractures of the tibia, which may require an open

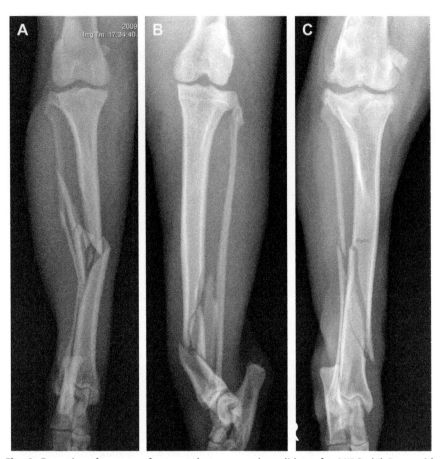

Fig. 4. Examples of common fractures that are good candidates for MIPO. (*A*) Dogs with highly comminuted diaphyseal fractures can be treated with MIPO technique reasonably easily due to minimal soft tissue covering over the medial surface of the tibia and ample healthy bone proximally and distally for screw placement. (*B*) MIPO can also be used effectively for comminuted fractures in cats. (*C*) Less comminuted fractures can also be treated effectively using MIPO technique.

approach to ensure accurate anatomic reduction of the joint surface to reduce the risk of future osteoarthritis. Even in this instance, MIFR can be used under fluoroscopic guidance. MIFR is particularly advantages in comminuted, open, and highly traumatic fractures associated with extensive soft tissue trauma.[12,13] The preservation of blood supply to the comminuted fragments not only speeds formation of bone callus, but also reduces the chance of infection. There are no specific contraindications to MIFR repair of tibial fractures. A recent study of 36 tibial fractures treated with MIFR found a very high rate of success regardless of size, species, or breed of patients.[10,12]

DECISION MAKING
Simple Versus Comminuted

Patients should be evaluated for the potential use of MIFR techniques versus a traditional open technique when treating tibial and fibular fractures. The contralateral leg should be radiographed preoperatively to assist in contouring of the plate and assessment of normal limb length.[12] MIPO is an excellent choice for minimally displaced fractures where little fracture reduction is needed (**Fig. 5**). MIPO also can be used in highly comminuted fractures when there is no chance of reconstructing the bone column (**Fig. 6**). Traditional open reduction and rigid stabilization using fundamental Association for Osteosynthesis principles can lead to successful healing with minimum morbidity. Simple transverse, long oblique and spiral fractures are examples of fractures that could be handled well with a traditional open approach. These simple types of fractures also can be handled using a minimally invasive technique with direct reduction if desired. Because MIPO of comminuted fractures relies heavily on biologic osteosynthesis, plates are often applied in a bridging fashion and secondary bone healing and large callus formation are expected (see **Fig. 6**).[12,13,25] External fixation is also an excellent option for bridging osteosynthesis of the tibia due to the minimal soft tissue coverage over the tibia (**Fig. 7**).[5]

With comminuted fractures, it is recommended to choose a bone plate that is at least twice the length of the fracture gap.[12,13] Longer plates with fewer screws are stronger than shorter plates with more screws.[13] A longer plate, with screws only at the ends, has increased compliance.[12,13] This relative stability can stimulate secondary bone healing and result in profound callus formation. Simple, transverse fractures have a small fracture gap, and consequently high interfragmentary strain.[26] If

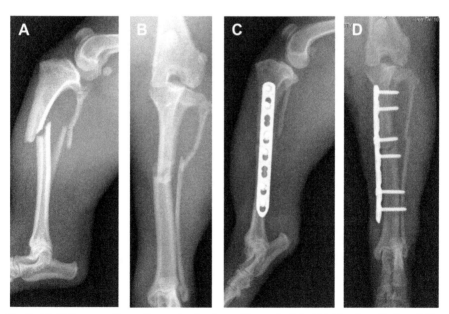

Fig. 5. (*A, B*) Preoperative radiograph of a dog with a reducible tibial fracture that could be repaired using a traditional open reduction technique. This type of fracture is also a good candidate for MIPO in an effort to reduce patient morbidity and preserve blood supply to the fracture zone. (*C, D*) Postoperative radiograph showing use of a locking plate with MIPO technique. The goals of stabilization are to apply a long plate along the shaft of the tibia. Screws are typically inserted at the proximal and distal aspect of the plate. Additional screws are inserted near the fracture when the fracture is simple and when using direct reduction.

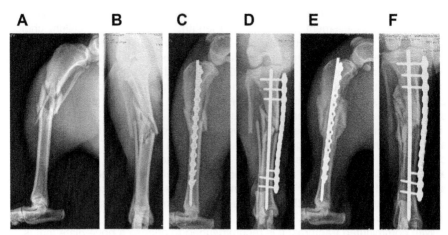

Fig. 6. (*A*, *B*) An open comminuted mid-diaphyseal fracture in a 42-kg mixbreed dog was evaluated for surgical repair. MIPO was selected over an external fixator due to patient management concerns postoperatively. (*C*, *D*) The fracture was repaired using a plate-rod technique in MIPO fashion. The intramedullary pin was placed first to establish partial stability and regain limb length and alignment. A locking plate was placed next, increasing axial, bending and rotational stability. (*E*, *F*) Healing is seen 7 weeks after surgical stabilization using MIPO technique. The dog was gradually returned to normal activity over a 4-week period.

MIPO is used for these fractures, it is necessary to place additional screws near the fracture site (see **Fig. 5**).[12,13] This adds stiffness to the construct, reducing motion and interfragmentary strain. Regardless of the application of the bone plate, it is recommended to span as much of the bone as possible with the plate.[12,13] See Simon Roe's article, "Biomechanics of Fracture Fixation," in this issue for further details of biomechanics.

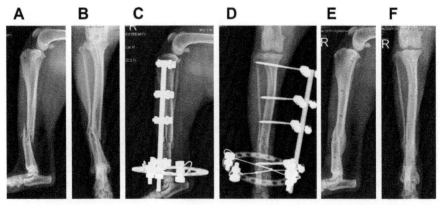

Fig. 7. (*A*, *B*) A comminuted distal diaphyseal fracture in a 13-kg mixbreed dog was evaluated for surgical repair. (*C*, *D*) A hybrid external fixator was applied using minimally invasive technique. External fixators are a good option for stabilizing comminuted fractures of the tibia due to the ability to place fixator pins easily without disruption of soft tissues overlying the tibia. (*E*, *F*) Healing is seen 6.5 weeks after surgery at the time of removal of the external fixator. The dog was gradually returned to normal activity over a 4-week period.

Immature Versus Mature

External coaptation may be considered in young puppies and kittens having minimally displaced tibia fractures. External coaptation provides less stability but preserves the soft tissue envelope of the bone. A splint or cast can provide adequate stability because of the minimal displacement and robust healing in the immature puppy or kitten (**Fig. 8**). MIPO can be used effectively in immature and mature dogs. Elastic osteosynthesis is a technique to reduce the chance of screw pull-out in thin, soft bone found in puppies when using cortical screws.[27] Typically, VCP plates are used to span the entire tibia

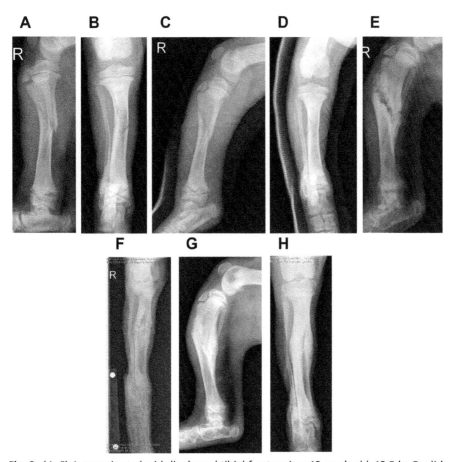

Fig. 8. (*A, B*) A comminuted mid-diaphyseal tibial fracture in a 12-week-old, 13.5-kg English mastiff was evaluated for fracture stabilization. (*C, D*) A lateral fiberglass splint was used to stabilize the fracture due to the minimally displaced nature of the fracture and the young age of the puppy. Activity was prevented for 3 weeks after applying the splint. The splint was changed weekly. (*E, F*) Good bridging callus is seen 3 weeks after stabilization of this fracture using a lateral fiberglass splint. Good stability of the tibia could be appreciated on palpation. The fracture appears healed on the anteroposterior view, but healing is incomplete on the lateral view. The splint was removed at this time and the dog was gradually returned to normal activity over a 4-week period. (*G, H*) Good healing and remodeling of the callus is seen 6 months after fracture stabilization with a lateral splint. Good alignment and continued growth of the bone was achieved.

and are attached with 2 to 3 screws at the end of the plate on the proximal and distal aspect of the bone (**Fig. 9**). A very thin plate is used to allow elasticity and decrease the tendency for screw pull-out.[27] This technique had a favorable outcome in all but 1 patient in a recent study.[27] Healing was typically seen as bridging callus in approximately 5 weeks.[27] Mature dogs that are expected to heal require slightly heavier plates, but healing with bridging callus also occurs quickly, usually in 4 to 6 weeks.[9,12]

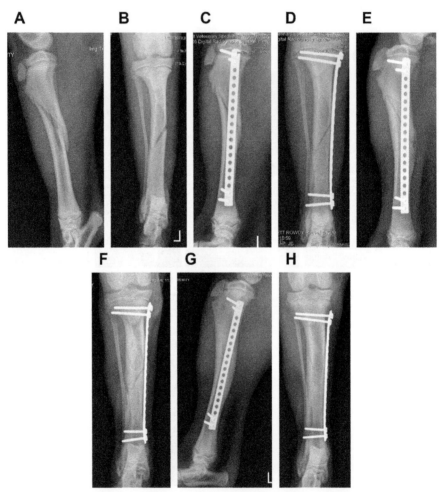

Fig. 9. (*A, B*) A spiral mid-diaphyseal tibial fracture in a 13-week-old, 14.5-kg Labrador retriever puppy was evaluated for fracture stabilization. (*C, D*) Elastic plating technique was used to stabilize the fracture due to the minimally displaced nature of the fracture and the young age of the puppy. A plate is applied along the entire length of the medial tibia and 2 screws are placed proximally and distally in MIPO fashion. Activity was limited to leash walk for 2 weeks postoperatively. (*E, F*) Good bridging callus is seen 2 weeks after stabilization of this fracture. Good stability of the tibia could be appreciated on palpation. The dog was allowed increased walking exercise for 2 additional weeks then a gradual return to normal activity over a 2-week period. (*G, H*) Good healing and remodeling of the callus is seen 6 weeks after fracture stabilization. Good alignment and continued growth of the bone was achieved.

Diaphyseal Versus Metaphyseal

Metaphyseal fractures are seen less commonly than diaphyseal fractures. Metaphyseal fractures may be simple or comminuted and may extend to the articular surface. Fractures having an articular component require anatomic reduction for that component. This portion of the reduction can be accomplished using open or minimally invasive technique. If an open approach is used to reduce and stabilize the articular portion of the fracture, the remaining portion of the fracture can be repaired using MIFR technique. Diaphyseal fractures of the tibia and fibula are particularly well suited for MIFR techniques because the medial surface of the bone is readily accessible and has little soft tissue covering. Fracture stabilization can be accomplished with minimal disturbance of the fracture site. Distal metaphyseal fractures may provide for little room distal to the fracture site to gain screw purchase. Care must be taken not to interfere with the stifle joint when placing screws proximally or the talocrural joint when placing screws distally. The risk of placing a screw in the joint when stabilizing metaphyseal fractures is increased when using locking screws due to the necessity to place the screws perpendicular to the plate. Typically the most proximal or distal screw is at greatest risk. Two options exist to avoid placement of the screw into the joint. A cortical screw can be angled away from the joint surface or a short locking screw can be used (**Fig. 10**). It is generally recommended to have at least 2 bicortical screws in each of the major fracture segments, although 3 screws are preferred if allowed by the fracture configuration. MIPO technique has been found to be an equally effective method of treating metaphyseal and diaphyseal fractures of the tibia in dogs and cats.[10,12]

Acute Versus Chronic

MIFR is best applied to acute fractures that have a fresh hematoma. MIFR can be used very successfully in fractures of duration less than 2 weeks. With chronic fractures that require significant reduction to regain length and alignment, muscle contracture and preexisting callus formation may not allow for adequate indirect reduction. In these cases, it may be necessary to open the fracture site to help achieve appropriate length and acceptable alignment. The exception may be chronic fractures with minimal displacement and little need for reduction, as these fractures respond well to MIFR technique. Many of these cases may heal appropriately with external cooptation as well. Chronic fractures treated with MIFR may benefit from percutaneous injection of biological catalysts of healing, such as platelet rich plasma or stem cells. Adjunctive techniques, such as shock-wave therapy or magnetic therapy, may also help to stimulate the biological status of fracture healing. MIPO using locking plates can also be successful in clinical patients previously having complicated fracture repair. MIPO helps preserve fracture biology in patients having failed fracture repair leading to osteomyelitis and nonunion (**Fig. 11**).

Locking Versus Nonlocking Plates

Locking plates have several advantages over nonlocking plates when stabilizing tibia and fibular fractures using MIPO, particularly in the metaphyseal regions.[13] Although the authors prefer locking plates for many fractures of the tibia and fibula, it should be emphasized that conventional plating systems can and have been used for many years to successfully treat simple and comminuted fractures of these bones. A recent study showed no difference in outcome when treating tibial fractures in dogs and cats with MIPO technique using VCP, LCP, or LCDCP plates.[12] The density of bone in the proximal metaphyseal region of some large and giant breed dogs such

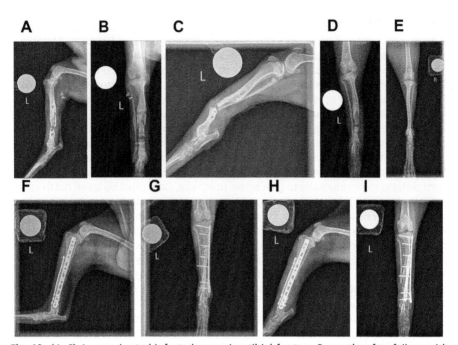

Fig. 10. (*A, B*) A comminuted infected nonunion tibial fracture 3 months after failure with external fixation in a 9-month-old malti-poo Note the lack of callus and presence of a sequestrum. (*C, D*) The patient was initially treated with debridement, sequestrectomy, antibiotic therapy, and external coaptation. (*E–G*) All evidence of infection had resolved 3 weeks postoperatively. Stabilization was performed using MIPO technique with the aid of fluoroscopy and precontouring of the medial plate to match the opposite tibia. The fracture was stabilized with orthogonal plates (2.0 VOI locking plate and 1.7 mm micro Fixin plate). Cancellous bone graft was mixed with demineralized bone matrix allograft and placed in the fracture gap. (*H, I*) The fracture has healed 2 months postoperative and no complications were encountered. Patient outcome is excellent. Abbreviation: VOI, veterinary orthopedic implants.

as the German shepherd, mastiff, and great Dane can be low. Locking screws provide increased protection against backing out of screws in soft bone. Very proximal and distal metaphyseal fractures of the tibia may not be amenable to placement of 3 screws. Use of 2 locking screws in these fractures improves stability and the risk of implant failure. Locking screws provide fixed-angle stability and are unlikely to loosen. Cortical screws are more likely to loosen, particularly when only using 2 screws in a bone segment. Instability may ensue, increasing the possibility of delayed bone healing or loss of limb alignment. Nonlocking or locking bone plates can be used successfully for diaphyseal fractures of the tibia and fibula. Anatomic plate contouring of the bone plate is required at the site where nonlocking screws are placed. The plate contour can be approximated preoperatively using radiographs of the contralateral normal limb. If the plate is not contoured properly in the regions where cortical screws are placed, loss of alignment will occur as the bone is drawn toward the plate during screw tightening (**Fig. 12**). The need to anatomically contour the plate adds surgical time and increases the technical difficulty. Precise contouring of locking plates is not needed because the head of the screws lock into the plate, preventing the lag effect on the bone as the screw is tightened (**Fig. 13**). Fracture alignment is thus maintained despite

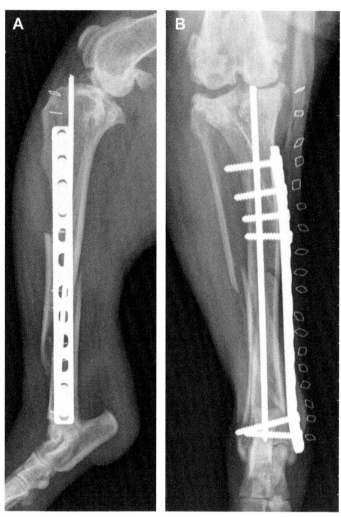

Fig. 11. (*A, B*) A cortical screw can be angled proximally away from the distal tibial articular surface to avoid penetrating the tibiotarsal joint. The medial malleolus can be used as a landmark to help estimate the needed angle for the screw.

the presence of small gaps between the plate and the bone. It is recommended that the gaps between the plate and the bone be kept to 2 mm or less to prevent significant loss of construct stability.[28] The lack of need for precise contouring of the plate with MIPO is a tremendous advantage because of the lack of accessibility to the surface of the bone due to the minimally invasive nature of the technique. The disadvantages of using fixed-angle locking screws are an inability to angle the screws and the increased cost. The surgeon must be careful to avoid placing screws into the stifle or tarsus when inserting locking screws proximally or distally if the plate is contoured to match the flared surface of the bone. The contouring of the plate proximally or distally directs the holes of the plate toward the joint. Fixed-angle locking screws are presently placed perpendicular to the plate with most of the present systems available, and thus accidental placement of the screw into the joint can occur if this

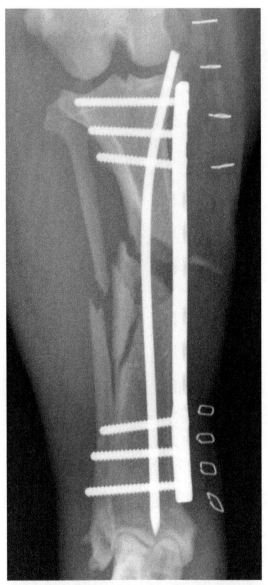

Fig. 12. If the plate is not contoured properly in the regions where cortical screws are placed, loss of alignment will occur as the bone is drawn toward the plate during screw tightening. The proximal tibial fragment was drawn up to an inadequately contoured bone plate causing valgus deformity.

possibility is not anticipated. The surgeon typically can use a short screw in this situation to avoid penetration into the joint. By contrast, polyaxial locking plate systems allow the surgeon to insert screws with 10° to 15° of angulation, which can be helpful in avoiding articular surfaces and fracture lines.

The increased cost of locking screws is greater than nonlocking screws; however, it is minimal especially when considering the time savings from not having to precisely

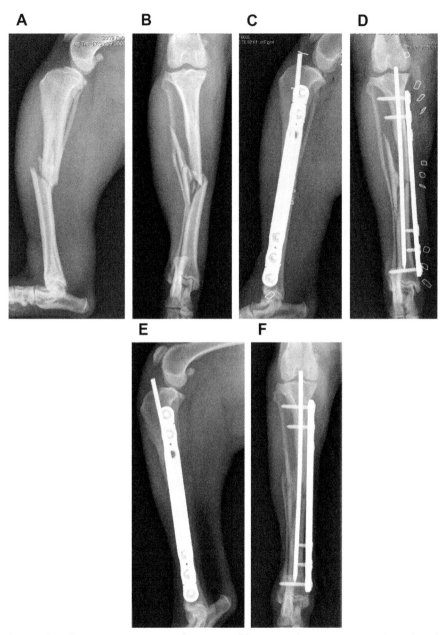

Fig. 13. (*A, B*) Preoperative views of a 4-year-old Spitz with an open comminuted mid-diaphyseal tibial fracture. (*C, D*) The fracture was repaired with a plate-rod implant using MIPO technique. Precise contouring of locking plates is not needed because the head of the screws lock into the plate, preventing the lag effect on the bone as the screw is tightened. The advantages of not anatomically contouring the plate distally are decreased surgical time and ability to place the most distal locking screw in bicortical fashion without being directed toward the joint. (*E, F*) Good bridging callus is seen 7 weeks after stabilization of this fracture. Monocortical screws were needed due to the intramedullary pin present. Locking screws are less likely to loosen and back out compared with traditional cortical screws.

contour the plate and cost savings should a revision surgery be needed. In addition, surgeons typically use fewer screws when using locking systems. Another advantage of using locking screws is the increased stability achieved when using screws in a monocortical fashion. The use of a plate in combination with an intramedullary pin for fixation (plate-rod construct) of tibial fractures has become very common due to the ease of application and increased resistance to bending forces.[10,12,26] The intramedullary pin may interfere with placement of some of the screws, requiring use of a monocortical rather than a bicortical screw. It is also possible to use a combination of nonlocking and locking screws. Use of both types of screws reduces the cost and provides a combination of methods of fracture stabilization (traditional plate and internal fixator). When using a combination of locking and nonlocking screws, it is important to place the cortical screws first to create the desired compression between the plate and the bone to increase the frictional forces that supply the stability. If a locking screw is placed before the cortical screw, the plate is unable to be pulled against the bone, creating this frictional force. It should be emphasized that nonlocking screws should be placed in areas in which good plate-bone contact is present to avoid undesirable displacement of bone fragments when the screw is tightened. Many different locking plate systems are available. Because of the lack of soft tissue covering over the medial aspect of the tibia, a low-profile plate is desirable. If a thin plate is used, supplemental stability can be provided using an intramedullary pin or a second plate on the cranial surface (**Fig. 14**). Bone plates are typically applied to the medial surface of the tibia where most tensile forces occur during weight bearing. The cranial surface of the bone is also an acceptable site when applying a second plate to the distal two-thirds of the bone.

PATIENT POSITIONING

The leg is clipped and prepped in routine fashion from the mid-femur to the metatarsophalangeal joints. It is helpful to have the stifle and the tarsus in the surgical field to facilitate evaluation of limb alignment and to give access for placement of an intramedullary pin if needed. The patient is usually positioned in dorsal recumbence. This allows good access for fracture repair using MIFR technique as well as an optimal view to assess limb alignment. A hanging limb preparation should be used. It is helpful to hang the leg under tension to fatigue the muscles to aid reduction. An effective means of providing tension is to hang the leg, placing tension while securing to an anchor point above the table. Lowering the table a short distance while leaving the leg suspended increases the amount of tension on the limb, thus adding reduction by distracting the fracture further. The leg can be left suspended during closed reduction and fixation using external fixation. The leg is typically lowered from its suspended position when using the MIFR technique.

INDIRECT REDUCTION FOR MINIMALLY INVASIVE PLATE OSTEOSYNTHESIS

Fracture reduction is attained indirectly in most comminuted tibial fractures repaired with MIFR. Sustained distractive forces are applied across the fracture to fatigue muscles causing overriding of the fragments to regain limb length. Distraction can be applied manually, by suspending the leg from above, using a distraction table, using a fracture distractor or a temporary external fixator with linear motors.[12,13,21,29] As limb length is regained, the fracture fragments are drawn more closely toward their original position because of the preservation of muscle attachments. Limb length was restored to 99% of normal length following indirect reduction in tibial fractures treated with MIFR.[12] Indirect fracture reduction can lead to very good reduction if

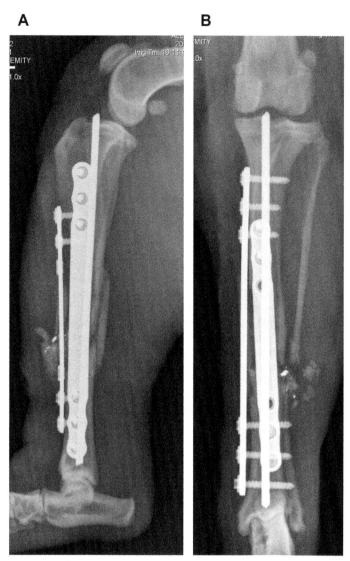

Fig. 14. (A, B) A second plate was added to the cranial surface of the tibia in this dog after stabilizing this comminuted tibial fracture with a plate-rod MIPO technique. Adding a second plate to the cranial surface of the tibia added additional stability to this very excitable dog with a very unstable fracture.

the fracture is treated early. Reduction of fragments can be assisted using bone-holding forceps through the proximal and distal incisions (**Fig. 15**).[12] Guiot and Dejardin[12] achieved good or adequate reduction in all patients after MIPO repair of tibial fractures in 36 dogs. Once the limb length is restored to as normal as possible, axial and rotational alignment must be restored. Axial alignment is assessed by evaluating the limb along the sagittal and frontal planes. It is important for the joint surfaces of the stifle and tarsus to be aligned properly. The alignment of the joint surfaces can be evaluated by flexing and extending the stifle and the tarsus and ensuring that the

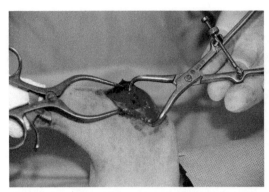

Fig. 15. Pointed reduction forceps can be used with MIPO technique to manipulate fragments when using indirect reduction or to temporarily stabilize the fracture with direct reduction.

plane of motion of both joints is in the same direction The alignment of the joint surfaces can be evaluated by flexing and extending the stifle and the tarsus. Rotational or varus/valgus malalignment can lead to suboptimal function and increase the risk of osteoarthritis. It is often helpful to place an intramedullary pin in normograde fashion to assist in restoring length to the limb and to help attain proper axial alignment. The pin provides temporary stabilization and facilitates application of the plate in MIPO. Any rotational malalignment can easily be resolved by rotating the fracture fragments around the pin. The pin can be either left in place when using a plate-rod construct, or it can be removed after the plate is partially secured to the bone. The intramedullary pin is typically placed normograde from the medial aspect of the tibial plateau, midway between the medial collateral ligament and patellar tendon. The pin should be carefully directed down the medullary canal to avoid accidental penetration of the lateral cortex. Fracture reduction can be assessed by palpation, using fluoroscopy or through a small incision over the fracture (observation portal).[10,12,13,21] See Bruno Peirone and colleagues' article, "Minimally Invasive Plate Osteosynthesis Fracture Reduction Techniques in Small Animals," in this issue for further information on reduction techniques.

SURGICAL APPROACH

A medial surgical approach has been previously described for MIPO of the tibia.[10,12,21] The location of the proximal and distal incisions is based on the plate selected for MIPO.[21] Typically the incisions will be near the proximal and distal extent of the bone because most comminuted fractures treated with MIPO use a plate that spans the entire bone (**Fig. 16**). The authors prefer to make the proximal incision first when using a plate-rod technique or an intramedullary pin for alignment purposes. The distal incision is made second at the site of the intended position of the distal end of the plate. Occasionally a third incision is made over the fracture to confirm accurate placement of the intramedullary pin or to assess fracture alignment (see **Fig. 15**). This incision, if used, is termed the observation portal. It should be emphasized that this portal should not be used to excessively manipulate the fragments and risk disturbing blood supply. The incisions are typically 2 to 4 cm in length. This is usually ample length for placement of 2 to 3 screws proximally and distally. There is very little risk of disturbing muscular of neurovascular structures when using MIPO for tibial fracture repair. An

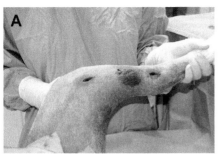
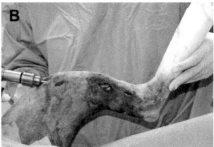

Fig. 16. Typically the incisions for placement of screws will be near the proximal and distal extent of the bone because most comminuted fractures treated with MIPO use a plate that (*A*) spans the entire bone. (*B*) A third incision can be made over the fracture zone to allow a view of the medullary canal of the distal fragment to aid placement of the intramedullary pin when using an MIPO plate-rod technique.

epiperiosteal soft tissue tunnel is developed below the subcutaneous tissues by passing Metzenbaum scissors or a periosteal elevator from the distal to proximal incision. Elevation of the periosteum is not necessary or desired.

SURGICAL PROCEDURE

The intramedullary pin is inserted initially if a plate-rod construct is planned (**Fig. 17**). If using a pin, it is important that the diameter of the pin be 40% of the diameter of the isthmus of the medullary cavity of the tibia.[10,12,26] This will allow ample room for placement of bicortical plate screws without interference by the pin. After fracture reduction is confirmed, the plate is applied. The plate is contoured as needed. Contouring can be facilitated using a radiograph of the opposite normal limb. Limb alignment and fracture reduction should be assessed immediately before plate insertion. The stifle and tarsus should be flexed and extended, making sure the sagittal plane of motion is the same for both joints. Fracture reduction is assessed by palpation, by direct visualization through an observation portal, or with fluoroscopy. The precontoured bone plate is inserted through one of the insertion incisions and slid along the medial surface

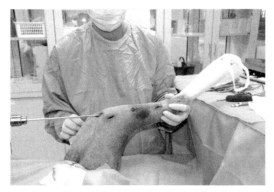

Fig. 17. The intramedullary pin used for a MIPO plate-rod technique is placed initially to help align the fracture and provide bending stability. The pin is placed in normograde fashion through a stab incision over the medial aspect of the tibial plateau midway between the patellar tendon and the medial collateral ligament.

of the tibia through the epiperiosteal tunnel that was previously created until the end of the plate is appropriately positioned in the second incision. It is often easiest to insert the plate through the distal incision and slide the plate toward the proximal incision. If a locking implant is used, it is useful to insert the drill guide in the end plate hole as a handle to insert and position the bone plate on the tibia. The position of the bone plate on the tibia can be checked with direct observation and digital palpation. A screw is inserted through the most distal hole in the bone plate into the distal tibial segment. The screw is centered in the distal tibia unless a plate-rod construct is being used. In this case, it may be necessary to adjust the position of the plate slightly more cranial or caudal to allow screw insertion past the intramedullary pin. The screw should be tightened enough to hold the position of the plate on the distal tibia, but still allow adjustment of the plate on the proximal tibia. Proper limb alignment and fracture reduction should be confirmed and adjusted as needed before insertion of the first proximal screw. The bone plate is adjusted so that the proximal end of the plate is positioned slightly caudal to the center of the proximal tibia. The caudal half of the proximal tibia is wider, therefore provides optimal bone purchase by the screw. The position of the plate should be adjusted as needed to avoid screw interference with an intramedullary pin if used. The first screw is then inserted into the proximal tibial segment through the most proximal hole in the bone plate. The proximal screw is tightened securely and then the first screw that was placed in the distal end of the plate is also tightened securely. Limb alignment and fracture reduction is again assessed. One or 2 additional screws are then sequentially inserted into both the most proximal and the most distal holes in the bone plate. Typically, we insert 3 screws in the proximal segment and either 2 or 3 (length of the segment permitting) screws in the distal segment of the tibia. All screws should obtain bicortical bone purchase if possible. If a combination of screws is used, nonlocking screws should be placed first in each bone segment, followed by locking screws. Typically, the 2 incisions are sufficient for placing all the necessary screws, as a Senn retractor can be used to shift the end of the incision either proximally or distally as necessary to expose additional holes in the bone plate. If a screw needs to be placed in a plate hole that cannot be accessed through the insertion incisions, then a stab incision can be created over the desired plate hole using digital palpation or fluoroscopic guidance. The incisions are closed in routine fashion after the plate is applied.

Occasionally, the MIPO technique can be used to combine direct and indirect reduction in patients having multiple fractures. Indirect reduction can be used to address the comminuted portion of the fracture, whereas direct reduction can be used for the simple portion of the fracture. This is particularly useful when the simple portion of the fracture is located near the end of the bone.

IMMEDIATE POSTOPERATIVE CARE

Immediate postoperative radiographs should be obtained in the anesthetized patient. Fracture apposition and limb alignment should be assessed. The proper alignment of the stifle and tarsal joints is confirmed by checking for proper angulation and rotational orientation. Excessive varus/valgus or rotational deformity should be revised immediately if the patient is stable. The position of the bone plate and screws, as well as the intramedullary pin if used, should be assessed. If screw purchase is inadequate, the screws should be replaced by opening the appropriate incision. If screws have inadvertently penetrated the stifle or tarsal joints, the offending screws should be removed and replaced with a shorter screw. The position of the intramedullary pin should be adjusted as needed to obtain optimal position. The pin is then bent over at its proximal end and cut, or it is cut short and countersunk based on surgeon preference. The authors place a soft-padded bandage as the patient is recovered from anesthesia. Pain management is as needed to keep the patient calm and pain-free.

MANAGEMENT DURING THE POSTOPERATIVE CONVALESCENT PERIOD

If a soft-padded bandage is placed, it is typically replaced with a nonadherent bandage applied over the incision the morning after surgery. Most patients with tibial fracture treated with MIPO are sent home the day after surgery. The patients are treated with postoperative analgesics as needed for 5 to 10 days. Postoperative antibiotic treatment is determined on a case-by-case basis. Activity should be restricted to short leash walks to urinate and defecate for the initial 2 weeks after surgery. Walks can be increased to 3 to 4 five-minute walks after suture removal 10 to 14 days after surgery. Running and jumping are strictly prohibited. Patients will benefit from rehabilitation exercises provided by a trained physiotherapist. Patients can typically walk up and down stairs beginning 6 weeks postoperatively. Swimming can begin 6 weeks after surgery in most patients, depending on the status of the individual patient. Animals

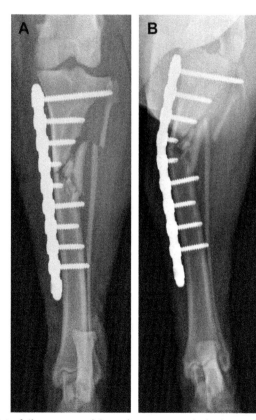

Fig. 18. (*A, B*) Plate failure occurred 3 weeks postoperatively due to cyclic bending loads. Use of a plate-rod technique would have significantly reduced the chance of this complication. Addition of an intramuscular pin 40% the diameter of the medullary canal increases implant life 10 times. The addition of an intramuscular pin helps provide initial alignment and makes placement of the plate and screws easier.

should be confined to a crate after surgery if needed to achieve the activity goals. Owners may assist walking using a sling as needed. Activity is restricted as described until clinical and radiographic documentation of bone healing has been obtained.

ASSESSMENT OF REPAIR AND OUTCOME

Recheck orthopedic examinations should be performed at 2, 4, 6, and 8 weeks. Follow-up radiographs should be obtained at 4 and at subsequent 3-week to 4-week intervals until radiographic evidence of bone union is obtained. Radiographs should consist of orthogonal views of the tibia. Limb alignment, fracture apposition, and integrity of the implants should be assessed and compared with the immediate postoperative radiographs. Fractures are considered healed when bony bridging is evident across the fracture zone on the medial-lateral and cranio-caudal views (see **Fig. 6**). Bridging callus is expected in 3 to 5 weeks in immature patients and 4 to 6 weeks in mature patients.[10,12,13,] The animal is allowed to return to normal activity gradually over a period of several weeks. Complications can also occur with MIPO similar to open reduction internal fixation. The most common complications with MIPO repair of tibial fractures include implant failure or inadequate limb alignment (**Figs. 18** and **19**). Use of an intramuscular pin with bone plates should be considered to reduce strain on the plate and screws because of the presence of a large gap at the

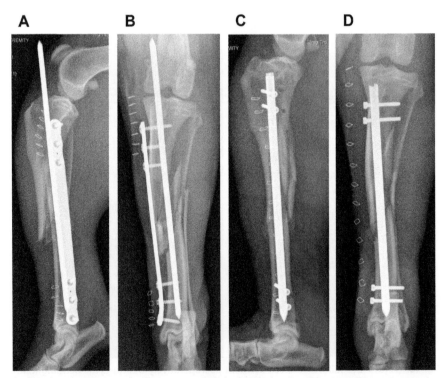

A   **B**   **C**   **D**

Fig. 19. (*A, B*) Suboptimal alignment and limb shortening is evident on this postoperative radiograph. Poor placement of the intramedullary pin led to poor axial alignment. (*C, D*) The patient was taken back to surgery and revised using an interlocking nail, leading to improved axial and torsional alignment and normal limb length.

fracture site. It is important to ensure proper limb alignment at the time of MIPO. Limb alignment should be carefully assessed intraoperatively and postoperatively, and corrected as needed. It is important to achieve both axial and torsional alignment to produce optimal outcome. Fluoroscopy and precontouring of the bone plate to match the opposite normal tibia can help prevent inadvertent limb malalignment.

SUMMARY

Tibial fractures can be repaired successfully using the MIFR technique with little risk of complication. The authors believe tibial fractures are the least complicated to repair using the MIFR technique and thus is an ideal starting point for novice MIFR surgeons. The ability to readily palpate the medial surface of the tibia, due to the lack of soft tissue covering, greatly aids indirect reduction of the fracture and placement of implants. The success of MIFR for repair of tibial fractures is dependent on adequate indirect fracture reduction, appropriate selection of an implant that will provide adequate stability until bridging callus has developed, proper contouring of the plate, preservation of soft tissues and blood supply, and appropriate postoperative management of the patient.

REFERENCES

1. Harasen G. Common long bone fractures in small animal practice—part 1. Can Vet J 2003;44:333–4.
2. Harasen G. Common long bone fracture in small animal practice—part 2. Can Vet J 2003;44:503–4.
3. Piermattei DL, Flo GL, DeCamp CE. Handbook of small animal orthopedics and fracture repair. 4th edition. St Louis (MO): Saunders Elsevier; 2006. p. p359–81.
4. Schwarz G. Fractures of the tibial diaphysis. In: Johnson AL, Houlton JEF, Vannini R, editors. AO principles of fracture management in the dog and cat. Davos (Switzerland): AO Publishing; 2005. p. 319–31.
5. Palmer RH. Biological osteosynthesis. Vet Clin North Am Small Anim Pract 1999; 29:1171–85.
6. Schmokel HG, Hurter K, Schawalder P. Percutaneous plating of tibial fractures in two dogs. Vet Comp Orthop Traumatol 2003;16:191–5.
7. Schmokel HG, Stein S, Radke H, et al. Treatment of tibial fractures with plates using minimally invasive percutaneous osteosynthesis in dogs and cats. J Small Anim Pract 2007;48:157–60.
8. Baroncelli AB, Peirone B, Winter MD, et al. Retrospective comparison between minimally invasive plate osteosynthesis and open plating for tibial fractures in dogs. Vet Comp Orthop Traumatol 2012;25:410–7.
9. Nicetto T, Longo F. Supercutaneous plating for the treatment of injuries of the appendicular skeleton in dogs. Vet Comp Orthop Traumatol 2019;32:149–57.
10. Reems MR, Beale BS, Hulse DA. Use of a plate-rod construct and principles of biological osteosynthesis for repair of diaphyseal fractures in dogs and cats: 47 cases (1994-2001). J Am Vet Med Assoc 2003;223:330–5.
11. Hortsman CL, Beale BS, Conzemius MG, et al. Biological osteosynthesis versus traditional anatomic reconstruction of 20 long bone fractures using an interlocking nail: 1994-2001. Vet Surg 2004;33:232–7.
12. Guiot LP, Dejardin LM. Prospective evaluation of minimally invasive plate osteosynthesis in 36 nonarticular tibial fractures in dogs and cats. Vet Surg 2011;40: 171–82.

13. Hudson CC, Pozzi A, Lewis DD. Minimally invasive plate osteosynthesis: applications and techniques in dogs and cats. Vet Comp Orthop Traumatol 2009;22: 175–82.
14. Johnson AL, Smith CW, Scheffer DJ. Fragment reconstruction and bone plate fixation versus bridging plate fixation for treating highly comminuted femoral fractures in dogs: 35 cases (1987-1997). J Am Vet Med Assoc 1998;213:1157–61.
15. Tong G, Bavonratanavech S. AO manual of fracture management minimally invasive plate osteosynthesis (MIPO). Clavadelerstrasse (Switzerland): AO Publishing; 2007.
16. Krettek C, Muller M, Miclau T. Evolution of minimally invasive plate osteosynthesis (MIPO) in the femur. Injury 2001;32:SC14–23.
17. Farouk O, Krettek C, Miclau T, et al. Effects of percutaneous and conventional plating techniques on the blood supply to the femur. Arch Orthop Trauma Surg 1998;117:438–41.
18. Farouk O, Krettek C, Miclau T, et al. Minimally invasive plate osteosynthesis: does percutaneous plating disrupt femoral blood supply less than the traditional technique? J Orthop Trauma 1999;13:401–6.
19. Borrelli J Jr, Prickett W, Song E, et al. Extraosseous blood supply of the tibia and the effects of different plating techniques: a human cadaveric study. J Orthop Trauma 2002;16:691–5.
20. Johnson AL, Houlton JEF, Vannini R. AO principles of fracture management in the dog and cat. Davos (Switzerland): AO Publishing; 2005.
21. Pozzi A, Lewis D. Surgical approaches for minimally invasive plate osteosynthesis in dogs. Vet Comp Orthop Traumatol 2009;22:316–20.
22. Schutz M, Sudkamp NP. Revolution in plate osteosynthesis: new internal fixator systems. J Orthop Sci 2003;8:252–8.
23. Baumgaertel F, Buhl M, Rahn BA. Fracture healing in biological plate osteosynthesis. Injury 1998;29:C3–6.
24. Evans HE, Christensen GC, editors. Miller's anatomy of the dog. 2nd edition. Philadelphia: W. B. Saunders; 1979. p. 210–5.
25. Pozzi A, Hudson CC, Gauthier CM, et al. A retrospective comparison of minimally invasive plate osteosynthesis and open reduction and internal fixation for radius-ulna fractures in dogs. Vet Surg 2013;42(1):19–27.
26. Hulse D, Hyman W, Nori M, et al. Reduction in plate strain by addition of an intramedullary pin. Vet Surg 1997;26:451–9.
27. Sarrau S, Meige F, Autefage A. Treatment of femoral and tibial fractures in puppies by elastic plate osteosynthesis. A review of 17 cases. Vet Comp Orthop Traumatol 2007;20:51–8.
28. Stoffel K, Dieter U, Stachowiak A, et al. Biomechanical testing of the LCP – how can stability in locked internal fixators be controlled. Injury 2003;34(Suppl 2):11–9.
29. Rovesti GL, Margini A, Cappellari F, et al. Clinical application of intraoperative skeletal traction in the dog. Vet Comp Orthop Traumatol 2006;19:14–9.

Meta-bone Fracture Repair via Minimally Invasive Plate Osteosynthesis

Charles S. McBrien Jr, DVM, MS*

KEYWORDS

- MIPO • Fracture • Metacarpal • Metatarsal

KEY POINTS

- Traditional open methods of fracture repair for metacarpal and metatarsal (meta-bone) fractures in small animal patients have no proven benefit in outcome as compared with external coaptation alone.
- Minimally invasive plate osteosynthesis shows the most promise of currently available techniques to improve outcome in small animal patients.
- The anatomy of meta-bones lends itself particularity well to minimally invasive plate osteosynthesis.

INTRODUCTION

Metatarsal and metacarpal (meta-bone) fractures are commonly seen in veterinary practice and result in lameness or pain in 18% to 70% of the patients who suffer them. Up to 11.9% of all fractures presented are of the meta-bones,[1,2] and nearly half of patients who present with meta-bone fractures have 3 or more fractured bones.[3] Recommendations for the treatment of meta-bone fractures have largely been adopted from the practices of physicians in human patients. These time-honored guidelines include surgery

1. If more than 2 meta-bones are fractured in the same manus or pes
2. If the fractures involve both primary weight-bearing bones (III and IV)
3. If a fracture is articular
4. If fracture segments have suffered greater than 50% displacement
5. If the fracture involves the base of meta II or V (because this will lead to medial and lateral instability and varus or valgus deviation)
6. If the patient is large, giant, an athlete, a working dog, or a show dog[4]

Disclosure Statement: The author has nothing to declare.
MedVet Cleveland West, Cleveland, OH, USA
* 14000 Keystone Parkway, Brook Park, OH 44135.
E-mail address: Charles.mcbrien@medvet.com

Vet Clin Small Anim 50 (2020) 207–212
https://doi.org/10.1016/j.cvsm.2019.08.011
0195-5616/20/© 2019 Elsevier Inc. All rights reserved.

vetsmall.theclinics.com

Despite the relative importance to humans of injuries to the hands or feet (a common outcome measure is days of work missed), physicians also suffer from a paucity of high-level evidence to guide decision making for treatment, with meta-analysis concluding as much.[5] The rigorous application of the scientific method has therefore not really been applied to pets or people, and current veterinary studies have rightly questioned the logic of conventional wisdom. More recent analysis has suggested that surgery via the traditional means of open reduction and internal fixation is not associated with a better outcome than external coaptation alone and is associated with a higher rate of complication.[3] It is important to note that in this study, synostosis is considered a complication, and although undesirable, this outcome is typically of neutral clinical consequence. In addition, open reduction and internal fixation of meta-bone fractures are almost always paired with external coaptation, thus eliminating one of the greatest benefits associated with surgery, namely a faster return to weight-bearing without bandages and bandage-associated costs, management, and complications. Surprisingly, one study found that open reduction and internal fixation were associated with a convalescence period of nearly twice as long in surgical patients than in patients managed conservatively.[6] Because veterinary surgeons aspire to transition from empirically based to evidence-based practices, it is clear that more evidence is needed to make the best recommendations for meta-bone fractures. It is equally clear by the current lack of an unmistakably demonstrated benefit of open surgical repair over external coaptation alone, that better outcomes with new and pioneering techniques must be developed. Although no longer new, minimally invasive plate osteosynthesis (MIPO) is a prime candidate to advance patient care and outcome in the area of meta-bone fractures and potentially to allow these fractures to be treated without concurrent external coaptation.

SURGICAL ANATOMY OF THE META-BONES

Meta-bones II through V are suitable candidates for surgical repair. Each bone is composed of a base proximally that articulates with its correlating numbered carpal or tarsal bone. The base of each meta-bone is in intimate association with adjacent meta-bones. Traveling distally, the base becomes a shaft and terminates at its head. The head of meta-bones articulates with its corresponding phalange. Meta-bones II and III have a slight medial reflection as they travel distally. Meta-bones IV and V likewise gently spiral away from midline as they travel distally and face more laterally. The obliquity of the distal portion of the bone relative to the proximal portion is of particular importance when plating. In addition, the proximal aspect of meta-bones is square, whereas the distal aspect is more rounded. Because meta-bones travel distally, they "fan out." This phenomenon is exaggerated in the cat as compared with the dog.

Extensor tendons run along the dorsal aspect of the metacarpal bones, whereas the vascular bundles are found parallel to them. The common dorsal digital vasculature may be encountered between the base of metacarpals II and III, where it branches to course parallel to the shafts of metacarpals II, III, and IV. The situation is slightly different in the metatarsus, where the tendon of the long digital extensor runs over the entire dorsal aspect of the metatarsus, and the vasculature is generally more numerous and more frequently encountered along the dorsal aspect of the bone.

When considering various strategies for repair, the surgeon should consider that the small size of meta-bones relatively decreases their medullary canal, giving the feeling of more cortical bone and a relatively "harder" bone in most patients. These factors combine to make fracture repair here somewhat technically demanding because the bone is less forgiving, and overall, there is a narrow margin for error, particularly when placing screws that may split the bone and worsen the fracture.

INSTRUMENTATION

Necessary instrumentation includes general surgery instrumentation for execution and closure of stab incisions as well as creation of an epiperiosteal tunnel, small reduction forceps, and the surgeon's choice of internal fixation implants.

Increased options in veterinary orthopedic implants offer the surgeon many choices for MIPO of meta-bones. The Synthes (Solothurn, Switzerland and West Chester, Pennsylvania, United States) Veterinary cuttable plate (1.5/2.0 cortical or 2.0/2.7 cortical), Intrauma (Rivoli, Italy and Hoboken, New Jersey United States of America) Fixin cuttable plates (1.3-1.7 locking, 1.9–2.5 locking), Kyon (Zurich, Switzerland) Advanced locking plate system (also cuttable, 1.5 cortical, 2.4 locking or cortical, 2.7 cortical, 3.2 locking, or 4.0 locking), Liberty Lock (Everost Veterinary Orthopedics, Sturbridge, Massachusetts, United States of America) 2.4 cuttable, as well as a vast array of dynamic compression (DCP), limited contact DCP, and locking compression plates all may be used for MIPO of meta-bones. Given the successful use of the veterinary cuttable plate in MIPO, a locking construct is not considered to be necessary, although their biomechanical preeminence is elsewhere described. The superiority of plate-screw constructs over other commonly used minimally invasive constructs in human metacarpal fractures has also been recently documented with plates assessed as 11 to 15 times stronger in 3-point bending than other constructs.[7]

As in many MIPO applications, fluoroscopy can be a great advantage when repairing meta-bones. However, given their sparse soft tissue coverage and ready palpation paired with MIPO's goal prioritizing alignment over anatomic reduction, intraoperative imaging is not always necessary.

PREOPERATIVE ASSESSMENT AND CARE

Complete physical examination and treatment of the more important injuries associated with trauma are prioritized as usual. When present, open fractures are not ideal candidates for MIPO, although many surgeons operate grade 1 open fractures with plates. Evaluation of meta-bone fractures is readily achieved with lateral and dorsopalmar or plantar radiographs (**Fig. 1**). Sedation or general anesthesia is helpful to obtain quality diagnostic images especially with small fractures at the base or communicating with a joint. When available, imaging of the contralateral normal meta-bones allows the surgeon to use orthopedic templating software to preplan surgery, including selection and length of implants. Preplanning in this way also allows precontouring of plates.

Standard aseptic orthopedic preparation of the patient is performed. Most surgeons operate meta-fractures with the patient in dorsal recumbency, but some find an advantage to positioning the patient sternally ("superman").

OPERATIVE CARE

Fracture alignment is often best achieved by traction. In some fractures, reduction may be palpable, and application of a reduction forceps percutaneously is possible. For meta-bones, stab incisions at the proximal and distal aspect of the bone are executed. Epiperiosteal tunnels are performed through gentle elevation, creating a tunnel between the 2 stab incisions. With tendons retracted, implants are then inserted. Depending on fracture configuration, repair is most easily achieved

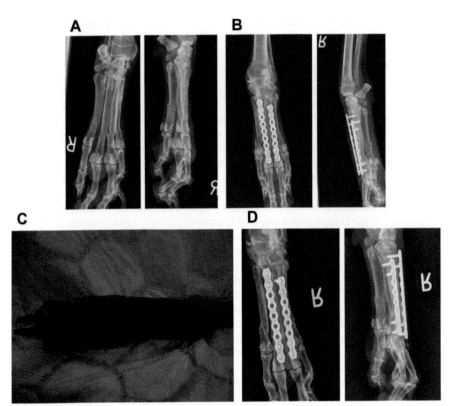

Fig. 1. *(A)* DP and ML radiographs of the right carpus and metacarpus of a 13-year-old Borzoi showing diaphyseal fractures of metacarpal bones II to IV. The carpal joint was partially fused because of a previous trauma unrelated to the actual fractures. *(B)* DP and ML postoperative radiographs after reduction and stabilization of Mc III and IV with 2 ALPS 8-mm plates positioned via dorsally performed tunnels. Good alignment and reduction are observed. Plates were not precontoured, and the most distal screws were applied monocortically to avoid interference with the sesamoid bones. *(C)* Picture taken immediately postoperative showing the sutures where the skin incisions were performed between Mc III and IV to position the plates. Skin incisions were displaced medially and laterally to fix both metacarpal bones. *(D)* DP and ML radiographic follow-up 6 weeks after surgery. Clinical bone union is documented. The implants were not removed because they did not affect performance of the dog. (*From* A. Piras, T. G. Guerrero. Minimally Invasive Repair of Metabones, Veterinary Clinics: Small Animal Practice, 2012; 42:5; with permission.)

by placing the most proximal screw first and then reducing the fracture via traction. Having an assistant apply traction to either the distal aspect of the meta-bone or the phalange with a small point-to-point reduction forceps, or simply digitally, is a useful technique when the fracture cannot be palpated or is too small to practically apply bone reduction forceps to at the fracture site. Once alignment is achieved, the most distal screw is then placed. In placing the distal screw, recall that the distal aspect of the meta-bone is not directly parallel to the proximal aspect and that either subtle plate contouring or angling of the screw will be necessary. In larger meta-bones, there may be enough bone to place a screw in the more lateral or medial aspect if the surgeon is imperfect in implant contouring or screw angling. This potential error is magnified in meta-bones II and V, which generally have greater torsion and demand more precise implant contouring. With all meta-bones, placement of the proximal screw first is imperative because the most proximal aspect of the bone is squarer than the rounded distal aspect. Placing the distal screws first is more likely to lead to malalignment and poor reduction secondary to torsion of the bone as the proximal screw is tightened (dorsal proximally will not be aligned with dorsal distally). In meta-bones, 2 screws (4 cortices) are often all that can be achieved, although more are obviously desirable.

POSTOPERATIVE CARE

Depending on surgeon preference, external coaptation consisting of a soft padded bandage and either cast or caudal splint is applied for 2 to 4 weeks. To date, there are no published cases that have avoided concurrent external coaptation. Patient reevaluation is performed as for most fractures with radiographs at the end of a rest period, around 6 weeks after surgery.

DISCUSSION

MIPO shows the most promise of all techniques for improving the outcome in cats and dogs with meta-bone fractures. External skeletal fixation has fairly clear limitations in meta-bones given their size and general lack of bone to accommodate an appropriate number of pins proximal and distal to fractures. A technique of external skeletal fixation "tied-in" to intramedullary pins has been described for meta-bone fractures in dogs and cats.[8] This open reduction technique has been advocated for juxtaarticular fractures but also raises a concern for morbidity at the metacarpal or metatarsalphalangeal joint. Other minimally invasive techniques that bear investigation but to the author's knowledge have not yet been reported in veterinary patients include "bouquet" pinning, simple crossed K-wire pinning, percutaneous inter-meta-pinning, and flexible intramedullary nail. These techniques are currently used in human patients. Although promising, the main disadvantage of these techniques is similar to external skeletal fixation: care and maintenance associated with implants that are outside of the skin and the necessity for a second procedure for implant removal. Once a familiarity with the principles of MIPO have been achieved and used successfully in larger bones by a veterinary surgeon, its use in meta-bones is considered a viable method of therapy and shows the most promise for improved outcome as compared with open strategies or conservative management.

REFERENCES

1. Ness MG, Abercromby RH, May C, et al. A survey of orthopedic conditions in small animal veterinary practice in Britain. Vet Comp Orthop Traumatol 1996;9:43–52.
2. Phillips IR. A survey of bone fractures in the dog and cat. J Small Anim Pract 1979; 20:661–74.
3. Kornmayer M, Failing K, Matis U. Long-term prognosis of metacarpal and metatarsal fractures in dogs. Vet Comp Orthop Traumatol 2014;1:45–53.
4. Wernham BGJ, Roush JK. Metacarpal and metatarsal fractures in dogs. Compend Contin Educ Vet 2010;32:E1.
5. Zong SL, Zhao G, Su LX, et al. Treatments for the fifth metacarpal neck fractures: a network meta-analysis of randomized controlled clinical trials. Medicine (Baltimore) 2016;95(11):e3059.

6. Kapatkin A, Howe-Smith R, Shofer F. Conservative versus surgical treatment of metacarpal and metatarsal fractures in dogs. Vet Comp Orthop Traumatol 2000; 13:123–7.
7. Curtis BD, Fajolu O, Ruff ME, et al. Fixation of metacarpal shaft fractures: biomechanical comparison of intramedullary nail crossed k wires and plate-screw constructs. Orthop Surg 2015;7:256–60.
8. Fitzpatrick N, Riordan JO, Smith TJ, et al. Combined intramedullary and external skeletal fixation of metatarsal and metacarpal fractures in 12 dogs and 19 cats. Vet Surg 2011;40:1015–22.

Minimally Invasive Osteosynthesis Techniques for Articular Fractures

Grayson Cole, DVM[a],*, Brian Beale, DVM[b]

KEYWORDS

- Minimally invasive osteosynthesis • Articular • Fracture • Dog • Cat

KEY POINTS

- The repair of articular fractures requires anatomic reduction, rigid fixation, and early return to mobility.
- Minimally invasive approaches decrease morbidity and allow an earlier return to function.
- Minimally invasive approaches include mini-arthrotomy, arthroscopic-assisted, and percutaneous techniques.
- Minimally invasive articular fracture repair is performed using implant systems similar to open approaches.

INTRODUCTION

Articular fractures occur commonly in dogs and cats. Articular fractures can occur in any diarthrodial joint, but the most commonly affected joints are the elbow and hip. Repair of articular fractures requires anatomic reduction and rigid fixation to reduce the chance of osteoarthritis and joint dysfunction. Traditional arthrotomy can be used to accomplish these goals, but anatomic reduction can be difficult with certain fractures because of an inability to adequately view the joint surfaces. Minimally invasive osteosynthesis (MIO) using a minimally invasive or mini-arthrotomy approach, arthroscope-assisted approach, or percutaneous techniques have been used to treat articular fractures in humans and in dogs and cats.[1–11] Arthroscope-assisted surgery has the advantages of superior visualization and less invasiveness, improved outcome, and accurate reduction, in addition to the diagnosis and repair of related injuries.[1–3,10] Disadvantages of arthroscopic repair of articular fractures include a

Disclosure Statement: No conflicts of interest to disclose.
The article is an update of "Beale BS, Cole G. Minimally invasive osteosynthesis technique for articular fractures. Vet Clin North Am Small Anim Pract. 2012;42(5):1051-68."
[a] Department of Surgery, Gulf Coast Veterinary Specialists, 8042 Katy Freeway, Houston, TX 77055, USA; [b] Beale Veterinary Specialist and Emergency, 3804 Houston Highway, Victoria, TX 77905, USA
* Corresponding author.
E-mail address: drcole@gcvs.com

learning curve, and possible increase in anesthesia time and initial expense of the needed equipment.

GOALS OF REPAIR OF ARTICULAR FRACTURES

The goal of surgical repair of articular fractures is a return to pain-free motion and to decrease the likelihood and/or progression of osteoarthritis. The principles of articular fracture repair include the following:

1. Anatomic reduction of the articular surface
2. Rigid stabilization
3. Early surgical repair
4. Early mobilization of the joint

Adherence to these important principles is critical to giving the patient the greatest opportunity of maintaining a healthy articular surface, viable hyaline cartilage, normal periarticular supporting connective tissues, and less muscle atrophy and fibrosis. Deviation from the principles will likely lead to a poor outcome characterized by osteoarthritis, joint fibrosis, muscle atrophy, and chronic pain.

FRACTURE ASSESSMENT

Articular fractures involve disruption of the articular surface of the joint within the synovial cavity. Articular fractures are most common in the elbow and hip, but they can also occur in the shoulder, carpus, stifle, and tarsus. Fractures of the joint surface have a greater likelihood of the development of osteoarthritis as compared with fractures that do not involve the joint surface. Many of these fractures also occur in growing dogs and cats. The physis is a common site for fracture because of the relatively weak zone of hypertrophied chondrocytes. Fractures through the physis have been classified by Salter and Harris into 6 types.[12] The severity of physeal fractures increases with the increasing numerical type of Salter-Harris fracture. Some Salter-Harris fractures occur within the joint but do not involve the articular surface. Salter III and IV fractures invade the joint surface and result in an articular fracture. Increased severity of physeal fracture is associated with increased chance of growth disturbance of the physis, potentially leading to limb shortening or angular limb deformity. Identification of an articular component, presence of preexisting orthopedic conditions, presence of physeal involvement, fracture classification, duration of injury, and expected patient and owner compliance are important to consider in the decision-making process for the treatment plan for articular fractures.

INDICATIONS FOR MINIMALLY INVASIVE OSTEOSYNTHESIS

The type of surgical approach for articular fractures should be considered carefully before the start of surgery. Traditional surgical approaches to the joints of the dog and cat have been previously reported and can be used to treat all articular fractures.[13] A minimally invasive surgical approach using an MIO technique is optimal for repair of certain articular fractures, particularly fractures that are minimally displaced, simple (2 pieces), and acute. This may be accomplished using arthroscopy and percutaneous placement of implants or using an arthroscope through a mini-arthrotomy to better view the articular fracture.[1-3,10] The use of an arthroscope within an arthrotomy incision is known as arthroscopic-assisted arthrotomy.[14] The mini-arthrotomy incision is much shorter than the arthrotomy incision used to treat articular fractures using traditional open reduction and stabilization techniques. The mini-arthrotomy incision can be extended as needed to apply implants to stabilize the fracture. An MIO technique can be used for articular fractures of the glenoid, humeral head, humeral condyle, anconeal process, carpus, acetabulum, femoral head, femoral condyle, and tarsus. An MIO technique improves the surgeon's view of the articular surface and results in a more precise repair as a result of the magnification provided by the arthroscope.[2,3] In addition, traumatic cartilage damage that may affect prognosis can be diagnosed at that time. Fluoroscopy also can be used to improve the surgeon's spatial orientation and for assessment of fragment alignment and implant position.[4,6–8] Treatment of articular fractures with arthroscopy and an MIO technique has a significant learning curve. The technique should be practiced on cadavers if available. Novice surgeons can shorten the learning curve by assisting more experienced surgeons who are familiar with the MIO technique and by participating in minimally invasive plate osteosynthesis or MIO short courses that have lecture and laboratory components.

Shoulder

Supraglenoid fractures are uncommon and occur as traumatic or pathologic articular fractures.[2,15] The bicep brachii tendon originates from the supraglenoid tuberosity. Fractures of the supraglenoid tuberosity typically result in a weight-bearing forelimb lameness and shoulder pain. Swelling may be seen over the craniolateral aspect of the shoulder in some patients. Radiographic examination is usually diagnostic. The fracture line is usually clearly seen on the lateral shoulder view because of a distal displacement of the supraglenoid fragment caused by traction by the biceps brachii muscle. This articular fracture involves the cranial aspect of the glenoid cavity (**Fig. 1**). Supraglenoid fractures should be repaired because of the intra-articular nature and potential for chronic pain and future osteoarthritis. The fracture can be repaired using traditional open reduction and internal fixation (ORIF), but anatomic reduction is difficult without using an extensive surgical approach.[13,15,16] Supraglenoid fractures are amenable to a MIO technique.[2,11] Supraglenoid fractures are usually repaired by applying compression with pins or lag screws following anatomic reduction and percutaneous placement of implants (see **Fig. 1**; **Fig. 2**). The fracture can be initially reduced through percutaneous manipulation of the fragment using digital pressure with the surgeon's fingers or by application of a pointed reduction forceps. The ability to reduce the fracture should be confirmed arthroscopically, radiographically, or fluoroscopically. A traditional lateral scope portal or mini-arthrotomy is used when an arthroscope is used. Pointed-reduction forceps should be used to achieve fracture reduction when using imaging techniques to document temporary fracture reduction. It is often difficult to maintain fracture reduction while inserting implants used for stabilization. Final reduction is often performed after placement of a percutaneous Kirschner wire (k-wire). The k-wire is used to achieve temporary fracture stabilization. The fracture should be stabilized using an implant that will provide compression across the fracture line. Implants that are useful for supraglenoid fractures include lag screws, headless compression screws, and cannulated lag screws. An antirotational pin can also be used to provide adjunctive stabilization. Some surgeons perform a proximal biceps tenotomy to remove the distractive force on the fragment before reduction and stabilization of supraglenoid fractures. The reason for this is to ease reduction of the fragment and remove the risk of a potential distractive force postoperatively. The disadvantage of this practice is the potential for creating shoulder instability.[17] Arthroscopic biceps tendon release, however, has been found to result in clinical improvement in dogs with chronic tears of the tendon of origin of the biceps brachii muscle.[18,19]

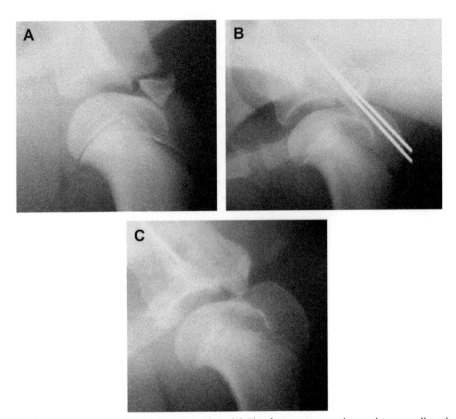

Fig. 1. (*A*) A supraglenoid fracture in a dog. (*B*) The fragment was deemed too small and fragile to place a lag screw. Stabilization was achieved using percutaneous divergent k-wires and a proximal biceps tendon release to remove the distractive force of the biceps. (*C*) Healed supraglenoid fracture following pin removal 8 weeks later.

Fractures of the glenoid cavity of the scapula involving other weight-bearing regions of the scapula occur uncommonly.[15] These fractures should be accurately reduced and stabilized with lag screws or compression pins when involving substantial regions of the glenoid and when fragments are of adequate size for fixation.[15] Reduction can be aided using fluoroscopy, arthroscopy, or arthroscopic-assisted arthrotomy. Surgical stabilization can also be accomplished using these MIO techniques by placing implants in a percutaneous fashion. Caudal glenoid fracture or fragmentation is typically treated with good outcome by arthroscopic excision of the small fragments.[2,20] Extensive or chronic fractures of the glenoid may necessitate shoulder arthrodesis. Excision arthroplasty of the shoulder has also been reported.

Fractures of the humeral head are uncommon. Occasionally, proximal humeral physeal fractures can lead to displacement of the humeral head. MIO technique can be used to repair minimally displaced humeral head fractures. Fluoroscopy or arthroscope-assisted arthrotomy can be used to facilitate fracture reduction and placement of surgical implants. The fracture should be reduced anatomically and stabilized with a suitable implant, applying compression across the articular component of the fracture line. Compression should be avoided across the physeal component of the fracture if there is significant remaining growth potential. Lag screws, headless compression screws or pins are commonly used for this type of fracture. Typically,

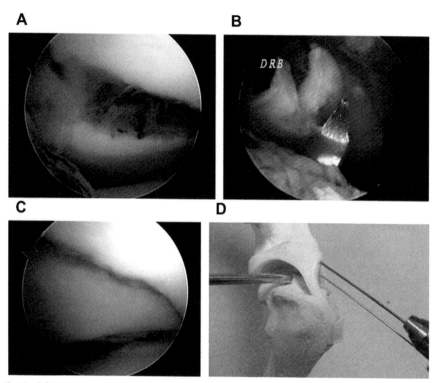

Fig. 2. (A) Arthroscopic view of a supraglenoid fracture in a dog seen in **Fig. 1**. (B) A percutaneous k-wire is placed in the supraglenoid fragment. The fragment is reduced by digital manipulation and use of the k-wire as a joystick. (C) The supraglenoid tuberosity is reduced under arthroscopic visualization using a lateral scope portal. Anatomic reduction is confirmed. (D) MIO technique for treatment of supraglenoid fractures is demonstrated on a bone model. A percutaneous k-wire is placed initially after anatomic reduction to provide temporary stabilization. A cannulated drill bit is used to drill a hole for placement of a cannulated lag screw.

physeal fractures are repaired using k-wires or pins to decrease the chance of developing compression across the physis, leading to premature closure and disruption of growth.

Elbow

Fractures of the lateral or medial humeral condyle are common, especially in growing dogs. Humeral condylar fractures require accurate anatomic reduction and rigid stabilization to achieve a favorable functional outcome. Complications are common if reduction is poor, if implant position is improper, or if surgical time is excessive.[4,21] Unicondylar humeral fractures can be repaired using a MIO technique, especially if minimal displacement is present. Lateral condyle fractures are much more common because of the forces acting though the relatively thin lateral epicondyle. Most lateral condyle fractures in immature dogs are Salter-Harris type III or IV physeal fractures. An MIO technique is easier to perform and recommended in fractures having mild or moderate swelling and a duration of less than 48 hours.[2,4] Traditional ORIF is recommended if substantial displacement has occurred because of the difficulty in achieving anatomic reduction. An MIO technique is not recommended for bicondylar fractures. These fractures are much more unstable and difficult to reduce without direct observation and open manipulation of the fragments. Closed reduction and stabilization of condylar fractures was found to result in minimal disruption of soft tissues and blood supply, decreased risk of infection, and earlier return to function.[4] Fluoroscopy was an effective method for evaluating the type of physeal fracture, assessing fracture reduction, and assisting in positioning implants used to stabilize the fracture.[4] Implants typically used to stabilize lateral or medial condyle fractures include traditional or cannulated lag screws, headless compression screws, or self-compression pins.[2,4–6,21] Reduction is performed using a combination of distraction, digital manipulation, and grasping with bone forceps placed in a percutaneous fashion. Vulsellum forceps, pointed reduction forceps, or a condyle clamp are often used to provide temporary stabilization. If reduction is accurate, both the condylar and epicondylar components should be anatomically aligned. Reduction is confirmed arthroscopically or fluoroscopically (**Fig. 3**).

Stabilization is achieved in most patients with a transcondylar screw and an antirotational pin placed across the epicondylar fracture line in percutaneous fashion. It has also been reported to use pins only for stabilization using multiple transcondylar pins and an antirotational pin in juvenile animals.[22] There is evidence that lateral condylar fractures with comminution are best treated with an epicondylar plate rather than an antirotational pin and therefore comminuted lateral condylar fractures may be treated with an open approach or a minimally invasive plate osteosynthesis technique.[23] Some surgeons prefer to repair the epicondylar portion first, whereas others choose to place the transcondylar screw first (**Fig. 4**). The transcondylar lag or self-compressing screw is percutaneously placed to compress and stabilize the condylar component of the fracture. The most prominent aspect of the lateral and medial epicondyles can be palpated and used as a landmark to place the screw in a proper position. Ideally, the screw is placed parallel to the humeroradial joint near the center of the condyles. The physis should be avoided if possible, to reduce the chance of growth disturbances in growing animals. The largest diameter screw that is appropriate for the patient should be used to decrease the chance of the screw breaking or loosening. Toy breed dogs and cats commonly require a 2.0-mm or 2.4-mm screw. Small, medium-size, large, and giant breed dogs typically require a 2.7, 3.5, 4.5, or 6.5-mm screw, respectively. A washer should be considered if the bone of the condyle is expected to be too soft to withstand the pressure of the screw head as it is tightened and compression is applied. Alternatively, intercondylar stability can be supplied using self-compressing screws or pins (**Fig. 5**).[5,6] An adjunctive antirotational k-wire can also be placed across the condyles to gain additional stability if room permits. It is essential to achieve accurate reduction to lessen the chance of future osteoarthritis. Rigid stabilization is required to prevent shifting of the fragments and proper healing. Early return to joint mobility is critical to maintaining normal elbow range of motion and a successful outcome. A non–weight-bearing sling or carpal flexion bandage can be used postoperatively to protect the repair for the first 1 or 2 weeks after surgery but allow range of motion of the elbow. Physical rehabilitation exercises should be considered starting 2 weeks postoperatively by a trained physiotherapist if possible. See also Karl C. Maritato and Gian Luca Rovesti's article, "Minimally Invasive Osteosynthesis Techniques for Humerus Fractures," in this issue for additional MIO techniques of humeral condylar fractures.

Incomplete ossification of the humeral condyle (IOHC) is a relatively common condition found in spaniel breeds (particularly the Brittany spaniel), but it has also been identified in other breeds including the rottweiler and mixed-breed dogs.[5] IOHC predisposes the dog to condylar fracture with minimal trauma. The condition

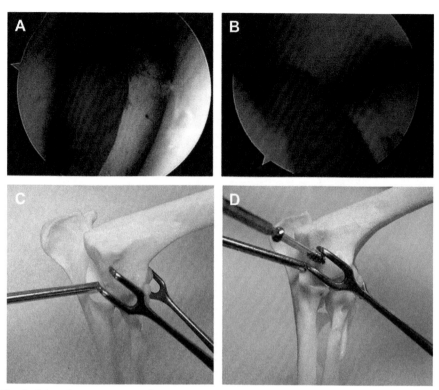

Fig. 3. (*A*) Arthroscopic view of a lateral condyle fracture is present in a dog. The intercondylar fracture gap is filled with the fracture hematoma. (*B*) The fracture is reduced with digital manipulation and compression with a Vulsellum forceps. Reduction may be facilitated by slightly extending the elbow. Excellent reduction of the articular surface has been achieved and the fracture hematoma can be seen protruding from the compressed fracture gap. (*C*) MIO technique for treatment of humeral condyle fractures is demonstrated on a model. The arthroscope is placed through a medial portal to confirm anatomic reduction of the articular surface and compression of the fracture. The Vulsellum forceps can be used to provide temporary stabilization. (*D*) A transcondylar lag screw is placed to apply compression and stabilization. A transcondylar pin can be placed first if desired to provide adjunctive stabilization and to help prevent rotation of the fracture during tightening of the lag screw.

has also been associated with lameness without obvious fracture. IOHC is associated with a zone of incomplete ossification at the mid-portion of the humeral condyle. Fibrous tissue is found in this region. The adjacent bone of the condyle is more dense than normal. IOHC is diagnosed using radiographic examination, computed tomography, or arthroscopy.[2,6,24,25] IOHC is commonly bilateral and is often diagnosed in the opposite asymptomatic elbow in dogs that have sustained a Y-fracture of the distal humerus as a result of minimal trauma. A transcondylar positional screw can be placed in MIO fashion in asymptomatic or symptomatic dogs with IOHC in an attempt to prevent future fracture and resolve lameness if present (see **Fig. 5**).[2] The goal of the screw is simply to buttress the zone of incomplete ossification to prevent fracture. Compression should not be applied across this area as this may actually increase the chance of fracture because of tension placed on the thin lateral epicondyle. The screw should have maximal diameter to prevent breakage of the screw because of

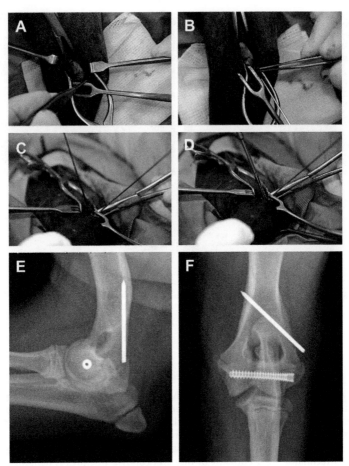

Fig. 4. (*A*) A small incision has been made over the lateral epicondyle of this dog with a lateral humeral condyle fracture. The epicondylar portion of the fracture is reduced. (*B*) A pin has been normograded across the epicondylar fracture and a Vulsellum forceps has been applied to reduce the intercondylar portion of the fracture. Reduction was confirmed using a C-arm. (*C*) A transcondylar guide wire was placed across the humeral condyle under fluoroscopic guidance. (*D*) A cannulated self-compressing screw is inserted across the fracture over the guide wire, providing compression and stability. (*E*) Lateral postoperative radiograph. The lumen of the cannulated screw is evident. (*F*) Anteroposterior postoperative radiograph. Anatomic reduction and stabilization have been achieved with a headless, self-compressing screw in the humeral condyle and a pin in the lateral epicondyle.

the effects of expected implant cycling and potential fatigue failure. Fitzpatrick and colleagues[6] have described an MIO technique to enhance healing in dogs with IOHC using an osteochondral autograft and a self-compressing screw.

Other intra-articular elbow fractures and disorders that can be occasionally treated using an MIO technique include anconeal fractures, medial coronoid fractures (jump-down syndrome), and radial head fractures.[2] The same principles of anatomic reduction and rigid stabilization apply to these fractures. Fractures with fragments that are too small to be reduced and stabilized, such as with the medial coronoid process, should be removed arthroscopically if possible.[2]

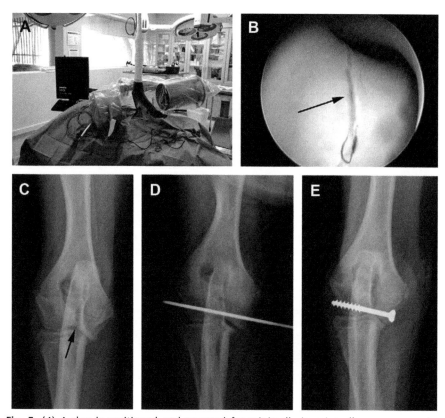

Fig. 5. (*A*) A dog is positioned and prepped for minimally invasive elbow surgery using fluoroscopy and arthroscopy. (*B*) Arthroscopic examination of the elbow confirmed IOHC (*arrow*). (*C*) IOHC (*arrow*) is seen in the dog with forelimb lameness. (*D*) A guide pin has been normograded across the humeral condyle using fluoroscopic guidance. (*E*) A cannulated screw has been placed across the humeral condyle over the guide pin. The screw is used to buttress the gap in the condyle. Lameness resolved in this dog and potential condylar fracture did not occur 6 years after surgery.

Ununited anconeal process (UAP) can also be stabilized using an MIO technique. This is best performed when the dog is immature and the fragment is minimally displaced and has viable hyaline cartilage and no evidence of radiographic remodeling. A distal dynamic ulnar osteotomy is initially performed through a small incision over the caudolateral aspect of the distal third of the ulna. The osteotomy gap is widened using distraction forceps or by levering with an elevator. The interosseous ligament can be disrupted as needed to free the ulna from the radius to allow less restricted movement of the ulna. The elbow is evaluated arthroscopically through a standard medial portal.[2] Many patients having UAP also have a concurrent fragmented medial coronoid process.[2,26] Treatment of the fragmented medial coronoid process should be performed in routine fashion at the discretion of the surgeon. The UAP fragment is identified and evaluated. A decision should be made whether to remove or reduce and stabilize the UAP fragment. If needed, fibrous tissue can be removed and debrided at the interface between the fragment and the olecranon using an arthroscopic shaver.[2] If the articular surface of the fragment seems to be in good condition a small threaded k-wire is percutaneously placed from the olecranon to the gap adjacent to the fragment (**Fig. 6**). This wire will be used for as a guide wire for a cannulated screw. The fragment is reduced and partially immobilized by placing the elbow in full extension. Placing the elbow in this position aids reduction and stabilization of the fragment. A caudal instrument portal can be created proximal to the anconeal process if needed to insert a freer elevator into the joint to lever the fragment against the olecranon.[2] This provides additional immobilization and resistance while the k-wire is driven into the fragment. Anatomic alignment is assessed using the arthroscope. The k-wire is driven into the fragment to provide initial stabilization. A small skin incision is made at the k-wire. An appropriate-sized cannulated drill bit is used over the guide wire to drill a hole in the olecranon and the fragment. A cannulated lag screw or headless compression screw is applied over the guide wire, compressing the gap between the fragment and the olecranon.

Carpus

Distal radial articular and radiocarpal bone fractures are occasionally seen. Diagnosis is achieved using radiography, computed tomography, or arthroscopy. If displacement is minimal, these fractures can be reduced closed and temporarily stabilized

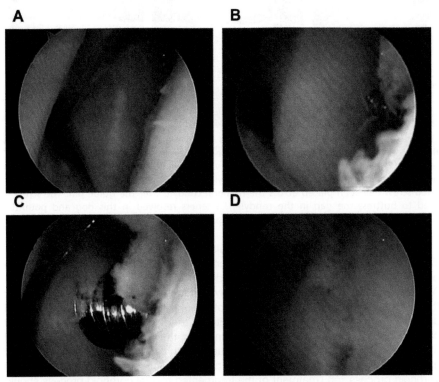

Fig. 6. (*A*) A UAP is seen in this dog. A proximal dynamic ulnar osteotomy was performed initially. (*B*) A threaded guide pin is percutaneously placed in the olecranon under arthroscopic visualization. The pin exits at the gap between the olecranon and the ununited fragment. The elbow is then extended to partially close the gap and stabilize the fragment. The pin is inserted into the fragment. (*C*) A cannulated lag screw is inserted over the guide pin into the fragment. (*D*) The screw is tightened, compressing the gap and stabilizing the fragment.

with a percutaneous pointed bone reduction forceps. Arthroscopic or fluoroscopic assessment is needed to accurately reduce the fracture when using an MIO technique. The fractures are typically stabilized using a lag screw, headless compression screw, or self-compressing pin through a small incision.[8,27] A cannulated screw is often used to facilitate the repair. Screws should be placed in compression mode. Headless compression screws have been found to be an effective means of stabilizing radiocarpal bone fractures.[27] Small chip fractures or avulsion fractures associated with collateral ligaments are generally not of adequate size for fixation, but they can be removed minimally invasively using arthroscopy.[28]

Acetabular Fractures

Acetabular fractures are relatively common pelvic fractures in dogs and cats and are categorized by their location (cranial, middle, and caudal). Caudal acetabular fractures and nondisplaced acetabular fractures in skeletally immature animals have been treated successfully with conservative management,[15,29,30] but all other acetabular fractures require surgical fixation to lessen the chance of osteoarthritis and a poor functional outcome.[31,32] These fractures are traditionally repaired via plating, screws and wire, or screws and polymethylmethacrylate.[31–33] Minimally invasive acetabular fracture repair has been reported in the human literature with assistance from computed tomography, fluoroscopy, arthroscopy, and, most commonly, a combination of fluoroscopy and arthroscopy.[10] Good candidates for percutaneous screw placement are articular fractures that are nondisplaced or minimally displaced. Use of an MIO technique for treatment of acetabular fractures in dogs and cats has not been reported to the authors' knowledge. The authors have used arthroscopy to assist in evaluation of the anatomic reduction of acetabular fractures in dogs. The arthroscope provides a magnified view of the articular fracture line along the dorsal acetabular rim so that optimal reduction can be achieved. Arthroscopy also gives a better view of the medial acetabulum to help ensure adequate reduction and ensure the absence of offending intra-articular fragments.

Capital Physeal Fractures

Capital physeal fractures are typically seen in dogs between the ages of 4 and 11 months of age.[15,33,34] However, spontaneous (atraumatic) capital physeal fractures have been described in cats as old as 16 months and are suspected to be to the result of delayed physeal closure.[35] Predisposed cats are commonly male, neutered, and overweight. Spontaneous capital physeal fractures have also been reported in dogs, humans, and rabbits.[33–36] Capital physeal fractures in dogs and cats are most commonly repaired via divergent or parallel k-wires in an effort to preserve the physis.[15,33] Parallel k-wire fixation has been shown to be stronger than divergent k-wire fixation in an in vitro study in dogs.[37] In mature animals, lag screw fixation can be used. In human children with capital physeal fractures, multiple k-wire fixation has been shown to have a higher complication rate than single cannulated screw fixation.[38] Prophylactic fixation of the contralateral hip, if unaffected, is recommended in children.[38] Feline capital physeal fractures are bilateral approximately 34% of the time according to one study; however, prophylactic fixation of the contralateral hip has not been reported in veterinary medicine.[35] The goals of capital physeal fracture fixation are anatomic reduction, restoration of stability, prevention of osteoarthritis, and avoidance of complications such as avascular necrosis and chondrolysis.[35–37] Femoral capital physeal closure also should be avoided in skeletally immature animals.[33,35,37] MIO repair can be used to treat minimally displaced femoral capital physeal fractures in dogs and cats (**Fig. 7**). Fracture reduction is usually accomplished by placing the hip in full extension while the patient is positioned in dorsal recumbency. Fluoroscopy or radiographic imaging is used to confirm adequate reduction. Fracture reduction can be adjusted slightly with manipulation of the proximal femur using percutaneous

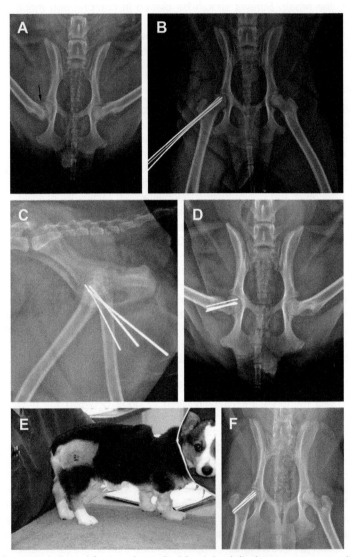

Fig. 7. (A) A capital physeal fracture (*arrow*) with minimal displacement was seen in this dog with a right hindlimb lameness. The frog-leg view was necessary to make the diagnosis because minimal displacement was seen on the ventrodorsal view. (B) The fracture was reduced by placing the hip in extension. Reduction was confirmed radiographically, and 3 divergent pins were placed across the fracture through a small incision over the lateral aspect of the proximal femur. (C) Adequate pin placement is checked on the lateral view of the hip. (D) The ventrodorsal postoperative radiograph confirms good reduction, stability, and positioning of the implants. (E) A small lateral incision was used to place the pins across the fracture of the capital physis in this corgi. (F) Follow-up radiographs at 6 weeks confirm healing of the fracture.

pointed reduction forceps attached to the greater trochanter. Minimally invasive placement of k-wires or screws can be accomplished in small animals with the help of fluoroscopic guidance and percutaneous placement. Implants should be well seated in the epiphysis of the femoral head but not disrupt the articular cartilage or the round ligament, which contains a portion of the blood supply to the femoral head.[33] Arthroscopy, fluoroscopy, or radiography of the hip can be used to verify adequate bone purchase and that pins do not penetrate the joint when using an MIO technique. See also Michael P. Kowaleski's article, "Minimally Invasive Osteosynthesis (MIO) Techniques of the Femur," in this issue for additional MIO techniques of femoral head and neck fractures.

Femoral Head and Neck Fractures

Femoral neck fractures are most commonly seen in dogs younger than 1 year and are typically associated with trauma.[16,37–39] Femoral neck fractures are also seen in kittens.[40–42] Simple fractures are typically repaired with a lag screw and an antirotational k-wire or divergent k-wires. Comminuted fractures in dogs are best treated with femoral head and neck ostectomy or total hip replacement. Fluoroscopic guidance can be used to place implants across the femoral neck in a similar manner as discussed for capital physeal fractures; however, compression is recommended for fixation of femoral neck fractures. A cadaveric study reported that the stability of femoral neck fracture repair achieved with Orthofix Magic Pins (Orthofix, Lewisville, TX) has similar load to failure as traditional fixation methods.[37] Orthofix Magic Pins can be inserted under fluoroscopic guidance and can achieve compression without predrilling or pretapping. Cannulated screws or other self-compressing implants can be placed percutaneously in combination with fluoroscopy to evaluate reduction and proper implant placement. See also Michael P. Kowaleski's article, "Minimally Invasive Osteosynthesis (MIO) Techniques of the Femur," in this issue for additional MIO techniques of femoral head and neck fractures.

Femoral Condylar Fractures

Fractures of the femoral condyle are most commonly Salter-Harris type II fractures in immature dogs.[16,43] A variety of fixation methods have been described for these fractures including a single intramedullary pin, cross-pinning, and dynamic intramedullary pinning; however, the latter 2 methods have shown greater in vitro load to failure.[16,43] Slight overreduction of the distal segment during intramedullary pinning allows for greater pin purchase, especially in dogs. Femoral condylar fractures are typically good candidates for minimally invasive fluoroscope-guided repair if displacement is minimal because closed reduction is inherently stable as a result of the interdigitating pegs of the distal femoral physis. Cross-pinning and dynamic intramedullary pinning can both be performed percutaneously with fluoroscopic guidance; however, cross-pinning is less technically challenging. Cross-pins should be placed such that they cross proximal to the fracture site and do not penetrate the articular cartilage of the stifle.

Tibial Plateau Fractures

Tibial plateau fractures are also most commonly seen in immature animals and can be associated with femoral condylar fractures.[16] In human orthopedics, tibial plateau fractures are classified into 6 types with multiple subtypes according to the Schatzker system.[40] Salter-Harris fractures of the tibial condyle can be repaired using a minimally invasive cross-pinning technique similar to that discussed for the distal femur with use of fluoroscopic guidance. In immature dogs, care should be taken not to permanently close the physis. Compression of the physis should be avoided. Varus and valgus stress radiography may be helpful in the diagnosis of minimally displaced Salter-Harris fractures of the proximal tibia. Tibial physeal separations may also occur in combination with tibial tuberosity avulsions. Small terrier breeds may be overrepresented for this combination of injuries. This type of fracture can be managed with percutaneous cross-pins in the proximal tibial physis and 2 pins in the tibial tuberosity. The stifle should be immobilized in slight extension for 10 days. Pins may be removed when the fracture has healed in 3 to 4 weeks if desired. Some surgeons remove pins in an attempt to prevent compression of the physis caused by the cross-pins as the tibia grows. Successful management of proximal tibial physeal and tibial tuberosity fractures has been reported with pin and tension band fixation and crossed k-wires.[44] A side effect of using a stainless steel tension band across the physis of the tibial tuberosity is premature physeal closure, leading to distal displacement of the tibial tuberosity and possibly patella baja. The authors typically use large diameter nylon as a tension band rather than stainless steel, to reduce the chance of physeal closure in dogs that have substantial remaining growth. This provides adequate stability to prevent displacement of the tibial tuberosity when stabilized with pins only but may result in less compression of the physis. When using this technique, strict exercise restriction is needed, and ideally the stifle is bandaged in relative extension for approximately 2 weeks. In addition, conservative management of minimally displaced tibial tuberosity avulsion fractures has been reported in 8 skeletally immature large breed dogs.[45]

Distal Tibia and Fibular Fractures

Surgical stabilization of fractures of the medial malleolus (of the tibia) and the lateral malleolus (of the fibula) is recommended because of their intra-articular nature and because these are the sites of origin of the collateral ligaments of the tarsus. Conservative management leads to continued tarsal instability and eventual osteoarthritis in most patients. Malleolar fracture repair has been reported with lag screw fixation, pin and tension band fixation, and k-wire fixation. Malleolar fractures are often associated with shear injuries, and fracture fixation may be complicated by open wound management and delayed stabilization. Collateral ligament instability of the tarsus can be repaired using a transarticular external fixator for 6 to 8 weeks or by ligament reconstruction and/or malleolar fracture stabilization. If minimal displacement is present, closed reduction can be performed and percutaneous self-compressing pins, lag screws, or headless compression screws can be used. Lateral malleolus fractures are usually repaired with a pin and tension band. Arthroscopic or fluoroscopic evaluation can be used to assess anatomic reduction of the articular surface. Comminuted fractures of the distal tibia frequently require open reduction or arthrodesis, and these patients are not good candidates for minimally invasive repair. Postoperative coaptation is recommended for 2 to 8 weeks following malleolar fracture repair or collateral ligament repair in most patients.

Central Tarsal Bone Fractures

Central tarsal bone fractures are most commonly fatigue fractures that are seen in the right hock of racing greyhounds, but they have also been reported in border collies and other breeds. Fractures of the plantar process of the central tarsal bone may look radiographically like luxations, with most of the central tarsal bone luxating in a dorso-medial direction. Repair of the central tarsal bone is associated with cartilaginous depressions and ligamentous injuries, thereby indicating the use of arthroscopy in diagnosing concurrent pathology and assessing reduction.

Talar Fractures

Fractures of the trochlear ridges of the talus are generally associated with a traumatic episode, but are uncommonly reported. Talar ridge fractures must be differentiated from osteochondritis dissecans lesions. Diagnostic imaging in this location is challenging because of the superimposition of other tarsal structures. A flexed dorsoplantar (skyline) view or plantaromedial dorsolateral radiograph can be useful in diagnosis; however, computed tomography is more sensitive and very helpful in evaluating the severity and configuration of the fracture. Fracture fixation is commonly performed with k-wires or lag screws, with the latter being preferred if the fragments are large enough to permit screw fixation. Traditional implants should be countersunk so that they do not protrude on the articular surface, or headless compression screws should be used. There are limited case reports of minimally invasive repair of talar fractures in humans but none, to the authors' knowledge, in animals. However, tarsal arthroscopy may be useful to assess concurrent pathology in the joint before surgery and may be helpful in evaluating reduction. Postoperatively, exercise should be restricted to leash walks only until the fracture has healed. A soft padded bandage can be used for 2 weeks postoperatively if desired, but early range of motion exercise is recommended to improve patient outcome.

Calcaneal Fractures

Calcaneal fractures are another common injury in the racing greyhound, but are also seen less commonly in other dogs and cats. They are frequently associated with either a central tarsal bone fracture or plantar proximal intertarsal subluxation. These fractures are traditionally approached laterally and fixed either with a plate or pin and tension band. Calcaneal fractures that have articular involvement typically require ORIF or arthrodesis. No reports of minimally invasive repair of calcaneal fractures exist in the veterinary literature. The human orthopedic literature typically recommends ORIF of intra-articular calcaneal fractures; however, there is recent literature regarding a new implant similar to an interlocking nail that has been used with the aid of fluoroscopy. As with other tarsal injuries, significant comminution may require arthrodesis.

POSTOPERATIVE CARE

The goal of fixation of articular fractures is to allow range of motion of the affected joint as soon as possible postoperatively to reduce joint stiffness and periarticular fibrosis. Damage to articular cartilage, especially in situations where larger segments of articular cartilage are damaged, should be protected from heavy weight bearing in the early stages, to allow for healing. However, joint motion is required to maintain health and promotes healing of injured articular surfaces. Early joint motion, while avoiding overloading, can be accomplished via several mechanisms. Non–weight-bearing bandages, such as a carpal flexion bandage, can be used to allow joint motion without weight bearing. Passive range of motion exercises can also accomplish this goal. Passive range of motion is especially recommended in patients that are not bearing weight and can be accomplished by owners at home with proper instruction. Underwater exercises and sling walking can also allow for joint motion without excessive loading on implants. Prolonged immobilization should be avoided to prevent bone atrophy, muscle atrophy, and articular cartilage damage. Movement is imperative for synovial fluid to nourish all cartilage within the joint. Articular cartilage changes resulting from immobilization may occur as soon as 2 weeks. In addition, immobilization can lead to periarticular adhesions between synovial folds and proliferation of fibrous connective tissue, all leading to decreased range of motion. Use of a canine rehabilitation specialist may be warranted for patients with a prolonged recovery or complications.

REFERENCES

1. Atesok K, Doral MN, Whipple T. Arthroscopy assisted fracture fixation. Knee Surg Sports Traumatol Arthrosc 2011;19:320–9.
2. Beale BS, Hulse DA, Schulz KA, et al. Small animal arthroscopy. Philadelphia: Saunders; 2003.
3. Miller J, Beale B. Tibiotarsal arthroscopy: applications and long-term outcome in dogs. Vet Comp Orthop Traumatol 2008;21:159–65.
4. Cook JL, Tomlinson JL, Reed A. Fluoroscopically guided closed reduction and internal fixation of fractures of the lateral portion of the humeral condyle: prospective study of the technique and results in 10 dogs. Vet Surg 1999;28:315–21.
5. Guille AE, Lewis DD, Anderson TP, et al. Evaluation of surgical repair of humeral condylar fractures using self-compress Orthofix pins in 25 dogs. Vet Surg 2004; 33:314–24.
6. Fitzpatrick N, Smith TJ, O'Riordan J. Treatment of incomplete ossification of the humeral condyle with autogenous bone grafting techniques. Vet Surg 2009; 38(2):173–84.
7. Hudson CC, Pozzi A. Minimally invasive repair of central tarsal bone luxation in a dog. Vet Comp Orthop Traumatol 2012;25(1):79–82.
8. Perry K, Fitzpatrick N, Johnson J. Headless self compressing cannulated screw fixation for treatment of radiocarpal bone fracture or fissure in dogs. Vet Comp Orthop Traumatol 2010;25:84–101.
9. Kregor PJ. Distal femur fractures with complex articular involvement. Orthop Clin North Am 2002;33(1):153–75.
10. Yang J, Chouhan DK, Oh K. Percutaneous screw fixation of acetabular fractures; applicability of hip arthroscopy. Arthroscopy 2010;26(11):1556–61.
11. Deneuche AJ, Viguier E. Reduction and stabilization of a supraglenoid tuberosity avulsion under arthroscopic guidance in a dog. J Small Anim Pract 2002;43(7): 308–11.
12. Salter RB, Harris WR. Injuries involving the epiphyseal plate. J Bone Joint Surg Am 1963;45:587–624.
13. Piermattei DL, Johnson KA. An atlas of surgical approaches to the bones and joints of the dog and cat. 4th edition. Philadelphia: Elsevier; 2004.
14. Beale BS, Hulse DA. Arthroscopy vs arthrotomy for surgical treatment. In: Muir P, editor. Advances in the canine cranial cruciate ligament. Ames (IO): Wiley-Blackwell; 2010. p. 23–7.
15. Johnson A, Houlton J, Vannini R. AO principles of fracture management. Clavadelerstrasse (Switzerland): AO Publishing; 2005.
16. Piermattei DL, Flo G, DeCamp C. Handbook of small animal orthopedics and fracture repair. 4th edition. St Louis (MO): Elsevier; 2006.
17. Sidaway BK, McLaughlin RM, Elder SH, et al. The role of the tendons of the biceps brachii and infraspinatus muscles and the medial glenohumeral ligaemtnin the maintenance of passive shoulder joint stability in dogs. Am J Vet Res 2004;65(9):1216–24.
18. Whitney WO, Beale BS, Hulse DA. Arthroscopic release of the biceps tendon for treatment of bicipital injury in the dog. Proceedings of the 28th annual conference of the Veterinary Orthopedic Society. February 24–March 1, 2001. Lake Louise (Canada): Veterinary Orthopedic Society; 2001. p. 3.

19. Wall CR, Taylor R. Arthroscopic biceps brachii tenotomy as a treatment for canine bicipital tenosynovitis. J Am Anim Hosp Assoc 2002;38(2):169–75.
20. Morgan OD, Reetz JA, Brown DA. Complication rate, outcome, and risk factors associated with surgical repair of fractures of the lateral aspect of the humeral condyle in dogs. Vet Comp Orthop Traumatol 2008;21:400–5.
21. Olivieri M, Piras A, Marcellin-Little D, et al. Accessory caudal glenoid ossification centre as possible cause of lameness in nine dogs. Vet Comp Orthop Traumatol 2004;17(3):131–5.
22. Cinti F, Pisani G, Vezzoni L, et al. Kirschner wire fixation of Salter Harris type IV fracture of the lateral aspect of the humeral condyle in growing dogs. Vet Comp Orthop Traumatol 2017;30:62–8.
23. Coggeshall JD, Lewis DD, Iorgulescu A, et al. Adjuct fixation with a Kirschner wire or a plate for lateral unicondylar humeral fracture stabilization. Vet Surg 2017;46:933–41.
24. Moores AP, Agthe P, Schaafsma IA. Prevalence of incomplete ossification of the humeral condyle and other abnormalities of the elbow in English springer spaniels. Vet Comp Orthop Traumatol 2012;15(3):211–6.
25. Marcellin-Little DJ, DeYoung DJ, Ferris KK, et al. Incomplete ossification of the humeral condyle in spaniels. Vet Surg 1994;25(6):475–87.
26. Meyer-Lindenberg A, Fehr M, Nolte I. Coexistence of ununited anconeal process and fragmented medial coronoid process of the ulna in the dog. J Small Anim Pract 2006;47:61–5.
27. Perry K, Fitzpatrick N, Yeadon R. Headless compression screw fixation for treatment of radial carpal bone fracture or fissure in dogs. Vet Comp Orthop Traumatol 2010;25(2):94–101.
28. Warnock JJ, Beale BS. Arthroscopy of the antebrachiocarpal joint in dog. J Am Vet Med Assoc 2004;244(6):867–74.
29. Brinker WO, Braden TD. Pelvic fractures. In: Brinker WO, Hohn RB, Prieur WD, editors. Manual of internal fixation in small animals. New York: Springer-Verlag; 1984. p. 40–52.
30. Denny HR. Pelvic fractures in the dog – a review of 125 cases. J Small Anim Pract 1978;19(3):151–66.
31. Boudrieau RJ, Kleine LJ. Nonsurgically managed caudal acetabular fractures in dogs: 15 cases (1979-1984). J Am Vet Med Assoc 1988;193(6):701–5.
32. Lewis DD, Stubbs WO, Neuwirth L, et al. Results of screw/wire/polymethylmethacrylate composite fixation for acetabular fractures in 14 dogs. Vet Surg 1997;26(3):223–34.
33. Moores AP, Owen MR, Coe RJ, et al. Slipped capital femoral epiphysis in dogs. J Small Anim Pract 2004;45:602–8.
34. Simpson DJ, Lewis DD. Fractures of the femur. In: Slatter D, editor. Textbook of small animal surgery. 3rd edition. Philadelphia: Saunders; 2003. p. 2059–89.
35. McNicholas WT Jr, Wilkens BE, Blevins WE, et al. Spontaneous femoral capital physeal fractures in adult cats: 26 cases (1996-2001). J Am Vet Med Assoc 2002;241(12):1731–6.
36. Knudsen CS, Langley-Hobbs SJ. Spontaneous femoral capital physeal fractures in a Continental giant rabbit. Vet Rec 2010;166:462–3.
37. Tilson DM, Roush JK, McLaughlin RM. Biomechanical comparison of three repair methods of proximal femoral physeal fractures in shear and tension. Vet Comp Orthop Traumatol 1994;7:136–9.
38. Azzopardi T, Sharma S, Bennet GC. Slipped capital epiphysis in aged children less than 10 years. J Pediatr Orthop B 2010;19(1):13–8.

39. Fisher SC, McLaughlin RM, Elder SH. In vitro biomechanical comparison of 3 methods for internal fixation of femoral neck fractures in dogs. Vet Comp Orthop Traumatol 2012;26(1):36–41.
40. Jeffrey ND. Internal fixation of femoral head and neck fractures in the cat. J Small Anim Pract 1989;30:674–7.
41. Beale B. Orthopedic clinical techniques femur fracture repair. Clin Tech Small Anim Pract 2004;19(3):134–50.
42. Markhardt BK, Gross JM, Monu JUV. Schatzker classification of tibial plateau fractures: use of CT and MR imaging improves assessment. Radiographics 2009;12(2):589–98.
43. Daly WR. Femoral head and neck fractures in the dog and cat: a review of 115 cases. Vet Surg 1978;7:29–38.
44. Pratt JN. Avulsion of the tibial tuberosity with separation of the proximal tibial physis in seven dogs. Vet Rec 2001;149(12):352.
45. von Pfeil DJ, Decamp CE, Ritter M, et al. Minimally displaced tibial tuberosity avulsion fracture in nine skeletally immature large breed dogs. Vet Comp Orthop Traumatol 2012;25(6):524–31.

Minimally Invasive Repair of Sacroiliac Luxation

James Tomlinson, DVM, MVSc

KEYWORDS

- Sacroiliac joint • Sacroiliac fracture/luxation • Fluoroscopy
- Minimally invasive repair

KEY POINTS

- Sacroiliac fracture-luxation is a common injury that is associated with ilial and acetabular fractures of the opposite hemipelvis.
- A minimally invasive technique for reduction and stabilization of sacroiliac fracture-luxation is a viable option for repair.
- A minimally invasive approach to reduce and stabilize a sacroiliac fracture-luxation is a viable method that equals or exceeds repair by an open method.
- Fluoroscopy is required to perform closed reduction and lag screw stabilization.

INTRODUCTION

Sacroiliac (SI) fracture-luxation is a common injury that is associated with ilial and acetabular fractures of the opposite hemipelvis.[1] SI fracture-luxation results in an unstable pelvis and potentially compromise of the pelvic canal. Bilateral SI fracture-luxations also occur without associate fractures of the ilium or acetabulum. Although conservative management of SI fracture-luxations is a treatment option, alignment and fixation is my preferred method of treatment. Surgery allows a quicker return to weight-bearing and prevents obstipation from pelvic canal collapse.[1]

The approaches for open reduction and methods of stabilization have been described.[1] Difficulty in finding the exact place for screw insertion, especially on the lateral side of the ilium, is a drawback to the open approach for stabilization. Another difficulty with an open approach is directing the screw across the sacrum so that the spinal canal and the lumbosacral disk space are not penetrated, yet allowing the screw to gain at least 60% purchase of the sacrum.[1,2] Angles for directing the screw across the sacrum have been described but may be difficult to execute during surgery.[3–5]

Disclosure Statement: None.

The article is an update of "Tomlinson J. Minimally invasive repair of sacroiliac luxation in small animals. Vet Clin North Am Small Anim Pract 2012;42(5):1069-77."

Department of Veterinary Medicine and Surgery, College of Veterinary Medicine, University of Missouri, 900 East Campus Drive, Columbia, MO 65211, USA

E-mail address: tomlinsonj@missouri.edu

A minimally invasive approach to the reduction and insertion of a screw for fixation of SI fracture-luxation using fluoroscopic guidance has been described.[6] The advantage of using this technique is that a small incision is made with minimal soft tissue disruption and reduced surgical time. Closed reduction of the SI fracture-luxation has been shown to be similar to an open repair technique.[2,6,7] Exact screw placement is facilitated by fluoroscopy to make sure that the disk space or vertebral canal are not penetrated yet, allowing an adequate length of screw purchase in the sacrum.[6,7] The big drawback to this procedure is that it requires the use of intraoperative fluoroscopy. Intraoperative fluoroscopy (C-arm) equipment is expensive and potentially exposes personnel to radiation.

SACROILIAC ANATOMY

The SI joint anatomy has been described.[8] Periarticular ligaments are located dorsal and ventral as the dorsal and ventral SI ligaments. Cranial SI ligaments are also present.[8,9] The dorsal SI ligament is the largest. The ligamentous portion and the synovial portion make up the two parts of the SI joint. The central and craniodorsal part of the joint is where the ligamentous portion of the joint is located.[8] The synovial part of the joint consists of the crescent-shaped articular surfaces of the ilium and sacrum lined with hyaline cartilage. A thin synovial membrane is present around the edge of the hyaline cartilage.[8,9]

When using a minimally invasive closed reduction repair technique with fluoroscopy, the five most important parts of the regional anatomy are (1) the sacral body, (2) the vertebral canal, (3) the lumbosacral disk space, (4) the ilial wings, and (5) the transverse processes of the sixth and seventh lumbar vertebra. These structures are easily seen by fluoroscopy (**Fig. 1**).

The sacrum consists of the sacral body, sacral wings, the vertebral canal, and the dorsal spinous processes. The sacrum is comprised of three sacral vertebrae that are fused together. The correct part of the sacrum for screw placement is the body of the first sacral vertebra (body). The surgeon needs to be aware of the vertebral canal and the lumbosacral disk space so that the screw is not inadvertently placed into these areas or out ventrally on the sacrum. The transverse processes of the sixth and seventh lumbar vertebra are also important landmarks for proper assessment of alignment of the sacrum in a true lateral position on the surgery table. From the lateral radiographic project of the caudal spine, the wings of the sacrum are not visible because of the overlap of the ilium. From the ventrodorsal projection, the wings of the

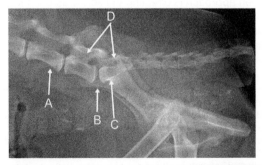

Fig. 1. Lateral view of the lumbar spine and pelvis in a true lateral position. *Arrow A* shows the superimposition of transverse processes of the seventh lumbar vertebra. *Arrow B* shows the lumbosacral disk space. *Arrow C* points to the first sacral vertebra. *Arrows D* points to the vertebral canal of the seventh lumbar and sacral vertebral canal.

sacrum are visible and can aid in determining if the SI joint is properly aligned (see **Fig. 1**).

PREOPERATIVE PATIENT ASSESSMENT AND DECISION MAKING

Preoperatively, standard orthogonal views of the pelvis are taken to assess the type and locations of the injuries that are present. Measurements of the length of screw that is needed to achieve at least 60% purchase of the sacrum are made. The total width of the sacrum is measured along with the thickness of the ilium at the point of screw insertion from a ventrodorsal image of the pelvis. In most cases, it is easier to measure from the nonluxated side than from the luxated side of the pelvis. A true ventrodorsal radiograph of this region of the pelvis and spine is required for accurate measurement of the ilial-sacral width.

In most instances, a fracture of the ilium or acetabulum is present on the opposite side of the pelvis from the SI fracture-luxation. Repair of the contralateral fracture decreases the displacement of the SI joint, making the final reduction of the SI joint easier. However, placement of a bone plate on the ilium potentially obscures the view of the sacrum thus making it more difficult to correctly place that screw. Using the C-arm, placement of the bone plate on the ilium is adjusted to prevent the bone plate from obscuring the sacrum in most cases. Repair of the SI luxation is performed as the first procedure as an alternative. However, exact reduction of the SI fracture-luxation is required if this is done first or it will make acceptable repair of a contralateral ilial or acetabular fracture more difficult or impossible.

ORTHOPEDIC EQUIPMENT, IMPLANTS, AND ANCILLARY EQUIPMENT

Performance of minimally invasive surgery for repair of SI fracture-luxation requires the use of a C-arm along with a radiolucent operating table. Proper radiation personal shielding devices (full aprons, leaded glasses, and thyroid shields) are also required to minimize radiation exposure.

Orthopedic instrumentation that is used for reduction of the SI luxation includes Kern bone-holding forceps (or other similar bone-holding forceps), and intramedullary (IM) pins. A Jacob's pin chuck is used as a handle on the IM pin during reduction of the SI fracture-luxation.

The most common implants used for joint fracture fixation include Kirschner (K) wires, screws, and washers. K-wires are used to locate the place for screw insertion and for temporary stabilization of the SI joint luxation after it is reduced. Tap sleeves, taps, screw driver, and drill bits of the appropriate size for the screw that is inserted are also required. Cortical screws are the implant most commonly used to stabilize the SI fracture-luxation. The appropriate-sized washer is used to increase the surface contact area of the implant to decrease the possibility of the screw head penetrating through cortex of the ilium.

PREOPERATIVE PREPARATION

A standard orthopedic aseptic preparation for surgery is performed. Just because a minimally invasive technique is being used does not reduce the importance of performing aseptic surgery. The one difference in draping procedure from performing an open repair is that a stockinette and/or adhesive drape is typically not used. The use of paper drapes that are attached to the skin with skin staples eliminates the need for towel clamps. Towel clamps tend to obstruct the field of view. In that the

C-arms typically are set for automatic exposure, the more metal present in the field decreases the quality of the image.

The patient is positioned in lateral recumbency so that the lower lumbar spine is in a perfect lateral position. It is important to position the patient in a perfect lateral recumbent position as possible to facilitate correct screw placement. A bean-bag that is suctioned out to conform to the patient may be useful to maintain this position. A cantilevered table that allows rotation of the table side-to-side is also useful for perfect lateral positioning of the lumbar spine. Superimposition of the lateral spinous processes of the sixth and seventh lumbar vertebrae is used to tell that the vertebrae are in a true lateral position. The lumbosacral disk space is used to judge if the sacrum is positioned correctly cranial to caudal. One should be able to look completely through the lumbosacral disk space without seeing an oblique view of the end plates of either vertebrae.

SURGICAL TECHNIQUE

Reduction of the SI fracture-luxation is performed. Three basic methods of reduction are possible (or in combination). The first method involves manipulation of the hemipelvis by controlling the ischium with either an IM pin or a Kern bone-holding forceps. This method requires that the hemipelvis is intact. If an ischial body fracture is present, this method does not work. A small approach to the ischium is performed to facilitate placement of a Kern bone-holding forceps. An IM pin is driven directly through the tuber ischium and used as a traction device. The second method of manipulation of the hemipelvis involves pushing caudally on the wing of the ilium with one hand while using the femur to apply caudal and lateral force to the pelvis with the other hand. This method works best for small, thin, and lightly muscled dogs or cats. If ipsilateral ischial body fractures are present, this method of reduction is tried. The third method (and my preferred method) of reduction involves pushing on the ilial wing using an IM pin. With this technique, the tip of the pin is inserted through the skin and driven into the cranial dorsal corner of the wing of the ilium. The pin is then used to push the ilium caudal and dorsal (ventral) as needed. The cranial aspect of the ilial wing is pushed medially to "wing" the caudal part of the hemipelvis laterally to widen the pelvic canal out to its normal position. Combining "pushing and pulling" is effective in reducing the SI joint in large dogs.

Assessment of reduction is estimated in the lateral view by superimposition of the two wings of the ilium and acetabuli. Comparison of the slope of the two sides of the pelvis gives an estimation of the angulation of the pelvis to the spine (normal ~45°) (**Fig. 2**). The C-arm is rotated 90° to assess reduction in the ventrodorsal projection. Once the SI joint appears reduced, a K-wire of appropriate size is driven across the SI joint caudal to the area that the lag screw will be placed to temporarily maintain reduction of the SI joint (see **Fig. 2**). A ventrodorsal view of the pelvis can also be taken, if desired, to assess appropriate reduction.

Two methods of screw application are available. For either technique, a K-wire is used to locate the proper place for insertion of the lag screw. Once the insertion site is found, a small (1 cm) incision is made through the skin, subcutaneous tissue, and muscle. The incision is made to parallel the direction of the gluteal muscle fibers. Instrumentation is passed through this incision to reach the bone.

Insertion of a cortical screw in lag fashion is performed in a routine manner except that the thread hole is drilled first because it generally is not possible to use the drill sleeve insert to center the glide hole and the thread hole. Once the correct position is found for insertion of the screw with a K-wire and viewing with the C-arm, a tap

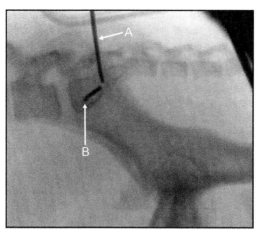

Fig. 2. Once the sacroiliac joint is reduced, a K-wire (*arrow A*) of appropriate size is driven across the SI joint caudal to the area that the lag screw will be placed to temporarily maintain reduction of the sacroiliac joint. *Arrow B* shows a K-wire that has been used to find the correct insertion position of the screw used to stabilize the sacroiliac joint.

sleeve is slid over the K-wire and pushed down to contact the ilium. The tap sleeve is positioned such that one can see directly down the center of the tap sleeve (only see a round circle when viewing from the lateral position) (**Fig. 3**). Insertion of a tap sleeve allows all of the drilling and tapping to be done without removal of the tap sleeve. If the sacrum is in a true lateral position and the tap sleeve is correctly centered on the sacral body, the thread hole is drilled completely across the sacrum without worry of penetrating the spinal canal, the disk space, or coming out ventrally. The glide hole is next drilled by finding the entrance to the thread hole in the ilium with the tip of the glide hole drill bit and enlarging it only through the ilium. One can usually feel the drill bit "drop" once it goes thru the ilium. The length of the screw is determined by measuring the difference between a K-wire inserted to the bottom of the screw hole and a K-wire inserted to the lateral aspect of the ilium next to the screw hole. From

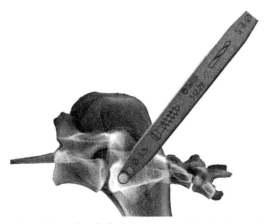

Fig. 3. The tap sleeve is positioned such that one can see directly down the center of the tap sleeve (only see a round circle when viewing from the lateral position).

preoperative measurements of the ilium and sacrum, the minimum length of screw that is acceptable (60% of sacral width) is determined. In most cases, because of the depth of the holed drilled into the sacrum, a screw that is longer than the 60% sacral width is used. A screw that is slightly shorter than the measured distance is inserted to make sure that the screw does not "bottom out" on the hole. If the screw "bottoms out," compression across the joint does not occur and there is a risk of stripping the screw threads. A washer is added to the screw to decrease the chance of the head of the screw tearing through the ilial cortex (**Fig. 4**). A second screw is added in some dogs. Typically, the K-wire is removed because it is difficult to cut it flush with the bone. A couple of sutures are placed to close the skin incision. For dogs with bilateral SI fracture-luxations, selection of the point of screw insertion is changed slightly. Instead of centering the screw on the sacrum, the screw insertion points are shifted so one screw is inserted slightly dorsal and cranial and the other ventral and caudal to the other.

The second method uses a cannulated drill bit to correctly position the screw hole. In this technique, a K-wire that corresponds to the size of the cannulated drill bit to be used is positioned and driven across the ilium and sacrum. If the sacrum is in a perfect lateral position, the K-wire should be viewed perfectly on end (a dot) when viewing from the lateral aspect. Once the K-wire is in place, the cannulated drill bit is slipped over the K-wire and the screw hole drilled. This is the thread hole for the screw in the sacrum. The appropriate size drill bit for the glide hole is then inserted down to the ilium and a glide hole drilled just across the ilium. The K-wire is removed. A cortical screw with an attached washer is then inserted through the tissue and tightened. A cannulated screw is not used because they are expensive and not as strong as regular cortical screws.

Postoperative care of a patient following closed reduction and lag screw fixation of SI fracture-luxation is the same as repair of any pelvic fracture-luxation case. Because most of these patients have contralateral pelvic injuries plus potentially other lower extremity fractures, restricted activity and weight support is required. Recheck radiographic examination at 4 and 8 weeks after repair is advised. In most cases, adequate healing is present at 4 weeks postoperatively such that the repair is unlikely to fail.

DISCUSSION

Closed reduction and screw fixation of SI fracture-luxation has been shown to be an effective method of treating this traumatic injury to the pelvis of dogs and cats.[6,7]

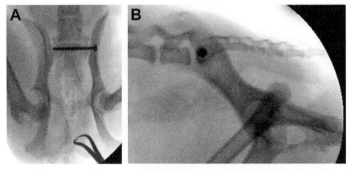

Fig. 4. Correct placement of the screw across the sacroiliac joint; (A) ventrodorsal view and (B) lateral view. The sacroiliac joint has been anatomically reduced and the screw goes completely across the sacrum.

Advantages of this procedure are minimal soft tissue disruption with less pain and chance for infection, good reduction of the luxation, precise screw placement, low percentage of screw loosening, and an early return to use of the leg on the luxation side. The minimally invasive technique for repair of SI fracture-luxations is fast, consistently more accurate, and much less traumatic for the patient than an open technique in my experience.

Accurate reduction of the SI joint is important for the success of the procedure. In a report on open reduction of SI fracture-luxation, screw loosening occurred in 22% of cases when greater than 90% reduction was achieved compared with 41% when less than 90% reduction was achieved.[2] In the first report of closed reduction and screw fixation of SI joint fracture-luxation repair, no screw loosening occurred with a mean reduction of 92% (range, 79.55%–100%).[6] In a subsequent report on closed reduction and screw fixation of SI joint fracture-luxation repair, the mean percent reduction of the SI fracture-luxation was 91% (range, 51%–100%).[7] In this report three cortical screws loosened and two of these SI joints had reduction of less than 90%. Five of the 24 SI joints had reduction less than 90%.[7] In a cadaveric study in cats using a minimally invasive osteosynthesis (MIO) technique, mean SI joint reduction was 98.33% (range, 90%–100%).[10] Reduction of greater than 90% should be easy to achieve with accurate fluoroscopic assessment.

Another method of assessing the adequacy of reduction is to measure the pelvic canal width. The mean pelvic canal diameter ratio has been reported to be greater than 1.1 (range, 1.07–1.82).[11] In the first report of closed reduction and screw fixation of SI fracture luxation, the mean pelvic canal width ratio was 1.2 immediately postoperatively and 1.11 at the last examination.[6] In the second report of closed reduction and screw fixation of SI fracture luxation, the mean pelvic canal width ratio was 1.17 immediately postoperatively and 1.06 at the last examination.[7] In a cadaveric study in cats using a MIO technique, the postoperative mean pelvic canal ratio was 1.25 (range, 1.09–1.42), which was not significantly different from preoperative measurements.[10] This indicates that the pelvic had been returned to close to its normal width and that stenosis of the pelvic canal did not occur.

Cortical screws are the implant of choice for most cases. In the two reports of closed reduction and screw fixation of SI fracture-luxation, one cancellous screw broke and one cannulated screw bent.[6,7] The cannulated screw that bent was associated with catastrophic failure of the bone plate repair of an ilial fracture on the opposite hemipelvis.[6] A screw of the proper diameter compared with the size of the sacrum is probably more important in preventing screw breakage than screw type. Percutaneous fluoroscopically assisted placement of a transiliosacral rod to stabilize SI fracture-luxations after limited open reduction has also been described.[12]

Screw length has been shown to be an important factor in screw loosening following repair of SI fracture-luxation using an open repair technique.[2] In this study, a 7% screw loosening rate was found when the cumulative screw depth/sacral width was greater than 60%.[2] A 48% screw loosening rate was found when the cumulative screw depth/sacral width was less than 60%.[2] In the 35 SI fracture-reductions that were repaired with a closed reduction and screw fixation technique, three (8.5%) screws loosened.[6,7] The mean screw length/sacral width was 79% and 64% postoperatively in these two reports of a closed reduction and screw fixation.[6,7] A significant difference between the open and closed techniques was that in the closed reduction technique only one screw was used, whereas in the open technique 22% of the cases had more than one screw placed.[2,6,7] In the open repair technique, placement of multiple screws was not believed to be important in screw loosening.[2] In a study evaluating static strength of SI fracture-separation repairs, two screws were stronger than one screw of similar size, two small screws were stronger than a single larger screw, and a reduction pin added no significant strength to a single screw repair.[13] In this study, failure of the implant occurred by pullout of the screws and not breakage. Considering the low loosening rate of one proper length and properly placed screw (1/33 or 3%) for a closed reduction and screw fixation technique, a single screw of the correct diameter is recommended.[6,7] In a cadaveric study in dogs comparing MIO and open reduction and internal fixation (ORIF) techniques, the mean length of the pilot hole in the sacrum was 97.1% for MIO and 67% for ORIF.[14] In a cadaveric study in cats using an MIO technique, mean screw purchase in the sacrum was 73.08% (range, 51%–100%).[10]

Correct location of the screw is also important in repair of SI fracture-luxations. The screw needs to be placed in the first sacral vertebral body. The location of the screw is easily visualized fluoroscopically. Use of a K-wire to find the spot on the first sacral vertebral body for screw insertion is easy accomplished. To allow the screw to be directed across the sacral body the proper depth (minimum of 60%), proper alignment of the sacrum in a true lateral position is required. A screw is placed across the entire width of the sacrum. It is important to not place the screw into the vertebral canal, the lumbosacral disk space or intervertebral foramen, the body of the seventh lumbar vertebra, or pelvic sacral foramina. In a cadaveric study in dogs comparing MIO and ORIF techniques, screw orientation was nearly perpendicular to the sagittal plane in all MIO specimens while screws were consistently oriented in a cranioventral direction in the ORIF group.[14] In a cadaveric study in cats using an MIO technique, 92% of screws were placed in a satisfactory location within the sacral body.[10]

The question arises as to the need to repair SI fracture-luxations. In the past, the "surgical wisdom" has been that SI fracture-luxations can adequately heal on their own without repair. Certainly some patients regain acceptable function without surgical repair. Some of the philosophy of not doing surgery probably comes from the difficulty that has been encountered in correct screw placement and reduction of SI fracture-luxations from an open technique. In our practice, just about all SI fracture-luxations are repaired because of the benefit to the patient and the ease of performing the procedure. Just about all of the patients have significant injury to the opposite hemipelvis that requires surgical repair. Some also have injuries to the lower extremities, such as fractures of the tibia or femur. My philosophy about repair of SI fracture-luxations is that we can provide stability to this part of the hemipelvis, which then translates into less pain and a quicker return to use and better function. In our first report of this technique, 9 of 13 dogs were willing to use the SI fracture-luxation side the day after surgery and one more dog was willing to walk on the leg 2 days after surgery. The only dogs (three) that did not walk on the leg soon after surgery had sciatic nerve injury caused by the original trauma that caused the fracture-luxation.[6] In most cases, we find that patients use the side with the SI repair before and better than the opposite side with an ilial or acetabular fracture repair. This all is in relationship to the patient's other types of injuries.

SUMMARY

A minimally invasive technique for repair of SI fracture-luxations is a viable option for repair of this injury and has considerable benefits. Reduction and fixation of a minimally invasive technique is comparable with an open technique without the associated morbidity of an open technique. However, a minimally invasive technique requires intraoperative fluoroscopy and associated possible radiation exposure.

REFERENCES

1. DeCamp CE. Principles of pelvic fracture management. Semin Vet Med Surg (Small Anim) 1992;7(1):63–70.
2. DeCamp CE, Braden TD. Sacroiliac fracture-separation in the dog a study of 92 cases. Vet Surg 1985;14(2):127–30.
3. Bowlt KL, Shales CJ. Canine sacroiliac luxation: anatomic study of the craniocaudal articular surface angulation of the sacrum to define a safe corridor in the dorsal plane for placement of screws used for fixation in lag fashion. Vet Surg 2011; 40(1):22–6.
4. Shales CJ, Langley-Hobbs SJ. Canine sacroiliac luxation: anatomic study of dorsoventral articular surface angulation and safe corridor for placement of screws used for lag fixation. Vet Surg 2005;34(4):324–31.
5. Joseph R, Milgram J, Zhan K, et al. In vitro study of the ilial anatomic landmarks for safe implant insertion in the first sacral vertebra of the intact canine sacroiliac joint. Vet Surg 2006;35(6):510–7.
6. Tomlinson JL, Cook JL, Payne JT, et al. Closed reduction and lag screw fixation of sacroiliac luxations and fractures. Vet Surg 1999;28(3):188–93.
7. Tonks CA, Tomlinson JL, Cook JL. Evaluation of closed reduction and screw fixation in lag fashion of sacroiliac fracture-luxations. Vet Surg 2008;37(7):603–7.
8. Gregory CR, Cullen JM, Pool R, et al. The canine sacroiliac joint. Preliminary study of anatomy, histopathology, and biomechanics. Spine (Phila Pa 1976) 1986;11(10):1044–8.
9. DeCamp CE, Braden TD. The surgical anatomy of the canine sacrum for lag screw fixation of the sacroiliac joint. Vet Surg 1985;14(2):131–4.
10. Fischer A, Binder E, Reif U, et al. Closed reduction and percutaneous fixation of sacroiliac luxations in cats using 2.4 mm cannulated screws: a cadaveric study. Vet Comp Orthop Traumatol 2012;1:22–7.
11. Averill SM, Johnson AL, Schaeffer DJ. Risk factors associated with development of pelvic canal stenosis secondary to sacroiliac separation: 84 cases (1985-1995). J Am Vet Med Assoc 1997;211(1):75–8.
12. Leasure CS, Lewis DD, Sereda CW, et al. Limited open reduction and stabilization of sacroiliac fracture-luxations using fluoroscopically assisted placement of a trans-iliosacral rod in five dogs. Vet Surg 2007;36(7):633–43.
13. Radasch RM, Merkley DF, Hoefle WD, et al. Static strength evaluation of sacroiliac fracture-separation repairs. Vet Surg 1990;19(2):155–61.
14. Déjardin LM, Marturello DM, Guiot LP, et al. Comparison of open reduction versus minimally invasive surgical approaches on screw position in canine sacroiliac lag-screw fixation. Vet Comp Orthop Traumatol 2016;4:290–7.

Percutaneous Plate Arthrodesis

Antonio Pozzi, DMV, MS[a],*, Daniel D. Lewis, DVM, MS[b], Caleb C. Hudson, DVM, MS[c], Stanley E. Kim, BVSc, MS[b], Emanuele Castelli, DMV[a]

KEYWORDS

- Minimally invasive • Arthrodesis • Plate • Percutaneous • Dogs • Cats • Carpus
- Tarsus

KEY POINTS

- Arthrodesis is an elective salvage procedure that eliminates pain and/or dysfunction by invoking deliberate osseous joint fusion.
- Traditional open arthrodeses require extensive surgical approaches that can cause vascular compromise leading to soft-tissue complications.
- Percutaneous plate arthrodesis is performed using limited surgical approaches and does not require joint disarticulation. Implants are applied through small plate insertion incisions and a limited approach is used to debride the affected joint.
- Intraoperative imaging is useful in guiding cartilage debridement and implant application.
- Percutaneous plate arthrodesis has been successfully used to address carpal and tarsal disorders.

INTRODUCTION

Perhaps one of the most useful applications of minimally invasive plate osteosynthesis (MIPO) in small animals is distal extremity percutaneous plate arthrodesis. Carpal and tarsal arthrodeses can be associated with the development of a substantial number of postoperative complications.[1] The risk of several specific postoperative complications can be decreased by performing these procedures in a minimally invasive fashion. Articular cartilage debridement is performed through limited approaches, and application of the plate is accomplished through small insertion incisions to minimize periarticular iatrogenic soft-tissue trauma. Preservation of the regional soft tissues mitigates

Disclosure Statement: None.
The article is an update of "Pozzi A, Lewis DD, Hudson CC, et al. Percutaneous plate arthrodesis in small animals. Vet Clin North Am Small Anim Pract 2012;42(5):1079-96."
[a] Vetsuisse Faculty, University of Zurich, Winterthurerstrasse 258c, Zurich 8057, Switzerland; [b] Department of Small Animal Clinical Sciences, College of Veterinary Medicine, University of Florida, 2015 Southwest 16th Avenue, Gainesville, FL 32610-0126, USA; [c] Gulf Coast Veterinary Specialists, 8042 Katy Freeway, Houston, TX 77024, USA
* Corresponding author.
E-mail address: apozzi@vetclinics.uzh.ch

disturbance of the extraosseous circulation to the arthrodesis site and facilitates tension-free closure. Consequently, using MIPO techniques when performing arthrodeses mitigates postoperative swelling, lowers the risk of wound dehiscence and distal limb ischemia, and potentially could lessen the occurrence of surgical-site infection and accelerate osseous union.

Arthrodesis is an elective surgical procedure that eliminates motion in a joint by promoting deliberate osseous fusion.[2–24] Arthrodesis is considered a salvage procedure. The primary indication for performing an arthrodesis is unremitting joint pain or dysfunction that interferes with daily activities and cannot be resolved by other treatment modalities, such as administration of analgesics, nonsteroidal anti-inflammatory drugs, weight loss, and physical rehabilitation or alternative appropriate surgical procedures. Arthrodeses are performed to relieve chronic joint pain, resolve irreparable joint instability, arrest progressive destructive arthropathies, and resolve postural dysfunction resulting from neurologic deficits.[15,18] Arthrodesis must be distinguished from ankylosis. Ankylosis is a process that eliminates effective joint motion secondary to severe, progressive articular degeneration. Although motion in the affected joint may become severely limited, the process does not progress to osseous fusion, and ankylosis is often associated with chronic pain and dysfunction.

There are 4 tenets to performing an arthrodesis[4,15,18]: (1) debridement of the articular cartilage, (2) placement of a bone graft,[25] (3) positioning the involved limb segment at a functional angle, and (4) application of stable fixation.[8,13] The articular cartilage needs to be debrided from the involved joint spaces to allow for eventual osseous fusion.[24] Debridement is typically performed using a high-speed pneumatic drill and a burr, but can be done manually with a curette.[15] After the cartilage has been removed to expose the underlying subchondral bone, the debrided joint spaces are packed with autogenous cancellous bone graft (allogenic grafts or other graft substitutes can be used in place of an autogenous cancellous bone graft) to expedite osseous union of the arthrodesis.[15,18] The involved limb segment should be stabilized in a functional position and maintained in that position with appropriate, stable fixation. The vast majority of arthrodeses are rigidly stabilized with plates[2,5,6,11,17,26]; however, transarticular external fixators, and in some instances transarticular pins or Kirschner wires, can be used to provide stable, but not rigid fixation.[10,16,27,28] These latter techniques are more useful in younger dogs and cats, which usually obtain osseous union in a relatively short period of time. Most skeletally mature dogs obtain functional union around 12 weeks following surgery.[14]

Owners must be informed before surgery that an arthrodesis is an involved surgical procedure and that there is considerable morbidity associated with the surgical approach, debridement of the affected joint, and implant application.[1] Extensive traditional open surgical approaches can cause vascular trauma leading to soft-tissue complications. Plantar necrosis has been reported following tarsal arthrodeses, most likely caused by iatrogenic trauma to the dorsal pedal or perforating metatarsal arteries.[1] In addition, bone plates are often applied on mechanically unfavorable bone surfaces when performing arthrodeses. Plates are frequently placed on the compressive rather than the tensile surface of the secured bone segments because the compressive surface is more readily accessible. These mechanical inadequacies can predispose to both early and late implant failure. The involved limb segment is often placed in a cast or splint, or an adjunctive external fixator may be used to supplement plate stabilization in an effort to prevent early implant failure. Owners must also be warned that fusion of one joint may place abnormal stress on adjacent joints, and the lack of mobility in the arthrodesed limb segment may predispose the limb to future trauma. Owners need to be adequately forewarned of possible adverse sequelae and complications before surgery[1,29]; however, the benefits of arthrodesis generally outweigh potential risks and possible complications, and the functional outcome can be excellent.[17,30,31]

Percutaneous plating has evolved to allow plates to be applied through small plate insertion incisions made remote to the articulation being stabilized. Although MIPO techniques were initially developed to stabilize fractures, these techniques can also be used when performing arthrodeses.[32] The MIPO technique conforms to the principles of biological osteosynthesis because there is limited disturbance of the adjacent soft tissues and vascular supply to the bones being stabilized.[33] Cadaveric studies have shown that periosteal vessels are preserved to a much greater extent when using MIPO in comparison with conventional open plating applications.[34,35] Conservation of the local circulation should accelerate osseous union with fewer postoperative complications.[34,36,37]

Minimally invasive arthrodesis techniques were first described for human patients to minimize soft-tissue complications and decrease the risk of postoperative infection. Percutaneous interphalangeal,[38] metatarsophalangeal,[39] sacroiliac,[40] vertebral pedicle,[41] and ankle[42] "arthrodesis" have been reported in humans. Cartilage debridement is not performed as extensively as in open approaches, and the implants are applied through small plate insertion incisions. One of the unique aspects of some described percutaneous arthrodesis procedures is that cartilage debridement is performed using fluoroscopic or arthroscopic guidance.[39,40,42–44] Successful fusion following ankle arthrodesis without cartilage debridement has been reported in human patients with rheumatoid arthritis.[43] Arthrodesis without cartilage debridement has also been investigated in experimental animal models.[45,46] Patellofemoral arthrodesis was performed in rabbits using 2 lag screws without cartilage debridement.[45] Histologic evidence of osseous fusion was found in most animals, demonstrating that compression and rigid fixation without cartilage debridement can result in successful joint fusion. The effect of synovial fluid depletion and immobilization on the articular surfaces was also evaluated in a rabbit patellofemoral model.[46] Synovial depletion in combination with drilling a hole through the cartilage and subchondral bone resulted in bone bridging across the joint, leading the investigators to recommend this technique for percutaneous arthrodeses without cartilage debridement.[46] A limited surgical approach that does not require joint disarticulation or complete articular cartilage debridement has been described to facilitate pastern arthrodesis in horses.[47] Pastern arthrodeses were performed in 12 limbs (11 horses) affected by chronic osteoarthritis. Limited cartilage debridement was performed by distracting the proximal interphalangeal joint and drilling holes through the articular surface. Good outcomes were obtained in 9 horses (10 limbs).[47] Although it is difficult to translate experimental data[45,46] or clinical data in human patients[43] and horses[32,47,48] to dogs with naturally occurring arthropathies, these studies suggest that a more conservative approach to cartilage debridement may be sufficient to promote successful joint fusion.

Although the high-motion joints such as the talocrural and antebrachiocarpal joints can be thoroughly debrided through a 2-cm incision, limited articular cartilage debridement of the other articulations may be performed, particularly the low-motion joints of the pes and manus. Aggressive open debridement of articular cartilage and application of a bone plate and screws can result in vascular compromise following both pantarsal and tarsometatarsal arthrodeses.[1] In addition, swelling and edema may make closure of the soft tissues over implants difficult when using a traditional open approach. Tension induced by closure can produce a constrictive, "tourniquet-like" effect that may further inhibit venous and lymphatic return from the paw. Preserving bridges of intact skin and underlying soft tissue between the plate insertion incisions, as well as any additional incisions required for articular debridement, are likely responsible for the nominal soft-tissue swelling the authors have observed following percutaneous plate arthrodeses. In addition, avoiding disarticulation of the joint to facilitate cartilage debridement may further decrease the risk of vascular compromise. The authors have observed minimal postoperative soft-tissue swelling and edema formation in tarsal arthrodeses performed using minimally invasive techniques in comparison with tarsal arthrodeses performed using a traditional open surgical approach.

Obtaining and maintaining compression across the debrided joint space is advantageous when performing percutaneous plate arthrodeses with limited cartilage debridement. The cartilage surfaces sustained in direct contact are deprived of nutrients normally provided by synovial fluid and may fuse secondary to chondrocyte death and ossification.[45] Compression of the joint space can be achieved using a plate, lag screws, pin and tension band fixation, or an external fixator. Maintaining articular surface congruence is important to obtaining intimate contact of the debrided articular surfaces and to achieving acceptable postoperative stability. When cartilage debridement is performed, it is important to preserve the underlying subchondral bone. Extensive subchondral bone debridement may increase the gap between the contiguous surfaces and delay osseous union.

TARSAL ARTHRODESES
Indications

Tarsal arthrodesis is often necessary to restore pelvic limb function in dogs or cats with severe traumatic or degenerative conditions affecting the talocrural, intertarsal, and/or tarsometatarsal joints.[2,5,6,9,11,18,27,28,49] Indications for tarsal arthrodeses include shearing injuries, particularly injuries with substantial osseous trauma, marked degenerative joint disease, which may be secondary to osteochondritis dissecans, chronic ligamentous instability or intra-articular fractures, irreparable Achilles' tendon injuries, and, in some instances, neurologic dysfunction associated with sciatic nerve damage.[18] Pantarsal arthrodesis is often performed to resolve pain and dysfunction affecting the talocrural joint irrespective of whether the pathology involves distal articulations of the tarsal joint. Partial tarsal arthrodesis, which typically refers to arthrodesis of the intertarsal and tarsometatarsal articulations, are performed in animals with pathologic conditions involving the intertarsal or tarsometatarsal joints without associated talocrural disorder. Animals should be thoroughly evaluated before committing to a partial arthrodesis because a pantarsal arthrodesis may be preferable in some instances whereby talocrural disorder initially appears minor.

Percutaneous plate arthrodesis can be performed in most situations whereby a traditional open plate arthrodesis would be considered. The signalment of the animal does not limit consideration of percutaneous arthrodesis. An open traditional arthrodesis might be more appropriate in animals with marked pre-existing conformational deformities, especially if a corrective ostectomy is indicated as a component of the procedure. In animals with chronic tarsal disorder, fibrous tissue may prevent proper alignment of the involved segments. Percutaneous rather than open plate arthrodesis may be preferable in animals with acute traumatic soft-tissue injuries of distal extremities. The circulation to the pes may already be compromised as the result of the inciting traumatic incident, predisposing the paw to vascular complications following surgery. The extent of iatrogenic soft-tissue trauma induced during a percutaneous plate arthrodesis is nominal compared with that of traditional arthrodeses using open plating techniques.

Surgical Anatomy

The talocrural joint is a modified hinge joint involving the articulation of the tibia, fibula, and talus.[50] The articular surface of the distal tibia is concave and conforms the contour of the talus. The congruity of this joint should be maintained when performing a pantarsal arthrodesis to improve the postoperative stability. The proximal surface of the talocrural joint is bordered medially by the medial malleolus, a protuberance of the tibia that projects distal to the talar trochlear ridges and articulates with the medial surface of the talus. Performing a malleolar ostectomy allows ready access to the talocrural joint for cartilage debridement and negates the need for extensive plate contouring when applying a medial plate to stabilize a pantarsal arthrodesis. Multiple extensor tendons cross the dorsal surface of the tarsus (**Fig. 1**A) and should be preserved, if possible, during tarsal arthrodesis surgery. The bones of the tarsus (**Fig. 1**B) articulate at several levels and are stabilized by a complex of ligaments on the plantar and dorsal surfaces. The medial and lateral collateral ligaments span the talocrural joint bilaterally. There are numerous short dorsal ligaments between the individual tarsal bones on the dorsal surface of the tarsus (see **Fig. 1**A). A large

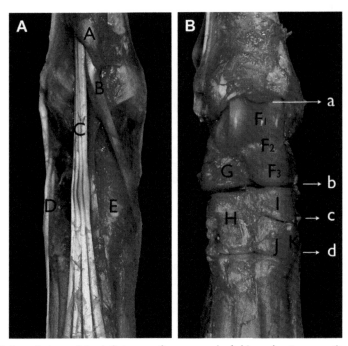

Fig. 1. (*A*) Dorsal view of the left tarsus after removal of skin, subcutaneous tissue, fascia, superficial veins, and nerves: A, proximal extensor retinaculum; B, tibialis cranialis tendon; C, extensor digitorum longus tendon; D, extensor digitorum lateralis, peroneus longus, and peroneus brevis tendons; E, short dorsal tarsal ligaments. (*B*) Dorsal view of the left tarsus after removal of ligaments and tendons: F_1, talus, trochlea; F_2, talus, neck; F_3, talus, head; G, calcaneus; H, fourth tarsal bone; I, central tarsal bone; J, third tarsal bone; K, second and first tarsal bones; a, talocrural joint; b, proximal intertarsal joint; c, distal intertarsal joint; d, tarsometatarsal joint.

ligament unites the talus with the third and fourth tarsal bones. Oblique ligaments support the central and second tarsal bones as well as the central with the third tarsal bone. The distal row of tarsal bones is joined to the base of the metatarsal bones by small ligaments. The plantar ligaments are thicker than the dorsal ligaments. A more distinct ligament extends from the body of the calcaneus to the fourth tarsal bone and distally inserts to the bases of the fourth and fifth metatarsal bones.[50]

Preoperative Planning

Tarsal arthrodeses are major elective procedures, and an extensive evaluation of the animal before surgery is warranted. Obtaining a thorough history is essential because pre-existing medical conditions such hyperadrenocorticism or diabetes may predispose the animal to delayed healing or increased risk of infection. A systematic orthopedic examination should be performed to identify conformational deformities and soft-tissue injuries, and to define the location and extent of the pathology necessitating arthrodesis. The animal should be evaluated for concurrent orthopedic abnormalities in the affected as well as the other 3 limbs to ensure that any existing concurrent orthopedic problems will not impair function following arthrodesis. A thorough neurologic evaluation should also be performed to identify neurologic dysfunction, which could impair function or predispose to pes ulceration.

Orthogonal radiographs of the distal tibia and fibula, tarsus and entire pes should be obtained for preoperative planning. Stress radiography may be used to identify level or levels of instability. The bone plate should be preselected and precontoured using the preoperative radiographs. The diameter of the metatarsal bones should be measured from a lateral-view radiograph to determine appropriate screw diameter. The diameter of screws to be placed in the metatarsal bones should not exceed 30% of the sagittal diameter of the metatarsal bones. Hybrid 2.0/2.7-mm or 2.7/3.5-mm hybrid plates (Veterinary Instrumentation, Sheffield, UK) can be used for proximal intertarsal and tarsometatarsal arthrodeses because these hybrid plates allow smaller-diameter screws to be inserted distal to the tarsometatarsal joints.[49] Newer locking-plate models (Intrauma, Rivoli, Italy) allow the surgeon to choose the screw size based on the dimensions of the distal metabones. Precontoured 2.0- to 2.7-mm or 2.7- to 3.5-mm angled plates are also available for medial plate application for performing pantarsal arthrodesis.[11] A medially applied plate has the mechanical benefit of being loaded through the plate's widest dimension during weight bearing.[51] Locking implants can be used for tarsal arthrodesis. There are several advantages to using an angle stable plate to stabilize an arthrodesis.[52,53] The angular stability provided by the screw head-plate locking mechanism decreases the risk of implant failure caused by screw pull-out. Another advantage of using a locking plate is that the implant does not need to be precisely contoured to the surface of the underlying bones if locking screws are used. The fixed angle of insertion of the locking screws can be problematic when placing screws in the metatarsus, and the plate must be torsionally contoured or appropriately aligned so that screws will effectively engage the metatarsal bones.

Patient Positioning

The animal is positioned in dorsal recumbence with both pelvic limbs positioned at the end of the table. The ipsilateral proximal humerus should be prepared and draped for procurement of an autogenous cancellous bone graft. Depending on which side of the limb the plate will be applied, the animal can be tilted slightly laterally and the affected distal pelvic limb rested on a Mayo stand. Positioning should take into account the need for intraoperative image acquisition, with the ability to obtain both craniocaudal and mediolateral projection images.

Surgical Technique: Pantarsal Arthrodesis Using a Medial Plate

The procedure is usually performed through 3 medial incisions. The plate is held next to the limb to determine the locations where the skin incisions should be made. Proximally, the incision parallels the long axis of the tibia and is centered over the anticipated location of the 2 most proximal holes of the plate. A 3-cm long intermediate incision is made, centered over the medial malleolus. The distal incision is made at the anticipated location of the 2 most distal plate holes over the second metatarsal bone. After elevating the soft tissue from the medial surface of the distal tibia, a medial malleolar ostectomy is performed (**Fig. 2**). The purpose of this ostectomy is to render the medial aspect of the distal tibia as flat as possible, which negates the need for extensive contouring of the plate. Excision of the medial malleolus also affords extensive exposure of the talocrural joint (see **Fig. 2**). The articular cartilage of the distal tibia and talus should be removed without extensively debriding the subchondral bone, especially on the talus, so as not to compromise stability of the arthrodesis. Metzenbaum scissors are used to develop an epiperiosteal tunnel joining the 3 skin incisions. This tunnel should be developed adjacent to the periosteal surface, deep to the overlying soft-tissue structures, without damaging the periosteum.

The intertarsal joints are debrided through the central incision (**Fig. 3**A) by retracting the commissure of the skin incision. The tarsometatarsal joints are debrided through 2 separate 3- to 5-mm linear incisions positioned both medially and laterally on the pes. Debridement performed through 2 incisions allows reasonable access to all 4 major tarsometatarsal articulations. A hypodermic needle is used to identify the joint spaces. Small individual incisions are made over the medial and lateral articulations, and a number 15 scalpel blade or tenotomy scissors are used to separate the soft tissues so that a burr can be inserted into the joint spaces. Fluoroscopy can be used, if available, to facilitate this process (**Fig, 3**). The intertarsal and the tarsometatarsal joints can be debrided with a modified fanning technique, as described for carpometacarpal arthrodesis in horses.[54,55]

Autogenous cancellous bone graft (or a suitable alternative) is packed into the debrided joint spaces. Alternatively, bone marrow or platelet-enriched plasma can be injected in joints that have not been sufficiently exposed for the placement of a bone graft.[56] The talocrural articulation is placed at the desired angle, which is typically between 135° and 145° in a dog and 115° to 125° in a cat,[18] and a Kirschner

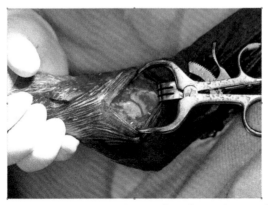

Fig. 2. A 2-cm linear skin incision was made over the talocrural joint. The incision is long enough to allow sufficient exposure to excise the medial malleolus. The ostectomy provides sufficient exposure of the talocrural joint to allow effective cartilage debridement.

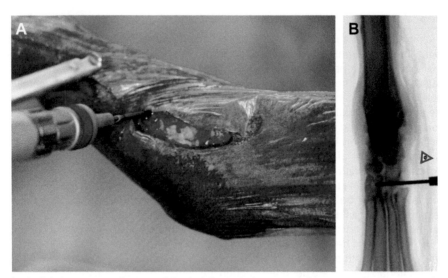

Fig. 3. (*A*) the intertarsal joint is debrided through the central skin incision by retracting the skin distally. Debridement of the tarsometatarsal joints is performed from the medial and lateral aspect through separate stab incisions. (*B*) Fluoroscopy is useful to evaluate the position and depth of the burr during debridement.

wire can be placed across the articulation to maintain this angle. The Kirschner wire should be inserted from the plantar surface of the calcaneus and emerge centrally on the cranial surface of the distal tibia. The position of this wire is evaluated with fluoroscopy. A tibiotarsal lag screw is then placed by overdrilling the Kirschner wire to ensure optimal interfragmentary compression. Placing 1 or 2 additional calcaneotibial Kirschner wires will help maintain the desired talocrural angle as the initial Kirschner wire is overdrilled with cannulated drill bits of appropriate diameter (Arthrex, Naples, FL, USA), allowing the screw to be inserted in lag fashion from the plantar surface of the calcaneus. A cannulated screw can be used if available. The plate is inserted through either the proximal or distal insertion incision and maneuvered through the epiperiosteal tunnel until the end of the plate emerges from the other insertion incision (**Fig. 4**). The pes must be properly aligned with respect to the proximal tibia and stifle before inserting screws through the plate. Fluoroscopy can be used if available to assess the position of the plate and alignment of the limb before screw insertion (**Fig. 5**A, B & 6A-F). The first screw is inserted through the central hole of the plate and into the talus. Two or more screws are inserted in the holes at each end of the plate via the insertion incisions. The remaining screws are inserted in the holes in the plate through the insertion incisions or through separate small incisions. All incisions should be closed routinely in 2 layers. Postoperative radiographs are obtained to assess the position of the implants and the alignment of the joint (**Fig. 6**C, D). Recheck radiographs are obtained at 3- to 4-week intervals until osseous union of the arthrodesis is confirmed (**Fig. 6**E, F).

Surgical Technique: Partial Tarsal Arthrodesis

The procedure is usually performed through 3 small lateral incisions. The plate is positioned over the lateral aspect of the pes and the location of the incisions on the skin is marked. The proximal incision is parallel to the long axis of and centered over the tuber calcanei. An intermediate 2- to 3-cm long incision is initiated over the calcaneoquartal

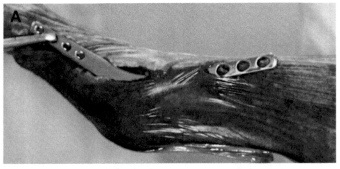

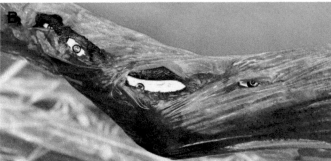

Fig. 4. (*A*) The plate is inserted through the middle incision, directed toward the proximal skin incision, and advanced distally (*B*). The minimally invasive surgical approach preserves bridges of intact skin over the medial aspect of the tarsus but still allows all holes in the medial pantarsal arthrodesis plate to be filled with screws.

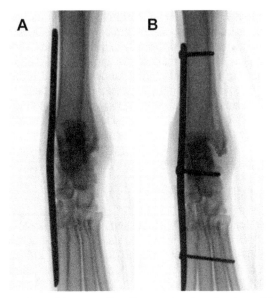

Fig. 5. (*A*) Fluoroscopy is used to assess the alignment and contouring of the medial pantarsal arthrodesis plate. Performing an ostectomy of the medial malleolus may eliminate or minimize the need for plate contouring. (*B*) The first screw is inserted in the talus, followed by screw insertion in the metatarsus and in the tibia.

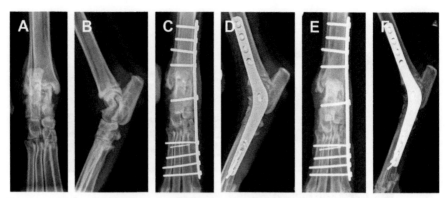

Fig. 6. (*A, B*) Tarsal preoperative radiographs. (*C, D*) Immediate postoperative radiographs. (*E, F*) Four-week postoperative recheck radiographs showing progress toward union of the pantarsal arthrodesis.

joint and extends distal to the tarsometatarsal articulation. The third incision is marked at the anticipated location of the 2 most distal plate holes, which should be located over the distal portion of the fifth metatarsal bone. After incising the skin and the subcutaneous tissues, the lateral intertarsal joints are identified through the central incision and debrided using a pneumatic drill and a burr (**Fig. 8A**). The protuberance located on the lateral aspect of the base of the fifth metatarsal bone is burred away, which decreases the amount of plate contouring required for plate application. Metzenbaum scissors are used to develop an epiperiosteal tunnel joining the 3 skin incisions (**Fig. 7**). The plate is then inserted proximal-to-distal or distal-to-proximal through the insertion incisions (**Fig. 8B**). The first screw is placed in the most distal plate hole. It is important to place this screw in the center of the fifth metatarsal bone to decrease the risk of metatarsal fractures. The hole can be initiated using a Kirschner wire, which is less likely to slip off the convex surface of the fifth metatarsal bone. The second screw is placed proximally in the calcaneus. At least 3 screws are placed in the calcaneus, with the third screw engaging the head of the talus. One screw is placed into the fourth and central tarsal bone and at least 3 screws into the metatarsi, with the most proximal screw engaging the base of 3 if not 4 of the metatarsal bones. The edges of the skin incisions may be retracted, if necessary, to allow all screws to be inserted (**Fig. 9**). The skin incisions are closed routinely. Postoperative radiographs are obtained to assess the position of the implants and the alignment of the pes (**Fig. 10A-G**). Recheck radiographs are taken every 3 to 4 weeks until the arthrodesis obtains osseous union.

PANCARPAL ARTHRODESIS
Indications

Although pancarpal arthrodeses are associated with fewer postoperative complications than tarsal arthrodeses, percutaneous plate pancarpal arthrodeses still afford many of the advantages previously alluded to for tarsal arthrodeses. Pancarpal arthrodesis is most commonly performed in dogs that sustain carpal hyperextension injuries or dogs with severe osteoarthritis.[4,7,10,14,15,19–22,57] Hyperextension injuries usually result in irreparable damage to the carpal palmar ligaments and palmar carpal fibrocartilage, which are the primary structures responsible for maintaining the carpus in a normal weight-bearing angle of 10° to 12° of extension. Medium and large breed dogs often sustain carpal hyperextension injuries as a result of falls or jumping. Acute

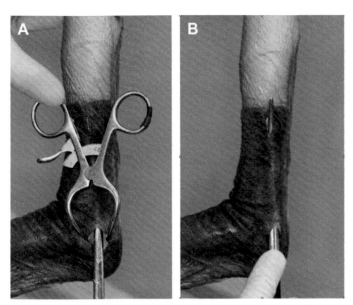

Fig. 7. (A) A 5- to 10-mm linear incision is made on the lateral aspect of the calcaneus just proximal to the calcaneoquartal joint. Debridement of the proximal intertarsal joint is performed through this incision and bone graft is inserted. A 5- to 10-mm longitudinal incision is then made over the lateral aspect of the fifth metatarsal at the level where the plate will be positioned distally. (B) The insertion tunnel is developed using straight Metzenbaum scissors, which are advanced until a tunnel is created between the proximal and distal incisions.

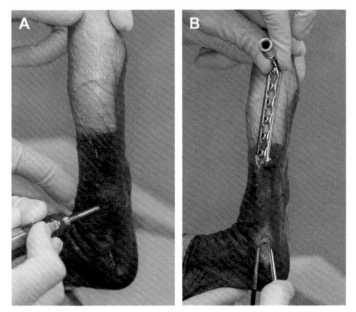

Fig. 8. (A) Articular cartilage debridement of the intertarsal and tarsometatarsal joints is performed with a high-speed pneumatic drill and a burr inserted through separate stab incisions made on the lateral and medial aspects of the tarsus. (B) The plate is inserted from distal to proximal through the epiperiosteal tunnel. Metzenbaum scissors can be used to facilitate the insertion of the plate.

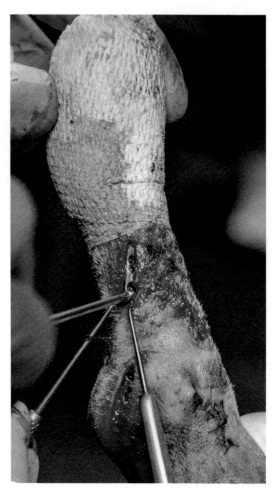

Fig. 9. Lateral aspect of the tarsus during partial tarsal arthrodesis. Skin hooks are being used to retract the distal skin incision edges proximally to allow insertion of a screw into the base of the metatarsal bones.

traumatic carpal hyperextension or luxation injuries result in a painful, non–weight-bearing lameness; however, most animals will attempt to bear weight on the affected limb within a few weeks of sustaining the injury. Animals with chronic carpal hyperextension injuries typically do not appear to be overly painful and will often bear weight on the affected limb. Pancarpal arthrodesis is generally necessary to resolve the lameness and dysfunction associated with hyperextension injuries because conservative management typically fails to result in a functional outcome.[15] Other indications for pancarpal arthrodesis include erosive arthropathies and fractures and/or traumatic subluxation or luxation of the antebrachiocarpal, intercarpal, and carpometacarpal joints. Most pancarpal arthrodeses can be performed using a percutaneous plating technique. A traditional open approach may be preferable to a percutaneous approach in animals with chronic osseous malalignment. For example, an ostectomy may be necessary to realign the manus before plating in an animal with a chronic luxation. For this reason, dogs with overt deformity may be better suited for a traditional open plate arthrodesis.

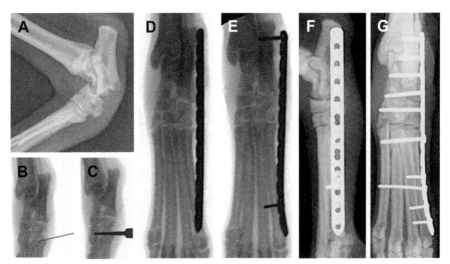

Fig. 10. (*A*) Preoperative lateral radiographic view of the tarsus showing a proximal intertarsal luxation, (*B, C*) Intraoperative fluoroscopic views showing identification of the lateral tarsometatarsal joints with a hypodermic needle and cartilage debridement using a high-speed drill and burr. (*D, E*) Fluoroscopy is used to estimate the amount of plate contouring needed and assess initial screw insertion proximally and distally. (*F, G*) Postoperative radiographs of a percutaneous plate partial tarsal arthrodesis performed with a 12-hole limited contact locking compression plate.

Surgical Anatomy

The carpus is composed of 3 joints: antebrachiocarpal, middle carpal, and carpometacarpal articulations (**Fig. 11**B). Several tendons and ligaments cross the joints (**Fig. 11**A). One of the unique anatomic features of the carpus is that the carpal collateral ligaments do not span all 3 joints. The ligaments of the carpus are generally short and most span only a single articulation, securing individual pairs of carpal bones. Palmar stability of the carpus depends predominantly on the integrity of the palmar carpal fibrocartilage and the numerous palmar ligaments.

Preoperative Planning

Evaluation of a potential candidate for a pancarpal arthrodesis is similar to what has been described for tarsal arthrodesis. Obtaining a thorough history and performing a systematic orthopedic examination are necessary to exclude underlying systemic disease or orthopedic abnormalities that might impair an acceptable return to function. Orthogonal radiographs of the carpus including the distal third of the antebrachium and the entire manus should be obtained to allow for preoperative selection of appropriate size implants. Selection of a plate of adequate length and screws of proper diameter can be problematic in some animals. The width of the third metacarpal bone is typically the limiting factor in selection of screw size because the diameter of the screw should not exceed 30% of the diameter of the bone. Hybrid plates designed specifically for pancarpal arthrodesis are available.[20,21,23] The plate should extend beyond the midpoint of the length of the third metacarpal bone to minimize the risk of postoperative fracture.[29]

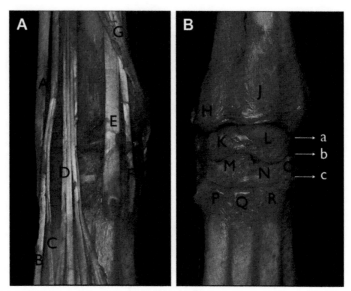

Fig. 11. (A) Dorsal view of the right carpus after removal of skin, subcutaneous tissue, fascia, superficial veins, and nerves: A, Extensor carpi ulnaris tendon; B and C, extensor digitorum lateralis tendons; D, extensor digitorum communis tendon; E and F, extensor carpi radialis tendons; G, abductor pollicis longus tendon. (B) Dorsal view of the right carpus after removal of ligaments and tendons: H, ulna; J, radius; K, ulnar carpal bone; L, radial carpal bone; M, fourth carpal bone; N, third carpal bone; O, second carpal bone; p, fifth metacarpal bone; Q, fourth metacarpal bone; R, third metacarpal bone; S, second metacarpal bone; a, antebrachiocarpal joint; b, intercarpal joint; c, carpometacarpal joint.

Patient Positioning

The animal is positioned in dorsal recumbence with the affected limb extended to allow the surgeon to access the dorsal aspect of the antebrachium and manus. The ipsilateral proximal humerus should be prepared and draped for the procurement of an autogenous cancellous bone graft. During the procedure, the limb may need to be suspended vertically to facilitate fluoroscopy imaging. The animal's position on the table should allow the C-arm of the fluoroscopy unit to be rotated around the limb to obtain orthogonal projection images.

Surgical Technique: Pancarpal Arthrodesis

Percutaneous arthrodesis is performed through 3 craniodorsal incisions. The central incision should be approximately 2 to 3 cm long and centered on the radiocarpal joint **(Fig. 12)**. The plate is held over the craniodorsal aspect of the limb and used to mark the location of the proximal and distal plate insertion incisions on the skin. After the central incision is made, the articular cartilage of the antebrachiocarpal and intercarpal joints are debrided with a high-speed pneumatic drill and burr through that incision. The carpometacarpal joints can usually be accessed through the central incision by retracting the skin distally, or through separate small isolated incisions positioned over the articulations. Once the articular cartilage has been debrided, the carpus is flexed and cancellous bone graft is placed in the debrided joint spaces. Placing the graft before plate application facilitates effective packing of the debrided joint spaces with graft. The flare of the cranial surface of the distal radius can be flattened by removing a small portion of the protuberance with a high-speed drill and burr, which

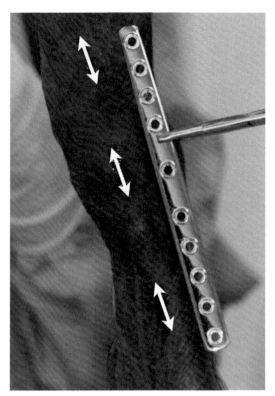

Fig. 12. Dorsal aspect of the distal radius, carpus, and proximal metacarpus. The white arrows indicate the locations of the 3 dorsal skin incisions used to perform a percutaneous pancarpal arthrodesis. The middle incision is centered over the radiocarpal joint. The proximal and distal skin incisions are located at the level of the proximal and distal ends of the plate.

reduces the amount of plate contouring necessary for the plate to conform to the cranial aspect of the distal radius. The plate should be contoured to produce approximately 10° of carpal extension. The plate should extend as distally as possible on the third metacarpal bone.[15]

The plate insertion tunnel is developed using Metzenbaum scissors and a periosteal elevator if necessary. Proximally, the plate is positioned under the extensor tendons. The tendons of the extensor carpi radialis muscle on the second and third metacarpal bones can be elevated percutaneously using a periosteal elevator. The general principles of plate application for pancarpal arthrodesis apply to percutaneous plate arthrodesis. The first screw is placed in the most distal plate hole to ensure that the plate is well aligned over the third metacarpal bone. The screw hole should be in the center of the dorsal aspect of the third metacarpal bone. To ensure that the hole is drilled in the center of the bone, the plate is removed, 2 needles are inserted on the medial and lateral aspects of the third metacarpal bone, and a Kirschner wire is used to predrill a pilot hole for screw placement. Intraoperative fluoroscopy may also be used to ensure that the distal plate holes are centered over the third metacarpal bone (**Fig. 13**). The second screw is placed in the radial carpal bone, but this screw is not tightened initially. The craniomedial proximal plate insertion incision allows placement of the more proximal screws in the distal radius. A screw can also

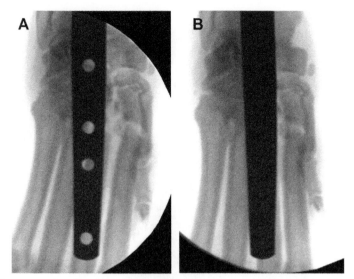

Fig. 13. Intraoperative fluoroscopy images of the carpus and metacarpals. (*A*) One of the distal third metacarpal screws is placed first to ensure that the hole is positioned in the middle of the metacarpal bone. Note the valgus angulation of the paw caused by the metacarpal fracture. (*B*) Before placing a second screw in the third metacarpal bone, valgus is corrected by direct manipulation of the paw. After correcting the malalignment, additional screws are inserted in the metacarpal bone and the radius.

be inserted in the distal radius through the central incision. The distal plate insertion incision is used to insert 2 or preferably 3 screws into the third metacarpal bone. An additional screw may be placed in the base of the third metacarpal bone through a separate small isolated incision. Once all screws are placed, the screw in the radial carpal bone is tightened. Postoperative radiographs are obtained to assess implant position and joint alignment (**Fig. 14**A-D). Recheck radiographs are obtained every 3 to 4 weeks until radiographic union is achieved (**Fig. 14**E, F).

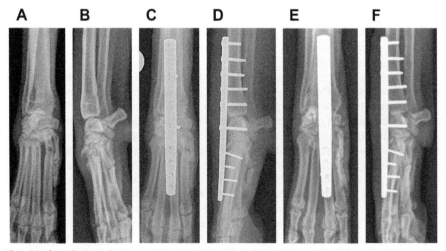

Fig. 14. (*A, B*) Carpal preoperative radiographs. (*C, D*) Immediate postoperative radiographs. (*E, F*) Four-week postoperative recheck radiographs showing that the pancarpal arthrodesis is in progress toward union.

IMMEDIATE POSTOPERATIVE CARE

Tarsal and carpal arthrodeses are protected by immobilizing the arthrodesed limb segment in an external coaptation splint for 1 to 3 months following surgery.[15,18] The duration of coaptation depends on the age of the animal and the progression toward radiographic union of the arthrodeses. A gradual return to normal activity is allowed over the subsequent 4 weeks following splint removal. Plate removal may become necessary in some animals following union because of screw loosening or extensor tendon inflammation. Motion between the metatarsal bones during weight bearing may cause loosening of the distal screws in animals that have undergone tarsal arthrodeses. Pancarpal arthrodeses are also predisposed to implant loosening as a consequence of the plate being applied cranially, which is the compression surface of the distal forelimb.[58]

CLINICAL RESULTS

We have performed percutaneous arthrodeses of the carpus and tarsus in our institutions since 2007 with excellent clinical results. Conditions necessitating arthrodesis include traumatic fractures and/or luxations, hyperextension injuries, shearing injuries, erosive arthritis, and advanced osteoarthritis. Partial tarsal arthrodeses were stabilized with a lateral plate and pantarsal arthrodeses were stabilized with a medial plate. Pancarpal arthrodeses were performed with either dorsal or medial plate applications. Intraoperative complications included breakage of the drill bits, burs and metatarsal or metacarpal bone fracture. None of the arthrodeses had severe soft-tissue swelling in

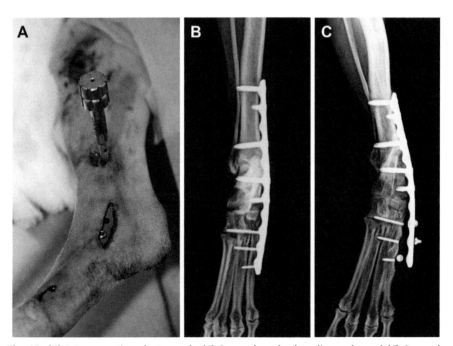

Fig. 15. (A) Intraoperative photograph, (B) 2-month recheck radiograph, and (C) 6-month recheck radiograph of a pantarsal arthrodesis performed in a 10-kg Bichon Frise that presented with an irreparable Achilles' tendon injury. The screws distal to the calcaneoquartal joint failed at the level of the lateral cortex of the second metatarsal bone.

the immediate postoperative period. Minor postoperative skin-related complications, such as erythema, pressure sores, interdigital dermatitis, and dermatitis secondary to the dog licking, occurred later in the convalescent period in some dogs. These complications were primarily attributed to splinting and all resolved with conservative management. None of the dogs developed vascular complications or plantar necrosis. Postoperative implant-related complications included screw breakage (**Fig. 15**), screw or plate loosening, and Kirschner wire migration, requiring implant removal in some dogs. Although clinical instability was not noted in any of these dogs, complete radiographic union was not always evident on follow-up radiographs. Plate removal was also necessary in some dogs that developed implant-associated infections, typically after effective arthrodesis had been confirmed on radiographs.

SUMMARY

Most dogs and cats are able to resume normal activity following arthrodesis of the tarsus and carpus; however, major complications can develop following traditional open plate arthrodeses, especially following tarsal arthrodeses. The percutaneous plate arthrodesis technique described herein offers several advantages compared with open plating techniques. When performing percutaneous plate arthrodeses, cartilage debridement is less extensive than with open plating techniques. High-motion joints such as the talocrural and antebrachiocarpal joints can be thoroughly debrided through a 2- to 4-cm central incision, which allows exposure to these articulations similar to that obtained with traditional open plating techniques. The other smaller, distal low-motion articulations can be effectively debrided through separate isolated incisions if necessary. Although cartilage debridement performed in this manner is conservative, we have noted a high rate of osseous union and a limited number of complications. Future comparative studies are needed to determine whether the percutaneous technique is superior to traditional open plate arthrodesis techniques and to develop recommended guidelines for patient selection for percutaneous plate arthrodesis.

REFERENCES

1. Roch SP, Clements DN, Mitchell RA, et al. Complications following tarsal arthrodesis using bone plate fixation in dogs. J Small Anim Pract 2008;49:117–26.
2. Allen M, Dyce J, Houlton J. Calcaneoquartal arthrodesis in the dog. J Small Anim Pract 1993;34:205–10.
3. Benson JA, Boudrieau RJ. Severe carpal and tarsal shearing injuries treated with an immediate arthrodesis in seven dogs. J Am Anim Hosp Assoc 2002;38: 370–80.
4. Buote NJ, McDonald D, Radasch R. Pancarpal and partial carpal arthrodesis. Compend Contin Educ Vet 2009;31:180–92.
5. DeCamp CE, Martinez SA, Johnston SA. Pantarsal arthrodesis in dogs and a cat: 11 cases (1983-1991). J Am Vet Med Assoc 1993;203:1705–7.
6. Dyce J, Whitelock RG, Robinson KV, et al. Arthrodesis of the tarsometatarsal joint using a laterally applied plate in 10 dogs. J Small Anim Pract 1998;39:19–22.
7. Guerrero TG, Montavon PM. Medial plating for carpal panarthrodesis. Vet Surg 2005;34:153–8.
8. Johnson A, Houlton J. Arthrodesis of the carpus. In: Johnson AL, Houlton JE, Vannini R, editors. AO principles of fracture management in the dog and the cat. Stuttgard (Germany): Thieme; 2005. p. 446–57.

9. Klause S, Piermattei D, Schwartz P. Tarsocrural arthrodesis: complications and recommendations. Vet Comp Orthop Traumatol 1989;3:119–24.

10. Lotsikas PJ, Radasch RM. A clinical evaluation of pancarpal arthrodesis in nine dogs using circular external skeletal fixation. Vet Surg 2006;35:480–5.

11. McKee WM, May C, Macias C, et al. Pantarsal arthrodesis with a customised medial or lateral bone plate in 13 dogs. Vet Rec 2004;154:165–70.

12. Muir P, Norris JL. Tarsometatarsal subluxation in dogs: partial arthrodesis by plate fixation. J Am Anim Hosp Assoc 1999;35:155–62.

13. Vannini R, Bonath K. Arthrodesis of the tarsus. In: Johnson AL, Houlton JE, Vannini R, editors. AO principles of fracture management in the dog and the cat. Stuttgard (Germany): Thieme; 2005. p. 464–71.

14. Michal U, Fluckiger M, Schmokel H. Healing of dorsal pancarpal arthrodesis in the dog. J Small Anim Pract 2003;44:109–12.

15. Piermattei DL. Fracture and other orthopedic conditions of the carpus, meta-carpus, and phalanges. In: Piermattei DL, Flo GL, DeCamp CE, editors. Hand-book of small animal orthopedics and fracture repair. Philadelphia: Elsevier; 2006. p. 382–428.

16. Rahal SC, Volpi RS, Hette K, et al. Arthrodesis tarsocrural or tarsometatarsal in 2 dogs using circular external skeletal fixator. Can Vet J 2006;47:894–8.

17. Worth AJ, Bruce WJ. Long-term assessment of pancarpal arthrodesis performed on working dogs in New Zealand. N Z Vet J 2008;56:78–84.

18. Piermattei DL. Fracture and other orthopedic injuries of the tarsus, metatarsus, and phalanges. In: Piermattei DL, Flo GL, DeCamp CE, editors. Handbook of small animal orthopedics and fracture repair. Philadelphia: Elsevier; 2006. p. 661–713.

19. Denny H, Barr A. Partial carpal and pancarpal arthrodesis in the dog: a review of 50 cases. J Small Anim Pract 1991;32:329–34.

20. Diaz-Bertrana C, Darnaculleta F, Durall I, et al. The stepped hybrid plate for car-pal panarthrodesis—part II: a multicentre study of 52 arthrodeses. Vet Comp Orthop Traumatol 2009;22:389–97.

21. Diaz-Bertrana C, Darnaculleta F, Durall I, et al. The stepped hybrid plate for car-pal panarthrodesis—part I: relationship between plate and bone surfaces. Vet Comp Orthop Traumatol 2009;22:380–8.

22. Haburjak J, Lenehan T, Davidson C. Treatment of carpometacarpal and middle carpal joint hyperextension injuries with partial carpal arthrodesis using a cross pin technique: 21 cases. Vet Comp Orthop Traumatol 2003;16:105–11.

23. Li A, Gibson N, Bennett D, et al. Thirteen pancarpal arthrodeses using 2.7/3.5 mm hybrid dynamic compression plates. Vet Comp Orthop Traumatol 1999; 12:102–7.

24. Johnson KA, Bellenger CR. The effects of autologous bone grafting on bone heal-ing after carpal arthrodesis in the dog. Vet Rec 1980;107:126–32.

25. Johnson K. A radiographic study of the effects of autologous cancellous bone grafts on bone healing after carpal arthrodesis in the dog. Vet Radiol 1981;22: 177–83.

26. Clarke SP, Ferguson JF, Miller A. Clinical evaluation of pancarpal arthrodesis us-ing a CastLess plate in 11 dogs. Vet Surg 2009;38:852–60.

27. Halling K, Lewis D, Jones R, et al. Use of circular external skeletal fixator con-structs to stabilize tarsometatarsal arthrodeses in three dogs. Vet Comp Orthop Traumatol 2004;17:204.

28. Shanil J, Yeshurun Y, Shahar R. Arthrodesis of the tarsometatarsal joint, using type II ESF with acrylic connecting bars in four dogs. Vet Comp Orthop Traumatol 2006;19:61–3.

29. Whitelock RG, Dyce J, Houlton JE. Metacarpal fractures associated with pancarpal arthrodesis in dogs. Vet Surg 1999;28:25–30.

30. Andreoni AA, Rytz U, Vannini R, et al. Ground reaction force profiles after partial and pancarpal arthrodesis in dogs. Vet Comp Orthop Traumatol 2010;23:1–6.

31. Jerram RM, Walker AM, Worth AJ, et al. Prospective evaluation of pancarpal arthrodesis for carpal injuries in working dogs in New Zealand, using dorsal hybrid plating. N Z Vet J 2009;57:331–7.

32. James FM, Richardson DW. Minimally invasive plate fixation of lower limb injury in horses: 32 cases (1999-2003). Equine Vet J 2006;38:246–51.

33. Hudson CC, Pozzi A, Lewis DD. Minimally invasive plate osteosynthesis: applications and techniques in dogs and cats. Vet Comp Orthop Traumatol 2009;22: 172–85.

34. Borrelli J Jr, Prickett W, Song E, et al. Extraosseous blood supply of the tibia and the effects of different plating techniques: a human cadaveric study. J Orthop Trauma 2002;16:691–5.

35. Garofolo S, Pozzi A. Effect of plating technique on periosteal vasculature of the radius in dogs: a cadaveric study. Vet Surg 2013;42(3):255–61.

36. Field JR, Tornkvist H. Biological fracture fixation: a perspective. Vet Comp Orthop Traumatol 2001;14:169–78.

37. Perren SM. Evolution of the internal fixation of long bone fractures. The scientific basis of biological internal fixation: choosing a new balance between stability and biology. J Bone Joint Surg Br 2002;84:1093–110.

38. Ruchelsman DE, Hazel A, Mudgal CS. Treatment of symptomatic distal interphalangeal joint arthritis with percutaneous arthrodesis: a novel technique in select patients. Hand (N Y) 2010;5:434–9.

39. Bauer T, Lortat-Jacob A, Hardy P. First metatarsophalangeal joint percutaneous arthrodesis. Orthop Traumatol Surg Res 2010;96:567–73.

40. Al-Khayer A, Hegarty J, Hahn D, et al. Percutaneous sacroiliac joint arthrodesis: a novel technique. J Spinal Disord Tech 2008;21:359–63.

41. Anderson DG, Sayadipour A, Shelby K, et al. Anterior interbody arthrodesis with percutaneous posterior pedicle fixation for degenerative conditions of the lumbar spine. Eur Spine J 2011;20:1323–30.

42. Mader K, Verheyen CC, Gausepohl T, et al. Minimally invasive ankle arthrodesis with a retrograde locking nail after failed fusion. Strategies Trauma Limb Reconstr 2007;2:39–47.

43. Lauge-Pedersen H. Percutaneous arthrodesis. Acta Orthop Scand Suppl 2003; 74:1–30.

44. Lui TH. New technique of arthroscopic triple arthrodesis. Arthroscopy 2006;22: 461–5.

45. Lauge-Pedersen H, Aspenberg P. Arthrodesis by percutaneous fixation: patellofemoral arthrodesis in rabbits without debridement of the joint. Acta Orthop Scand 2002;73:186–9.

46. Lauge-Pedersen H, Aspenberg P. Synovial fluid depletion: successful arthrodesis without operative cartilage removal. J Orthop Sci 2003;8:591–5.

47. Jones P, Delco M, Beard W, et al. A limited surgical approach for pastern arthrodesis in horses with severe osteoarthritis. Vet Comp Orthop Traumatol 2009;22: 303–8.

48. Panizzi L, Barber SM, Lang HM, et al. Evaluation of a minimally invasive arthrodesis technique for the carpometacarpal joint in horses. Vet Surg 2011;40:464–72.
49. Fettig AA, McCarthy RJ, Kowaleski MP. Intertarsal and tarsometatarsal arthrodesis using 2.0/2.7-mm or 2.7/3.5-mm hybrid dynamic compression plates. J Am Anim Hosp Assoc 2002;38:364–9.
50. Evans HE. Arthrology. In: Evans HE, Miller ME, editors. Miller's anatomy of the dog. Philadelphia: Saunders; 1993. p. 252–6.
51. Guillou RP, Frank JD, Sinnott MT, et al. In vitro mechanical evaluation of medial plating for pantarsal arthrodesis in dogs. Am J Vet Res 2008;69:1406–12.
52. Inauen R, Koch D, Bass M. Arthrodesis of the tarsometatarsal joints in a cat with a two hole advanced locking plate system. Vet Comp Orthop Traumatol 2009;22:166–9.
53. Chodos MD, Parks BG, Schon LC, et al. Blade plate compared with locking plate for tibiotalocalcaneal arthrodesis: a cadaver study. Foot Ankle Int 2008;29:219–24.
54. Lang HM, Panizzi L, Allen AL, et al. Comparison of three drilling techniques for carpometacarpal joint arthrodesis in horses. Vet Surg 2009;38:990–7.
55. Barber SM, Panizzi L, Lang HM. Treatment of carpometacarpal osteoarthritis by arthrodesis in 12 horses. Vet Surg 2009;38:1006–11.
56. Rao RD, Gourab K, Bagaria VB, et al. The effect of platelet-rich plasma and bone marrow on murine posterolateral lumbar spine arthrodesis with bone morphogenetic protein. J Bone Joint Surg Am 2009;91:1199–206.
57. Parker R, Brown S, Wind A. Pancarpal arthrodesis in the dog: a review of forty-five cases. Vet Surg 1981;10:35–43.
58. Guillou RP, Demianiuk RM, Sinnott MT, et al. In vitro mechanical evaluation of a limited contact dynamic compression plate and hybrid carpal arthrodesis plate for canine pancarpal arthrodesis. Vet Comp Orthop Traumatol 2012;25:83–8.

Unique Differences of Minimally Invasive Fracture Repair in the Feline

Karl C. Maritato, DVM[a,b,]*, Philipp Schmierer, med Vet[c],
Antonio Pozzi, med Vet[c]

KEYWORDS

- Minimally invasive fracture repair • Feline • Minimally invasive plate osteosynthesis
- Differences • Cat

KEY POINTS

- A thorough knowledge of skeletal anatomy is critical to performing minimally invasive techniques.
- Feline patients have unique anatomic and biomechanical differences that can affect outcome.
- Feline behavior creates unique challenges to postoperative care.
- Feline physiology places limitations on postoperative pain management.

GENERAL ANATOMY

The overall anatomic template is relatively similar among mammals. When performing surgery, however, being aware of anatomic differences that may have an impact on the performance of the surgery itself, as well as expected outcomes and complications, is important. Some of the anatomic features that differ from those of canines are listed and specific differences as they relate to surgical approaches are discussed later.

- The humerus of the cat is a less pronounced S-shape than the dog. This is particularly relevant in the use of minimally invasive fracture repair (MIFR) techniques, because the topography of the limb is that much more important for proper implant placement when not directly visualizing the bone (discussed later). The

Disclosure Statement: No conflicts of interest to disclose.
[a] Department of Surgery, MedVet Medical and Cancer Centers for Pets, 3964 Red Bank Road, Cincinnati, OH 45227, USA; [b] Department of Surgery, MedVet Medical and Cancer Centers for Pets, Dayton, OH, USA; [c] Department for Small Animals, Vetsuisse Faculty, Tierspital Zurich, Kleintierchirurgie, Winterthurerstrasse 260, 8057 Zurich, Switzerland
* Corresponding author. 3964 Red Bank Road, Cincinnati, OH 45227.
E-mail address: kmaritato@medvet.com

cat does not have a supratrochlear foramen like the dog; it has a supracondylar foreman proximal to the medial epicondyle through which the median nerve and brachial artery pass.

- The radius of the cat has marked lateral torsion significantly different from the dog. This is important when performing MIFR in regard to proper plate placement (discussed later)
- Cats have no straight medial collateral ligament of the carpus. This is important in understanding the normal range of motion and function of the carpus and its possible injuries.[1]
- A cat's retractable claw is made possible because of the dorsal elastic ligament attachment to the middle phalanx and the middle and distal phalanx shapes.[2] These are important mechanisms to remember with injuries to the distal forelimb, because they can affect the behavior of the cat and, therefore, owners should be made aware.
- The sacral wing notch, a highly consistent anatomic feature in the dog, is present in only 34% of cats and its location is variable and, therefore, undependable. This is important to understand given the commonality of sacroiliac fracture/luxations in cats.[3]
- The artery of the ligament of the head of the femur contributes to epiphyseal blood supply in the femoral head, which is not the case in the dog.[4]
- The medullary canal of the tibia is more uniform in diameter than in dogs. Given how amenable the tibia is to MIFR, knowledge of its shape and proper areas for pin, screw, and plate placement is important.[5]
- As with the carpus, the tarsal ligaments present are different from those in the dog. Only short collateral ligaments are found versus both short and long ligaments in the canine. The feline medial collateral ligament involves oblique tibiotalar and straight talocentral components, and the lateral collateral ligament involves calcaneofibular and talofibular parts. There is also greater range of motion of the feline tarsus (22° flexion to 167° extension vs 39° to 164°, respectively, in dogs).[6–8]

BIOMECHANICS

Cats are very agile creatures, particularly in comparison to dogs. A large proportion of the biomechanical, kinematic, and kinetic differences appear to occur in their distal forelimbs, particularly with regard to the importance of supination and protonation of the antebrachium.

According to studies summarized by Kapatkin and colleagues,[9] a kinematic study in cats showed that when walking, the peak antebrachiocarpal angle was 15° and the peak metacarpophalangeal joint angle was 60°. Another study compared the kinetics and qualitative motion of feline and canine gaits. Using high-speed video, it was noted that cats pronated their front paws during the beginning of the stance phase, until the paw reached a neutral position. At the end of the stance phase, the paw was supinated with the medial phalanx released first, followed by the other phalanges. Dogs, however, put all 4 weight-bearing phalanges on the ground at the same time. They ended the stance phase by moving the paw medially with supination beginning in the swing phase.[10,11]

APPROACHES TO THE DIFFERENT BONES

As discussed previously, thorough knowledge of the feline anatomy and anatomic landmarks for safe corridors is important to perform MIFR safely. Indirect reduction and plate application can be challenging in cats due to the small size of the bones. In addition, the anatomic differences between cats and dogs should be considered when performing MIFR.[12] A short overview of the MIFR approaches in cats as well as the major anatomic differences between dogs and cats is discussed.

Humerus

Humeral fractures can be treated with MIFR using a craniolateral or a medial approach. A craniolateral approach is recommended for proximal and mid-diaphyseal fractures. The medial approach is indicated in mid-diaphyseal and distal fractures. This approach is recommended in cases with limited distal bone stock and if double plating is planned.

The proximal anatomic landmarks for the craniolateral approach are the greater tubercle and the deltoid tuberosity. A skin incision is performed along the cranial border of the greater tubercle. The skin and subcutaneous tissues are retracted while preserving the omobrachial artery and vein. The incision is advanced through the deep fascia and, after elevation of the acromial part of the deltoideus muscle, the underlying bone can be exposed. The lateral epicondyle serves as a landmark for the distal incision. The skin is incised extending from the lateral epicondyle to approximately 1 cm to 2 cm proximally and continued through the deep fascia along the cranial border of the lateral head of the triceps. In comparison to the dog, this muscle is of larger size.[13] A window to the bone is created between the brachialis muscle and the origin of the extensor carpi radialis muscle after partial elevation of its origin. Care must be taken to avoid damage to the deep and superficial branches of the radial nerve. This can be avoided by creating the tunnel underneath the brachialis muscle in a distal to proximal direction while visualizing the radial nerve (**Fig. 1**). When placing bicortical screws in the distal humerus, in cats the potential risk of penetrating the supracondylar foramen must be considered. This could lead to injury of brachial artery and the median nerve.[12]

For the medial approach, the cat is placed in dorsal recumbency. The affected leg is abducted. The proximal incision is located approximately 1 cm caudal to the palpable cranial border of the greater tubercle and 2 cm distal to this point. The incision should be 2 cm to 3 cm long for adequate exposure.[12] Blunt self-retaining Gelpi retractors for careful retraction of the skin and soft tissue can be used to facilitate the approach as the proximal humerus is well covered by soft tissue medially.[12] After performing an incision between the brachiocephalicus muscle and the superficial pectoral muscle, the underlying neurovascular structures should be recognized and protected. The aponeurosis of the deep pectoral muscle is incised along the shaft of the humerus, allowing the proximal part of the biceps to retract cranially. This reveals the underlying broad tendon of insertion of the teres major muscle. This serves as an important landmark because dissection should not be continued distally to avoid iatrogenic damage to the musculocutaneous nerve and the brachial artery.[12] For the distal incision, the supracondylar ridge and the medial epicondyle are used as anatomic landmarks. After a 2-cm skin incision along the supracondylar ridge and incision of the deep fascia along the cranial edge of the long head of the triceps muscle, care must be taken to protect the brachial artery and the median and ulnar nerves (**Fig. 2**). Once visualized, the medial head of the triceps is separated from its short part overlying the supracondylar foramen and carefully elevated.[13] The supracondylar foramen is an important structure in the distal humerus of the cat because the brachial artery and the median nerve pass through it. If necessary for implant positioning, these neurovascular structures can be freed from the supracondylar foramen after removing its medial border with bone-cutting forceps.[12]

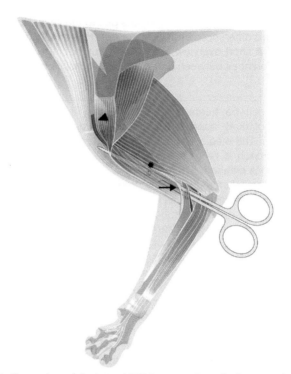

Fig. 1. Schematic illustration of the lateral MIPO approach to the humerus in a cat. The deep and superficial branch of the radial nerve (*arrow*) are in close proximity to the distal insertion incision. Extreme care must be taken to avoid damage to these structures. This can be achieved by creating the tunnel underneath the brachialis muscle (*asterisk*) in a distal to proximal direction while visualizing the radial nerve. Proximally, the omobrachial artery and nerve must be avoided (*arrowhead*).

Insertion of the plate from distal to proximal is advocated in order to avoid damage of the neurovascular structures and interference with the thoracic wall.

Radius and Ulna

The craniolateral approach to the radius is recommended for MIFR in cats because of the marked lateral torsion of the cranial radial surface.[12] Because of this torsion, the proximal approach is performed between the common digital extensor muscle and the lateral digital extensor muscle and the distal approach is done between the tendon of the extensor carpi radialis muscle and the tendon of the common digital extensor muscle (**Fig. 3**).[12]

If increased exposure is needed in the proximal approach, elevation of the supinator muscle might be necessary. Care must be taken to avoid the deep branch of the radial nerve during elevation. In the distal approach, the tendon of the abductor pollicis longus muscle can be transected to increase exposure (**Fig. 4**).[12]

The proximal ulna is approached through a lateral approach centered over the shaft. Elevation of the ulnaris lateralis muscle at the caudal border can be performed in order to increase exposure.[12] The distal approach starts just proximal to the styloid process between the palpable tendons of the lateral digital extensor muscle and the ulnaris lateralis muscle. The plate should be inserted in

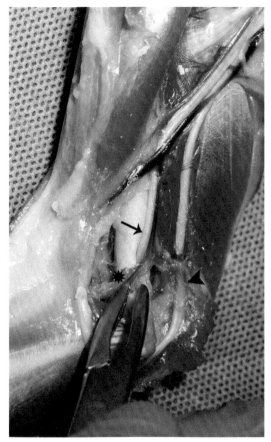

Fig. 2. Medial view on the distal humerus of a cat. The medial part of the supracondylar foramen (*asterisk*) can be removed with a rongeur to allow cranial retraction of the median nerve and the brachial artery (*arrow*). The ulnar nerve (*arrowhead*) should be preserved while performing the approach. The skin was removed to show the exact location of the neurovascular structures.

a proximal-to-distal direction because the styloid process can make implant insertion more difficult.[12]

Femur

The MIFR approaches for the femur have no major differences compared with those for a dog. A lateral approach is advocated with the proximal window located at the cranial aspect of the caudofemoralis and biceps femoris muscle. The caudal aspect of the vastus lateralis muscle can be elevated and cranially retracted after incision and retraction of the superficial and deep fascia lata.[12] The location of the distal approach depends on the planned position of the implants. Typically the approach is at the level of the patella. Identification of the biceps femoris muscle and incision of the fascia lata along its cranial border reveals the intermuscular septum connecting the vastus lateralis and biceps femoris muscle, which is subsequently incised.[12]

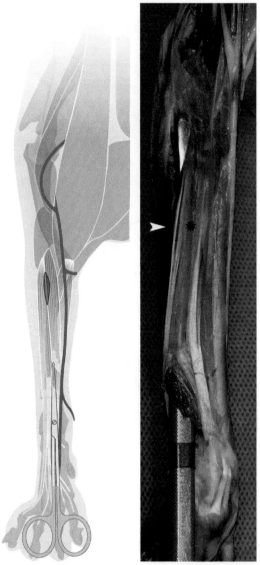

Fig. 3. Schematic of the cranial aspect of the antebrachium and Cadaver demonstrating the ateral muscles of the feline antebrachium. Note the lateral position of the approach between the common digital extensor muscle (*asterisk*) and the lateral digital extensor muscle (*arrowhead*). Care should be taken to preserve the cephalic antebrachial artery and vein (*arrow*). The skin was removed to show the exact location of the neurovascular structures.

Tibia

The MIFR approaches for the tibia have no major differences compared with those for a dog. The proximal approach is performed and centered over the medial proximal metaphysis, elevating the tendons of the sartorius, gracilis, and semitendinosus muscle to allow direct exposure of the bone. For the distal approach, an incision is

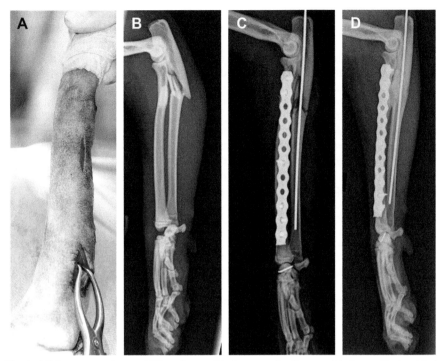

Fig. 4. (A) Intraoperative and (B) radiographic images of a 2-year-old, domestic short hair cat presented with radius-ulnar fracture and radial carpal bone luxation of the right forelimb after motor vehicle trauma. (A) A lateral MIPO approach was performed. The ulna fracture was reduced and stabilized with an intramedullary pin inserted in retrograde fashion through a small caudo-lateral approach. Consecutively the radius fracture was stabilized with a bone plate placed under fluoroscopic control. Note the lateral position of the plate (C, D). The cat returned to full function despite the radio-ulnar synostosis observed at the 8 weeks follow-up radiographs (D). The radial carpal bone luxation was treated with a trans fixation pin through an additional minimal medial approach (C, D).

performed just proximal to the medial malleolus. The medial saphenous artery and vein should be preserved.[12]

FRACTURE REDUCTION AND PLATE APPLICATION

Suitable techniques for indirect fracture reduction in cats include the hanging limb technique, intramedullary pinning, distraction with bone holding forceps, reduction with linear and circular external fixation, fracture distractors, and reduction through plate application.[14,15] One of the advantages of performing MIFR in cats is the limited soft tissue coverage and muscle bulk, which allows an excellent palpation of the anatomic landmarks. The hanging limb technique is indicated for distal extremity fractures. Final reduction is achieved manually or with bone forceps.[14] Bone forceps should be used carefully to avoid iatrogenic fissures. Intramedullary pinning is an easy and effective technique for indirect fracture reduction, helping to achieve distraction and to restore original limb length.

Plates can be used for indirect reduction, after anatomically contouring to the contralateral intact bone. In this case, the cortical screws are used to pull the fragments toward the plate. The proximal end of the plate is usually fixed first because the manipulation of the distal fragment is much easier.[15] Alternatively, locking plates can be contoured less accurately and the plate can be used for reduction at the contact points proximally and distally, based on preoperative planning. As in dogs, the plate is inserted via an epiperiosteal tunnel developed using a Freer periosteal elevator or Metzenbaum scissors.[12]

Specific types of fractures diagnosed more commonly in cats, such as distal tibial fractures, may require a particular choice of the implant and its position. In the authors' experience, these cases can be performed with the 2 incisions described for minimally invasive plate osteosynthesis (MIPO) in the tibia. Because the distal incision is practically over the fracture site, however, there is a necessary violation of MIPO principles. Regardless, these cases can be managed successfully with this partial MIPO approach.

POSTOPERATIVE CARE

Postoperative care is not very different from dogs; however, there a few points to note, one of which is pain control. In dogs, a mainstay of treatment of postoperative pain is nonsteroidal anti-inflammatory drugs. There are limited options for cats in this regard and, in the options available, compared with dogs, the labels call for shorter courses of treatment for safety reasons. The use of local analgesics with liposomal encapsulated bupivacaine suspensions and opioids, such as fentanyl patches, can be effective at keeping cats comfortable.

The other important difference is postoperative confinement methods. Unlike dogs, which can be kept in a small room, cats always should be kept in a large comfortable crate. This is because cats have a propensity to jump, and, therefore, it is best they have a roof over their heads. A small dog could easily be kept in a bathroom, but a cat would jump on the sink, toilet, tub, and so forth and potentially damage the repair. A crate large enough to place a litter box, food and water bowls, and bedding is the ideal setting for a cat.

REFERENCES

1. Shales CJ, Langley-Hobbs S. Dorso-medial ante-brachiocarpal luxation with radio-ulna luxation in a domestic shorthair. J Feline Med Surg 2006;8:197.
2. Gonyea W, Ashworth R. The form and function of retractile claws in the Felidae and other representative carnivorans. J Morphol 1975;145:229.
3. Burger M, Forterre F, Brunnberg L. Surgical anatomy of the feline sacroiliac joint for lag screw fixation of sacroiliac fracture-luxation. Vet Comp Orthop Traumatol 2004;17:146–51.
4. Culvenor JA, Black AP, Lorkin KF, et al. Repair of femoral capital physeal injuries in cats—14 cases. Vet Comp Orthop Traumatol 1996;9:182–5.
5. Newton CD, Nunamaker DM. Textbook of small animal orthopaedics. Philadelphia: JB Lippincott; 1985.
6. Voss K, Langley-Hobbs SJ, Montavon PM. Tarsal joint. In: Montavon PM, Voss K, Langley-Hobbs SJ, editors. Feline orthopaedic surgery and musculoskeletal disease. Philadelphia: Saunders/Elsevier; 2009. p. 507.
7. Jaegar GH, Marcellin-Little DJ, DePuy V, et al. Validity of goniometric joint measurements in cats. Am J Vet Res 2007;68:822.
8. Jaegar GH, Marcellin-Little DJ, Levine D. Reliability of goniometry in Labrador Retrievers. Am J Vet Res 2002;63(7):979–86.

9. Kapatkin AS, Garcia-Nolan T, Hayashi K. Carpus, metacarpus and digits in: veterinary surgery small animal. St Louis (MO): Elsevier; 2018. p. 920–38.
10. Corbee RJ, Maas H, Doornenbal A. Forelimb and hindlimb ground reaction forces of walking cats: assessment and comparison with walking dogs. Vet J 2014; 202:116.
11. Prilutsky BI, Sirota MG, Gregor RJ. Quantification of motor cortex activity and full-body biomechanics during unconstrained locomotion. J Neurophysiol 2005;94: 2959.
12. Schmierer PA, Pozzi A. Guidelines for surgical approaches for minimally invasive plate osteosynthesis in cats. Vet Comp Orthop Traumatol 2017;30(4):272–8.
13. Piermattei DL, Johnson KA. An atlas of surgical approaches to the bones and joints of the dog and cat. Oxford (United Kingdom): Elsevier LTD; 2017.
14. Hudson C, Pozzi A, Lewis D. Minimally invasive plate osteosynthesis: applications and techniques in dogs and cats. Vet Comp Orthopaedics Traumatol 2009;22(3):175–82.
15. Schmierer PA, Pozzi A. Minimally invasive plate osteosynthesis. In: Barnhart MD, Maritato KC, editors. Locking plates in veterinary orthopedics. Hoboken, New Jersey: Wiley Blackwell; 2018. p. 41–50.

Moving?

Make sure your subscription moves with you!

To notify us of your new address, find your **Clinics Account Number** (located on your mailing label above your name), and contact customer service at:

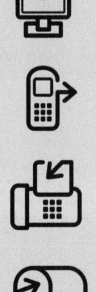

Email: journalscustomerservice-usa@elsevier.com

800-654-2452 (subscribers in the U.S. & Canada)
314-447-8871 (subscribers outside of the U.S. & Canada)

Fax number: 314-447-8029

Elsevier Health Sciences Division
Subscription Customer Service
3251 Riverport Lane
Maryland Heights, MO 63043

*To ensure uninterrupted delivery of your subscription, please notify us at least 4 weeks in advance of move.

Printed and bound by CPI Group (UK) Ltd, Croydon, CR0 4YY

03/10/2024

01040402-0012